AYURVEDA

# A Life of Balance

# NOTE ON THE COVER

The Puranas, a compilation of ancient stories of the Hindu tradition, are rich with descriptions of the struggle between good and evil. In one such story the contest between these two forces was so great that even the ocean was churned up into a raging sea. In the role of peacemaker, Lord Shiva offered the ocean's bounty equally to both. In gratitude, the ocean gave Shiva a pearl-white elephant boasting four trunks, which emanated the seven colors of the rainbow, named Airavata. He was claimed as the mount for Indra, Lord of the firmament.

The elephant, the oldest surviving mammal, is a symbol for both earth and space. The young, vital Airavata represents the foundation of the living universe. He is the symbol of the first subtle energy center, located at the base of the spine, known as the muladhara chakra. The four trunks are symbols of the human virtues of material wealth, continuous allurement, reverence for the laws of nature, and the pursuit of ultimate freedom of the spirit. The seven colors of the rainbow, along with the body of Airavata, symbolize the octave of creation, comprising earth, water, fire, air, space, mind, intelligence, and ego.

When the elements, the sense mechanism, and egoity are tamed into recognition of the One spirit, the four trunks of Airavata resolve into the single trunk of Gaja. Lord of the herbivores, Gaja represents the fifth chakra, known as Vishuddha, and thus the element of space. He bears knowledge of all the earth, herbs, and plants.

The elephant, as preserver of our sustenance, holds the memory of our beginning in space and our existence on earth. Space is the principle of vacuity, the resonance of sound. It is only because of space that we are able to vibrate in harmony with the earth. If these precious mammals become extinct, we will no longer be able to maintain the vital memory for sustenance of spirit or food on the planet. As it is, we are barely holding on to the frazzled threads of memory.

I chose the image of Airavata for the cover and took the liberty of placing on his back a lotus bowl of effervescent jade laden with fruits, vegetables, grains, and herbs. It is my fervent hope that we protect this species, which maintains our bountiful sustenance and vibratory link to the earth.

May the joyous Airavata transform our lives with health and gladness, and may the wise Gaja bless the earth with purity and firmness.

AYURVEDA

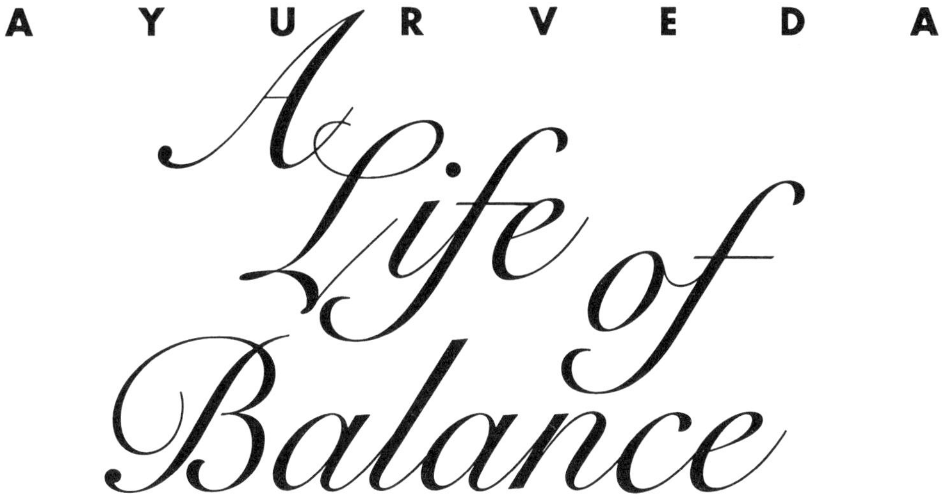

# A Life of Balance

THE COMPLETE GUIDE TO
AYURVEDIC NUTRITION AND BODY TYPES
WITH RECIPES

MAYA TIWARI

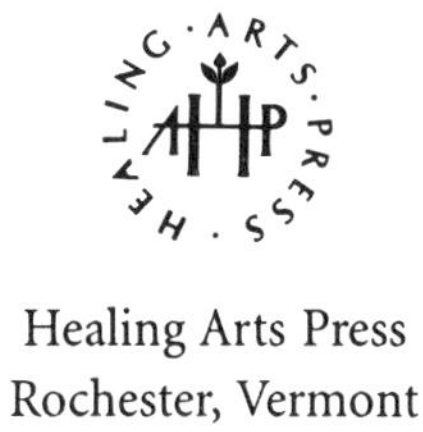


Healing Arts Press
Rochester, Vermont

Healing Arts Press
One Park Street
Rochester, Vermont 05767



***Note to the reader:*** *This book is intended as an informational guide. The remedies, approaches, and techniques described herein are meant to supplement, and not to be a substitute for, professional medical care or treatment. They should not be used to treat a serious ailment without prior consultation with a qualified health care professional.*

Library of Congress Cataloging-in-Publication Data

Tiwari, Maya.
Ayurveda: a life of balance / Maya Tiwari
p. cm.
Includes bibliographical references and index.
ISBN 0-89281-490-X
1. Nutrition. 2. Medicine, Ayurvedic. 3. Health. I. Title.
RA784.T58 1995 94-29178
613.2—dc20 CIP

Printed and bound in the United States

10 9 8 7 6 5 4 3 2

Text design by Virginia L. Scott
Line illustrations designed by Maya Tiwari and illustrated by Marnie Mikell
Cover image designed by Maya Tiwari and illustrated by Ellen John

This book was typeset in Minion with Hiroshige and Snell as display fonts

Healing Arts Press is a division of Inner Traditions International

Distributed to the book trade in Canada by Publishers Group West (PGW), Toronto, Ontario
Distributed to the health food trade in Canada by Alive Books, Toronto and Vancouver
Distributed to the book trade in the United Kingdom by Deep Books, London
Distributed to the book trade in Australia by Millennium Books, Newtown, N. S. W.
Distributed to the book trade in New Zealand by Tandem Press, Auckland
Distributed to the book trade in South Africa by Alternative Books, Randburg

*To my beloved teacher, Swami Dayananda Saraswati*

*May the universe never abuse food.*
*Breath is food,*
*The body eats food,*
*This body rests on breath.*
*Breath rests on the body,*
*Food is resting on food.*
*The one who knows this*
*becomes rich in food and great in fame.*

*Taittiriya Upanishad 11.7*

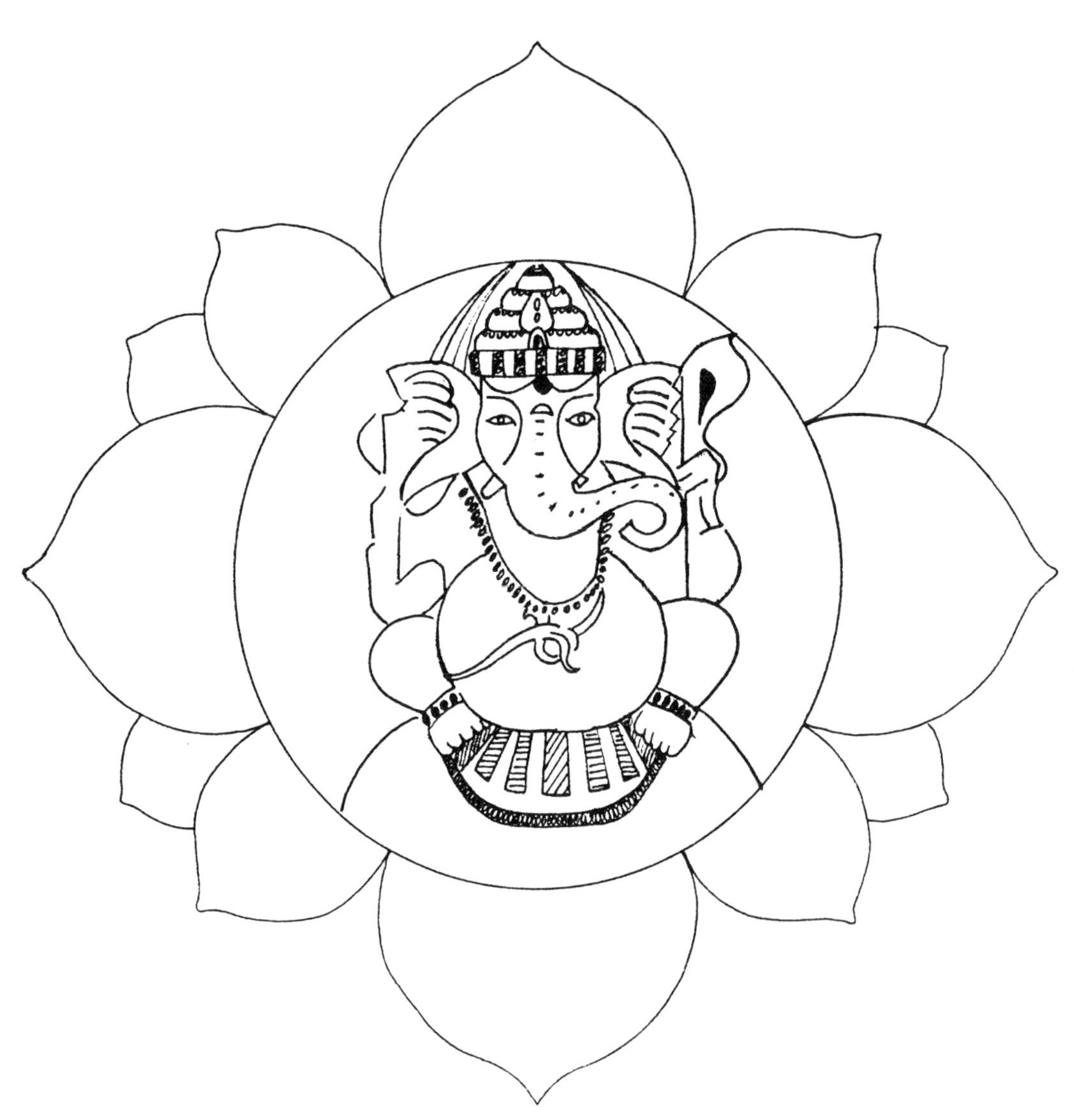

# CONTENTS

## PART THREE: UNIVERSAL RECIPES FOR EACH BODY TYPE

# FOREWORD

The concept of holistic health acknowledges that a human being is—and must be related to as—body, mind, and spirit. This concept has become an increasingly popular topic of conversation in Western culture over the last two decades. I began my personal journey to understand and embody it in the late 1960s and have been involved in public education on the subject since the mid-1970s. What I have noticed over the years is the frequent mistaking of "alternative" healing for "holistic" healing. Alternative simply means a method not ordinarily used in conventional treatment. A doctor may add herbal or vitamin therapy to a patient's treatment, thereby making it more gentle and less toxic (which is wonderful and needed) but still fail to take into consideration the patient's state of mind and lifestyle, which are inevitably contributing to the present manifestation of "disease."

Doctors may, through "alternative" treatment, be able to alter the body's chemistry and eliminate the symptoms of disease, but have they righted the imbalance in the body, mind, and spirit? If that imbalance is not addressed, we are not aligned with who we really are, and disease in one form or another will manifest once again.

So when we speak about healing or good health, we must look deeper and more fully at ourselves and at our methods of treatment than we generally do in this "make it easy, make it quick, and if at all possible make it something someone else can do for me" society.

The Vedas are the oldest and most complete body of knowledge to address the who, what, and why of human existence. They have covered the "how to" (using the current vernacular) through healing and attunement methods, coming from the understanding that we are body, mind, and spirit, innately and unalterably dependent on the rest of creation.

In *Ayurveda: A Life of Balance,* Maya introduces the Ayurvedic diet with universal flavor and shows how to awaken *ahamkara* (the memory of who we really are) through the proper use of wholesome foods. By understanding our individual body types, and by using foods that best support and enhance each type, we are employing a powerful and essential method of attunement.

I am truly grateful to Maya and the handful of other Vedic scholars who continue to devote their lives to sharing this knowledge with the rest of the world—a world that is in great need and that, we hope, may finally be ready.

Lindsay Wagner

# PREFACE

I met Maya almost two decades ago in the early morning light at Carl Shurz Park overlooking the East River in Manhattan. She was then a famous designer with a plush Madison Avenue store selling to the likes of Jackie Onassis. I was still a photographer working primarily for *Time Magazine* and NBC. Our friendship grew quickly. We spent endless hours discussing the overwhelming foreseeable plights of our planet. Maya is a great visionary whose spiritual fortitude was later to rescue her from her devastating war with cancer. (Her cancer was diagnosed as terminal, and she was given the vague possibility of six months to live.)

Maya became reclusive during that time and I traveled to various hospitals to bring her native Indian foods. They were all that she needed from the outside world. She confided that she chose to be reclusive since sympathy can kill someone faster than cancer. Her recovery was miraculous.

Maya returned to her life profoundly transformed and effected great changes in her personal lifestyle. She spent many years journeying and studying the sciences of holistic health, while successfully aiding numerous other cancer patients. Among her first studies was macrobiotics; later she studied the sciences of Ayurveda and yoga.

She has always carried the deep markings of a staunch Brahmin background. It was remarkable to watch her inherit the role of her true destiny. After the death of her beloved father, who was also her early teacher, Maya chose the life of a spiritual renunciate and embarked on the scholarly study of the Vedas, the original Hindu scriptures. Although we have since gone to different states and different pursuits, our shared vision has remained intact.

Like a pure white lily that is rooted in the mud of extensive personal experience, Maya is indeed that shining yogi. Her true work has only just begun. And I take great joy in watching the petals of her wisdom open to their full glory.

*Ayurveda: A Life of Balance* will bring benefit to everyone who is conscious of personal health and our global environment.

Barbara Y. E. Pyle
Vice President of Environmental Policy
Turner Broadcasting System, Inc.

# ACKNOWLEDGMENTS

My gratitude to the staff of Inner Traditions, and in particular to my editor Leslie Colket, for offering enormous encouragement and help; Sushila Blackman, for her editing of the work; Lindsay Wagner, for her foreword; Barbara Y. E. Pyle, an old friend, whose contribution in the form of the preface is appreciated; Dr. Robert E. Svoboda, for his excellent critical input; Dr. Wally Burnstein, for his kindred support and review comment; Deepak Chopra, M.D., the clearest voice in mind/body medicine, who has opened the doors for all to enter; Dr. Vasant Lad, for his many years of disseminating Ayurveda in the United States, for his availability to me during this project, and for the response of his kind staff to my needs; Scott Webb and Jeff Hollifield, for assisting me with the input of the manuscript; Beverley Viljakainen, my colleague, for editing the recipes; Don Davis, for computer assistance; Ellen John, for the final rendition of the cover illustration; Marnie Mikell, for the finished rendition of the line drawings; Nancy Bazaaz for the drawing of Lord Ganesha that opens the book; Roger Derrough and Earth Fare, for support with my natural foods needs; Bill White, for his endless support and assistance. Last, first, and always, my deepest gratitude to my family, for their courage, laughter, and wholesome hearts.

# INTRODUCTION

*Hope is nature's way of enabling us to survive*
*so that we can discover nature itself.*
***Swami Dayananda Saraswati***

The pervasive forces of protection are always at work. How else can a city like New York—my oasis of comfort for two decades—survive all the abuse, misuse, corruption, and decay rendered upon her? For years, I was washed clean by her pink northern lights at dusk. Her rivers absorbed my pain and the enormous collective pain of all her inhabitants. To live there was to know beyond a doubt that a power greater than the sum of humans exists and protects us, in spite of ourselves. Cosmic intelligence seeps through impenetrable walls; signs and symbols of life speak clearly, if only we would listen.

For many years I lived in Greenwich Village, across from a very small square. Each day as I walked past the park, the pigeons scurried about for scraps of bread fed them by the homeless and elderly. One day as I walked by all the pigeons flew away. That was the day I discovered that I had cancer. The journey that ensued took me through the darkly shadowed valley of my innermost self.

My purpose in writing this personal story is to share my discoveries as a seeker. Cancer has been my greatest teacher. Like a compass, it has guided me toward the path I have since been treading. It has given back to me my "memory," and the ability to make wholesome choices and to examine my motives. In short, it has taught me how to be alert to the significance of my being here.

I believe that no recovery is by chance. Mine was the result of a deliberate choice to live, to make peace with myself and to dissolve my cancer, which I had created inside of me. Before this resolve set in, I went through a dark period of fear followed by a longer stage of having blind faith in several well-recognized physicians and established medical institutions. Soon after being reassured that my

condition was benign, I learned it was not. It had migrated throughout the body and taken firm root in my liver; a malignant mass had also formed next to my kidneys. The pace of my physical failing was simply accelerated by the many rounds of radiation therapy. An array of baffled physicians began offering me various comfortable ways to exit the planet.

While in the warm, false embrace of morphine following my tenth surgical operation, I understood that I would most assuredly die unless I ran from what was then the fifth medical facility. The raw truth had impacted and, for the first time in my life, I felt lost. Years of anger and frustration, along with pain, surfaced. Anger at allowing myself to be thrown against those cold walls with no reprieve; frustration with those scientific chaps who had no regard for the cause of my condition; pain from realizing I had no choice but to audit my life and my agenda for it.

I knew that I would come face to face with my reasons for trying to kill myself at such a young age. Examining every detail of my past with a microscope was crucial to my new agenda—my recovery agenda. My biggest discovery in the process was that the real battles had begun long before my cancer surfaced. During this period of soul searching, I had to be extremely honest with myself and have consistency with my disciplines. I recognized that my cancer was born of me and because of me. *I* was the problem, and yet invariably also the solution.

Solitude was essential to the primal probing of my innermost self. That winter, I isolated myself for three months in a small cabin in the undifferentiated white of the Vermont winter. If I was going to die, I had to set certain things right with myself. As I kept the wood fires burning, I ceaselessly emptied myself of fears, pain, hopes, dreams, and disappointments. Days ran into nights unnoticed because of the tears. I understood how death had become an unconscious solution to my grief, and how all my actions had been channeled to that end. I saw how well I had manipulated my life, and how its successes had been founded on an enormous myth of my own construction.

I was guilty of tampering with the subtle forces of my primal self. I had been brought up in a traditional Hindu home in British Guiana, three generations removed from mother India. By the age of fifteen, I had decided to recarve my life to fit an image of my own choosing. This action was rooted in the false belief that I had the power to live separately from the circumstances of a painful childhood, that I could totally replace the family, the tradition, the lineage, and all the beauty and anguish that were an intrinsic part of my personal heritage. In sum, I had created a second life.

What I had not counted on was the factor of memory: the unerasable record of layer upon layer of both resolved and unresolved past impressions. The truths too painful to deal with; the unrealistic expectations of myself; the childhood agonies I had run from; the loose ends of family ties; the primal anger that stemmed from generations of being uprooted—all these were stored intact. They became the fodder for my recovery.

This division in myself, this second life, was the primary reason for my cancer. According to the Vedic scriptures, there are pursuits in life common to all human beings: *dharma, artha, kama,* and *moksha.* Dharma is one's alignment with what is right as defined by the universal laws of nature; artha is the natural pursuit of wealth; kama is the natural pursuit of pleasures; and moksha is absolute freedom or liberation from all actions of artha, kama, and even dharma. The cycle of rebirth can only end through moksha, when direct knowledge of the self is known. Moksha, freedom from human limitation, is considered the last accomplishment of human life. Although the pursuit of wealth and pleasure is admittedly a natural part of life, when the means defy the laws of universal dharma, that pursuit becomes a living hell. Dharma, the universal law of nature, is part of every society, every tradition, every religion, as it is part of every human being. By common sense, we are aware when we rub against the grain of what is right.

Through that Vermont winter, I cossetted myself in the warmth of a raging fire only to feel the desolate cold of my inner being. How many inner signals I must have missed to find myself confronted with this fatal situation. How wrong I was in trying to rewrite my destiny. For those few months, my nightmares became reality as I delved into all my unconscious agendas. Cancer, indeed, has a way of knocking us down in order to get us out of our own way.

According to the Vedas, the ancient sacred scriptures of India, six qualities are necessary to succeed in any venture: proper effort; perseverance; courage; knowledge of the given pursuit; skill and resources; and the capacity to overcome obstacles. While these qualities brought me great success in the material world, ironically I had neglected to apply them to my life as a human being. As a result, my shallow success inevitably had to collapse. I had tampered with universal forces and thus was deprived of their invincible protection.

Finally I reached the bottom and felt that to continue to live would be too brutal. Too tired to pursue answers to the great mysteries, I prayed to quietly slip away. In the agony of this prayer, a vision of my father appeared. I had severed all ties with my father and family twelve years earlier. As his image appeared to me my life began to turn inside out. The floodgates of cognition burst open, and memories of the past washed through my mind. All the closets were being emptied; all the monsters were pouring out. As I beheld his face—humbled by the years, seasoned with wisdom, quiet and compassionate—I was startled not to find the terrifying giant of my childhood. He seemed to know of my grief and was appearing to remind me of something I had forgotten since childhood. That something was *karma*. The word dropped like a bomb. The inescapable, the inevitable. What was death but a cosmic reaction to all actions in life, a notch in the wheel of life, and a guaranteed rebirth.

According to the Vedas, a human birth is not easy to achieve. Once the human body materializes, whether we understand it as due to karma or to natural selection, the factor of free will and the power of self-reflection come into play. The human birth is the only one endowed with the capacity to make choices. Each choice we make fuels the turning of the wheel of karma. Once we recognize this innate power, we must take responsibility for all our actions. I saw that to slip away silently would only compound my errors. I would then incur even more pain in the next life on the continuum of the life cycle. For death, according to the laws of karma, is but a brief silencing of memory. The Atman, which is the immortal spirit in each of us, continues, as do the collective memories of all our lives, which serve as essential guides through all time. Our choices and actions determine the nature of our rebirths. We are fully accountable for the choice to die, like the choice to live. If death was not the absolute resolution, what was my big hurry to stop spinning the wheel of life? I had to act according to the dharma. I had no choice but to see this birth through to its proper conclusion. Cancer showed me the false notions of my ways and the truth of the saying, *Dharma raksati raksatah:* if you protect dharma, it will protect you.

One day after three months, I left Vermont with the full knowledge that I would live. From that day on I felt death's grip loosen. Free of my old burdens, I had a lightness and a certain serenity. I took complete control of my life. Most of my recovery had in fact occurred during those few timeless months. Upon my returning to the world and having several tests, no sign of cancer was present in my blood. Prior to Vermont, the growth rate of my tumors had been rapid. Now only the tumor above one kidney remained, and it was about the same size as before. It was clear that my purging had arrested the disease, and that I was on the winning side.

Since the remaining tumor was inoperable, I was presented with a new set of options. A complete diet and lifestyle change was inevitable, but these changes would take a long time to finally rid my body of the tumor. Fears lingered, as I was still unable to trust that the intelligence of nature, my nature, would rid my body of all foreign matter as the connection to memory and my inner being strengthened. I looked into a course of chemotherapy treatment. Although I had lost faith in the scientific medical practices, I was still dependent on the scientists, with their obsession to achieve the end regardless of means. I understood that before my Vermont sojourn, I had been absent from my own healing process. Now I wanted to rid my body immediately of the tumor and confront the challenge of assuming full responsiblity for my actions. At least I was going to be very present and involved in the curative process. To rid myself of my residual enemy, I sought and found a doctor of great reason and science with whom I could work.

Under his supervision, three erudite diagnosticians were enlisted to review my biopsies, old and current. Everyone agreed on one point: it was a very rare strain of cancer. This was, at least, a good beginning. I implored them to tell me the exact nature of my condition; no more shots in the dark. I tested the patience and genius of my doctor and found his kindness and genius rare. Together, working with method, reason, and prayer, we eventually succeeded. My body was totally free of any signs of cancer. He quickly encouraged me to reunite with my family, who had since migrated to Canada due to the internal conflicts in British Guiana.

Upon returning from an embracing reconciliation with my family, I went back to sit in my park in Greenwich Village. This time the pigeons stayed and scrounged around uninterruptedly for food. I knew then that I was free of my cancer. I knew that I need never go back to the hospital for further blood tests. The cognitive memories of my past and future had become so powerful that they would guide me through this weave of form, motion, and sound called life, until in time even that weave would be erased by the eternal consciousness.

Now the real work was to begin. It was time to test my bravado, for it takes courage to live a simple, decent, and honest life. I learned to accommodate and forgive the people who caused me pain. I learned to forgive myself for my own trespasses. Little by little, I increased my quiet time.

As the daily routine became a daily discipline, the grace in my life increased. I began to aid fellow cancer patients, most of whom were left helpless by conventional therapies. I was asked to meet with a young man named Russell who had prostate cancer. His father, who strongly supported conventional therapy, was quite concerned that his son opted for the alternative course of macrobiotics. When I saw Russell in Newport, Rhode Island, two years later, his radiant health and good looks commanded my attention. He had cured himself of cancer through the use of wholesome foods and activities, and through the recognition of the oneness between his self and the supreme spirit.

I was beginning to understand that it is the spirit of light, air, soil, and the river which appears as this densely packed energy I call my body. As humans, we become so thickly absorbed in our separate and false realities that we lose our memory of being. In order to heal, we need to remember our being. Every action we perform flows from the immovable axis of our spirit.

I began to apply a constant alertness in my life. My practice of yoga asanas and meditation began. Studying natural means to good health became part of my daily life. While I continued to live and work in New York, with all its distractions, for years after my cancer bout, my focus was on the dharma and values important to my newly found freedom. My life became wholesome and conscious. I enjoyed the grace of my beautiful friends Aveline and Michio Kushi, pillars of the macrobiotic way of life. I began home studies in Oriental medicine, and finally my search led me to the discovery of Ayurveda, the mother of all healing sciences.

Perhaps it was my Hindu lineage that created such a deep desire in me to delve into this ancient wisdom of God, man, and nature. My studies of Ayurveda are based on the collected Sanskrit works, Samhitas, of Charaka and Sushruta, and an array of Ayurvedic works by masters such as Vaidya Bhagwan Dash, Pandit Shiv Sharma, Dr. Vasant Lad, and Dr. Robert E. Svoboda.

It has been twelve years since I began practicing and studying the general disciplines of naturopathy. This book is a synthesis of my life's discoveries. The unerasable truths and knowledge I found within myself lie within each of us. We can all tap this storehouse of cognitive memories. My story is one of how disease establishes itself in a body that refused to acknowledge its roots, that denied painful or unpleasant experiential memories. By severing part of my experiential memory, I had severed my deeper roots to the earth and my cosmic connection, as it were, in the form of my cognitive memory. I devote some of the first chapter in this book to examining the significance of cognitive memory in wholesome and healthful living.

Although this book is based on the Ayurvedic system of wellness, I have extracted and fused information from many systems and global practices. Most recently I have delved into the endless well of nectar, Vedanta—the end portion of the Vedas dealing with the study of self-knowledge.

After my father's death, the Lord's abiding and abundant grace blessed me with the arrival of my beloved teacher, His Holiness Swami Dayananda Saraswati. I lived with my teacher for several years and began my official studies in Sanskrit and Vedanta. Though I no longer live at the ashram, the presence of this great sage is continually with me as I study and imbibe his great wisdom and guidance in the daily dispensation of living.

I begin this book with a peace invocation from the Vedas.

*Svasti prajabhyah paripalayantam / nyajena margena mahim mahisah*
*Gobrahmanebhyah subham astu nityam / lokah samastah sukhino bhavantu*
*Kale varsatu parjanyah / prthivi sasya salini*
*Deso yam ksobha rahita / brahmanah santu nirbhayah*

May people be happy. May the peacemakers righteously rule the Earth.
Let there be welfare for animals and people of wisdom at all times.
May all be happy.
May it rain at the proper time. May the Earth produce grains.
May this world be free from famine. May people of contemplation be fearless.

I write this book to explore the nature of the human universe. From the beginning of time, the ancients referred to both the body and the universe as food. Christ, at the Last Supper with his disciples, shared the bread, which symbolized his body. In the Bhagavad Gita, Lord Krishna, in conversing with Arjuna, refers to his body as food and as the consumer of food. We are the air, water, soil, and light of this planet. Every grain of sand, every mountain range, every river, and every leaf contains the same elements. We celebrate nature in our very nature. We eat from nature what is within our nature. The food body of the universe is our personal food body. There is no difference.

I also write this book to refresh our cognitive memories. I use many ancient precepts from the Vedas to paint images that were originally transmuted in the fire of the universal mind. These pictures vivify the essence of being. They stir the cognitive memories of the *ahamkara,* the individual self, so that we may remember the Atman—our true timeless and boundless nature.

I explore the transformation of the five elements, which interlace the "material" of our being. Body types, or *doshas,* are a paradigm of the universal pattern. When we understand this microcosm, we are fully aware of reflecting the macrocosm. The foods, menus, and recipes given here are culled from the myriad of essential spices, herbs, grains, legumes, vegetables, fruits, and seeds of the planet, all woven in a state of balance by the Vedic principles of life.

Each body type has its own special practices or *sadhanas.* These are wholesome and abiding activities that are attuned to nature and that have been refined through the memory of all time. The sadhana inherent within each life form is prodded by memory. Every stirring within tree and animal, every stillness and transmutation within mountain and earth, every flow and confluence of streams and rivers, every leap of a kangaroo, flight of the deer, hop of a rabbit, gait of a tiger, fluttering of a sparrow, gliding of an eagle, every motion signifies sadhana. This is the pattern based on the memory of the universe. I propose we introduce sadhana into our lives as a wholesome guide to remembering nature. Sadhana stirs our cognitive memory and revives the lost art of beauty, grace, and accommodation. Through sadhana we are able to garner the vibrations of the universe to help us meld with the earth body.

PART ONE

# The Principles of Ayurveda

CHAPTER 1

# COSMIC ROOTS

Ayurveda is rooted in India's most cherished scriptures known as the Vedas, which date to about B.C. 1500. Of the four Vedas, two of them—the Rig Veda and Atharva Veda—give detailed information about healing, surgery, and longevity. The Rishis, the holy bards of ancient India who compiled the Vedas, received their instruction and information internally. The Rishis, which literally translates as "seers," would immerse themselves in contemplation and meditation and would "see" the truth. They culled their information from the cosmos. While we could say that Western medicine sprang from a microscopic examination of the microcosm, the physical world of amoebas and cells, Indian medicine arose from a microscopic examination of the macrocosm, the sublime embracing silence that contains all knowledge and the sacred memory of all time, our cognitive memory.

Ayurveda is not only the ancient Indian science of preventative health and healing but also a philosophy of living. Rarely treating the symptoms, Ayurveda cures by removing the cause of disease. From the rich legacy left us by the Rishis, we learn what we are now coming to know again in the West: transgressions against Nature's laws, against our own inner wisdom, are the cause of all disease. The disease may be either physical or karmic in origin. Physical diseases are due to engaging in excessive use of our senses, improper eating, or ignoring the cycles of the seasons or our age. Karmic diseases result from incorrect actions performed in this or previous lifetimes. Around the eighth century in India, when rebirth became recognized as a truth, it became understood that the physical body was the only part of us that dies. Our psychic instrument, or *antahkarana,* which is composed of the intellect, mind, and ego, or *ahamkara,* travels with us lifetime after lifetime until we attain final liberation, or *moksha.*

This book concerns itself with both types of transgressions because, in fact, they cannot be separated. As long as we are ignoring a karmic condition, we cannot be whole; as long as we are ignoring a natural law, we will remain fragmented.

Ayurveda removes the cause of disease by righting these transgressions and reestablishing balance

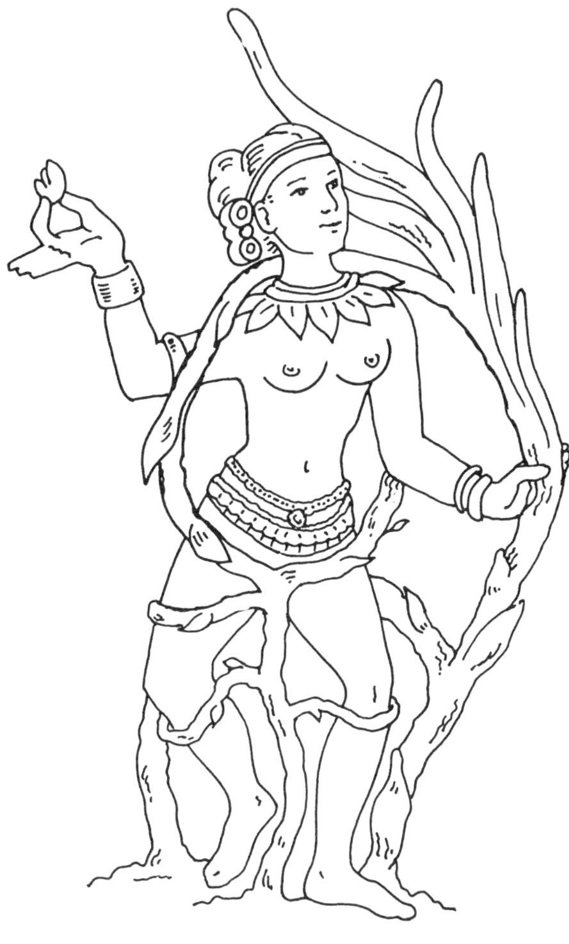

**Salabhanjika, the Tree Spirit.**
**Salabhanjika represents the primal forces of the wise Earth. She is intertwined with the tree whose vegetation represents Earth's fertility. The flow of her sap represents all of Earth's movements.**

to our system. To treat our entire cosmic nature, we must address all the component parts of a human being. According to Ayurveda, we are composed of three bodies: physical, astral, and causal. This translates into body, mind, and soul in Western terms. The antahkarana exists within the astral body. The physical form was given to us as a vehicle for practicing sadhanas, or wholesome activities. Through these practices we are able to understand our three bodies, or the three aspects of our nature. Food, which contains the memory of all time, is an extremely potent medium for bringing balance to our being.

According to the Rishis, from pure consciousness arose the sound of OM. In turn, the Five Great Elements took birth. These five elements take the form, in the human body, of the three doshas, or bodily humors. It is from these doshas that our individual constitution—our *prakriti*—is formed. As we come to identify ourselves with these primal elements, we create a bridge that allows us to climb back to the sky: we approach our cosmic roots.

*The self is the origin of all finite happiness,*
*But it is itself limitless, transcending definition.*
*It remains unaffected by deeds, good or bad.*
*It is beyond feeling and beyond knowledge.*
*It is the ever present in the meditation of a sage.*
***Brihadaranyaka Upanishad***

According to the Vedas, human birth is the most difficult to attain in the karmic cycle. It is the greatest act of transformation that a human being experiences. Free will is our divine birthright, as are our capacities for self-reflection and distraction. It is distraction that has, in part, created our present state of confusion and chaos. The earth existed billions of years before our arrival a mere three and a half million years ago. As the planet ages and we grow in universal wisdom and come to know the beauty of cosmic magnetism among all life-forms, we will begin to know ourselves. Presently we are preoccupied with our individual selves and external pursuits that distance us from the throb of planetary harmony. The universe is a cohesive entity held in majestic motion by space and her magic grasp. To be obsessed with our quest for personal uniqueness and excellence, while ignoring this life-giving space and all she contains, is to behave like immature adolescents. Conversely, to be obsessed with the woes of our planet and lose sight of the true self, which is consciousness and awareness, is equally immature.

Memory of life as unified and essential must begin to serve us again. Billions of atoms traveling throughout the universe become absorbed into billions of life-forms, including those of our own bodies. According to the Vedas, the entire body is totally renewed every seven years. Nevertheless, disease persists beyond the cycles of renewal because we are unable to make the transition from our separate and experiential selves into the whole state of cognition. We live in the past and future, prisoners trapped by concepts of time and space. In truth, the endless and timeless present is always with us and filled with possibility. We need only to remember this—to be still within our true nature, to be present in our activities and observations, to discard memories belonging to hearsay and beliefs that can't be verified, to simply be and to live.

This conscious self is referred to in the Vedas as the Atman, or the Indwelling Spirit. This self is the source of our true balance. Health is not the separate pursuit of the perfect body, or the forging of an intellectual mind, or even austere practices for the spirit. The life to which the sages refer in Ayurveda is the solid union of body, mind, and spirit. It is a balance of these three factors, and the further integration of each self with nature, family, and all living beings. When we recognize fragmentation to be the source of all illness, we may begin to benefit from the practices of a holistic life.

The word *dosha* literally means "that which has a fault," a system that is quick to change. This is the definition given by the ancients to our experiential nature. We were not meant to strive for perfection. Consciousness is the only perfection. Every manifestation is essentially endowed with change. It is through our fragmentary, imperfect existence that we can learn how to invite the cognitive self. As we come to reside more and more in the cognitive self, we are increasingly able to approach the conscious self, or Atman. Within the perimeters of our lives, we can strive to attain balance in our dynamic and quick-to-err nature, and in the unfolding process aspire to the knowledge of the self, as being unified with the nature of the absolute. This supreme, unfolding nature is the true character of our spirit. We can aspire to this perfection, for it is the only perfection. But it is erroneous and burdensome to attempt to maintain a perfect body, a perfect life, and perfect health, for the demands of such striving steal the vital force from life. What we can reasonably do is aspire to a life of balance, without desperate measures. It releases the harmful focus of a mind set in perfection and a will steeped in inimical reversals. Ayurveda is the pursuit of balance. A life of balance has no extremes and very little fragmentation.

## A HEALTHY AHAMKARA

The Vedas define ahamkara as the individual self, the vehicle bestowed upon each of us at birth to facilitate our particular life's journey. It is often referred to as the ego, but not in the Freudian sense of the word. Rather, ahamkara is the essence of the remembering self, an aspect of the Atman that is refined through the process of multiple rebirths. The ahamkara contains not only the individual self with its experiential memories of this life, but also the cognitive self with its collective memories of all time—past, present, and future. Each life is a journey toward the eventual attainment of knowledge of the Atman. The ahamkara—through cognitive memory—is our primary bridge to that knowledge.

To give an analogy, if one bead on a rosary represents your present lifetime, the rest of the beads on the thread of ahamkara are your past and future lives. The rosary as a whole, being more than the sum of its parts, holds the collective memories of all species in the cosmos. When we meditate or practice sadhanas—especially food sadhanas, which invoke cognitive memory—we can access this timeless past and future, and intrinsically know the present.

Ahamkara is conditioned from life to life through conception in the womb. The ego's identity is influenced by the maternal ovum, the paternal sperm, the time and season of conception, the state of the mother's womb, the foods and emotions of the mother, and the seasons through which the embryo grows.

The core of the Ayurvedic science of health is based on our inborn constitution, also called our prakriti. Karmic or causal factors also affect our individual birth. Ahamkara registers each and every behavior, whether conscious or unconscious, from the inception of each life. Ahamkara controls the millions of cells of the immune system. When both experiential and cognitive memory are fresh and clear, we are able to safeguard the organism against the invasion of mental and physical diseases. When the ahamkara, the individual ego, is displaced, fragmented, or shifted from its primal source of universal at-one-ment, it leaves the immune process vulnerable and volatile. This is the very first cause of ill health.

In the formative stages of life, when the ego is defenseless, protection by parents and teachers is necessary. When these primary guardians falter, the young mind, exercising its singular defense, insulates itself and blocks its natural outflow of expression. The result is the beginning of a weak ego, and oftentimes a lack of self-worth. As this life reaches early adulthood, certain patterns of defense and isolation have already formed. It is immensely difficult for this person to initiate the process of opening painful childhood wounds. These inflictions remain raw and unhealed within the gray shelters of the mind until that individual finds the courage to expose the damaged self, or is forced by providence through a difficult passage, like a deadly disease, to face and accept the fragmented ego. This marks the beginning of the healing process.

The practice of reparative sadhanas and a meditative life are necessary to become conscious and alive to each moment. Through sadhanas we can attain more and more constant awareness of the whole cognitive self. The process of healing may take many lifetimes, but the very process inspires the indweller to shine, and reflect its beauty on the world.

External pursuits of health are a waste of time and energy. They have created profitable mega-industries for those empowered by their own fragile sense of the holistic. They have also granted divergence to those who choose ever newer veils to shroud their pain. Essentially, there is no alternative to the process of achieving salubrious well-being. It is hard and dedicated work requiring great compassion for, and honesty with, ourselves. Our own healing begins with forgiving our protectors, who were also helpless prey to their own difficult circumstances.

Acceptance of ourselves as we are is the greatest health of all. For this, time stands still. The accomplishment of inner quiet, signifying peace of mind, removes years of aging. As we begin to nurture the wounds of the ego, we find that time actually reverses itself and we gain youth. Immortality is maintained by living in the present, without moments or minutes. This is the foundation of holistic health.

## OUR TIMELESS NATURE

There is a beautiful story in the Puranas that discusses the concept of time. Narada, in search of knowledge of the Self, approached Lord Krishna and asked "What is maya?" Lord Krishna replied, "Before I reveal maya, I need a drink of water."

Narada spotted a small village in the distance and made his way there to get water. When he knocked on the door of a small house in the village, a beautiful damsel opened the door, and he completely forgot his reason for being there. He was caught in the brake of love. The next day he returned, just to catch one glimpse of the exquisite creature. Still he had no memory of the thirsty Lord whom he kept waiting.

In time, Narada was wed to this damsel and she bore him three children. They lived a happy and contented life. After many years, his father-in-law died and Narada inherited his house. Twelve years passed. There was a great flood and Narada lost everything—his wife, children, and house. In his attempt to save his family, he was washed ashore. When he looked up, he beheld Lord Krishna in the same spot he had left him so many years ago.

"Narada, what took you so long?" asked the Lord. "I have been waiting here for you for half an hour!"

Twelve years of human time had been only a drop of half an hour in celestial time. That is the truth of *maya,* the material aspect of the universe. Physical time is different from the time that prevails over the spirit. How often have years elapsed between a visit to our loved ones, yet when we embrace them again, the time in between seems to never have happened.

Where is the truth of time in the dream state, when we lose ourselves in timelessness? Elaborate braids of dreams occur within split seconds of time as we know it. Cognition happens in a similar manner. Not organized sequentially within the time and space of existence, cognition is rather a split second opening into a vastness which has neither beginning nor end. We experience reality in a partial, self-absorbed manner, fluttering from the boughs of life. The truth of all time is refined within our memory. This cognitive memory is the entire creation held in stasis within a tiny seed. The seed is the self.

In terms of time and space, we live with a cosmic equation. On one side of the equation we exist in a time-bound reality, where our experiences are formed through cultures, traditions, families, and societies. We have charted the progress of the sun and moon and invented a time cycle of a three hundred-and-sixty-five day year, a twenty-four hour day, a seven day week, a sixty second minute, and so on. We continuously adapt to the seasons of the year; we have a light cycle in which we perform our activities and a dark cycle in which we rest and replenish our bodies and minds. This part of the equation I call our experiential time.

Experiential time varies for each species of the universe. The gods or superhumans experience time in a sweep much too vast for the human mind to fathom. In the puranic story, a half hour of celestial time was twelve years of human existence. It is said in the Upanishads that one night to Brahma the creator equals some millions of years of human time.

The time cycles for land and aquatic animals, as well as birds, are not confined to a precise schedule. These creatures adapt themselves to the light and dark cycles and to seasonal changes; they live more on the other side of the equation, that of timelessness. The dolphin traveling deep within the womb of the sea experiences a heightened pulse rate and vibratory frequency associated with a state of timeless awareness. The human experiences a similar vibratory fluidity during its embryonic state. While suspended in the water of life, an embryo sustains a heart rate of 160 beats per minute. On arrival into the time-bound atmosphere of external space, air, fire, water, and earth, the heart rate drops dramatically. In the process of birth, vibratory rate becomes less fluid and the timeless memories of creation become squelched. As a human species, we have adapted to charting our progress through the time-bound passage. We came equipped with mind and senses for proper navigation.

According to the wisdom shared in the Vedas, animals are considered the embodiments of the timeless spirit of consciousness. In the shamanic tradition, the dolphin is considered the one aquatic animal that knows of dream time, or the timeless nature of our cognition. The hawk, which soars beyond the time zone and returns to remind us of our timeless nature, is called the messenger of the Great Spirit.

If we want to know our timeless nature, we need to examine our unique attribute—our will, our power of choice and self-reflection. This divine human acquisition has in part been the source of much of our present confusion. Because of our composition—our physical body, mind, and senses—we feel compelled to live within a time-bound state. The body seems propelled by the mind, which is led by the senses, which in turn are influenced primarily by time-constrained perceptions. In reality, the senses are employed by the mind, and the mind is hired by the will, our great source of self-reflection. Of ten million species, we are the one species whose refinement, through the passage of some twenty billion years, yields a most stupendous reward: The ability to live fully within the balance of the time-bound and the timeless. It is only in our timeless nature that the source of full cognition prevails. And it is only through this time-bound journey of rebirths that we are able to inquire into our timeless nature.

At the end of every day we fall into slumber to be rejuvenated. When we are in deep sleep we resonate with our cosmic nature and are renewed in the bosom of silence. As a result, we are able to sustain our dream nature throughout the time-bound activities of the day.

Our cognitive memories are not the function of the sense organs, mind, or will. They are the result of recognizing our ageless and timeless nature. We do so through the practice of meditation, still observation, deep sleep, and food sadhanas, as revealed in this book.

## TAPPING COGNITIVE MEMORY

Often when we have a gut feeling, a sixth sense, or a deja vu, we dismiss it as a moment of misperception. Actually, it is during these moments that we are truly

conscious. The antics of body and mind have been quiet enough for a splinter of truth to unveil itself. For a moment we have been linked, ever so frailly, to another bead on the rosary, or *mala,* of cognitive memory. This memory guides us through the beads of all the lives, until the mala of all existence is complete and we merge with pure consciousness.We can permanently access this essential memory only when our actions become sadhanas connected to the earth.

During the last year of my bout with cancer, I had been anaesthetized eleven times. For this reason, my final operation was done without general anesthetic. I remember that, through my intense pain, the memories that came to comfort me were serene and simple. During the eight-hour procedure, I saw my guts pulled out of my stomach and smelled the deep brine and blood of being. I heard my father sing "Red River Valley," one of his old favorite tunes. I was taken back to the age of three or four and heard the plop, plop of shoes on smooth black mud, as my sister and I were carried on a long dirt path to visit my favorite aunt. I felt the coolness of her hut, which was daubed with cow dung. The eastern light streaming in through the small aperture of the dwelling enveloped me, and I was transported to the truth of my being. My sister and I must have spent many days in that faraway hut, surrounded by the brambles of gooseberry bushes and the briers of sweet white flowers. Swathed in cognition, time stood still.

This is an example of how we tap cognitive memory; it is by means of our deepest vibratory field, which lies within the element of space. The gravitational field of space is also the field of sound and prana, or breath. Our memory, held by ahamkara, resonates within this field. When the field of sound and space is distorted, it directly impinges the prana body and we begin to lose connection with our eternal vibrations. Humanity's misuse of the earth's resources directly relates to the slackening of the gravitational grasp of space. As a result, our capacity to hold eternal memory, which is received through cosmic vibration, is wearing thin.

In meditation, we are taught to silence the mind and sit in the self. In understanding this silence, we begin to understand the self. True meditation is dynamic; it goes far beyond sitting in silent postures. When it springs from a deeply conscious place within, meditation pervades every action.

The beauty of the self is that it shows us how to step out of our shadows and bask in its light, if we are alert and undistracted by the cacophony of living. This cognitive self is available to us through our daily sadhanas. These wholesome practices refine our vibratory powers and enable us to strengthen the spirit. Through our endless capacity for distraction and superficial countenances, we have lost access to our inner guide, cognitive memory. Without it, we are becoming a universe of living amnesiacs. Knowledge of the life force is not new. We have almost all known it at some time in our past, but we have forgotten. Now we need to strum the chords of ahamkara so that we may remember the immortal secrets of all life and health.

We must scrutinize the mechanism we employ in accepting something to be a truth. More than two-thirds of the information stored in our present-life (experiential) memory bank consists of invalid memories. Every moment of each day we form opinions based on inaccurately remembered or incomplete data. In this way we accrue false and useless information. These opinions, in their turn, are invariably filed into memory without resolve. We compile memory data with every breath. Sifting through the details of everything that comes to our attention is a stupendous task. That is why the ancients exhort us to listen with a discriminating heart and refrain from jumping to conclusions. As we begin to become more alert and observant of our intake, we will gradually store less invalid information in our memory banks.

A valid memory is one that can be verified as accurate and which, therefore, resonates with universal truth. If we refrain from condemnation and hasty conclusions, the truth usually reveals itself. All traditions were founded originally on universal truths. Unfortunately, the demise of many traditions is due, in part, to the karmas accumulated from corruption, personal greed, and selfish power. The mind of the universe is sustained in good health only when her memory holds the imprint of valid experiences. The human mind functions in the same manner.

Just as a lie cannot exist in honesty and a fish cannot survive in clay, so the invalid cannot be stored in an observant mind. The practice of sadhanas within the harmonic resonance of nature awakens us to these memories. They come through our vibratory field in a subtle and decisive way, without a big bang. These simple guides barely leave an impression, and yet the conviction of the choices we make as a result of this remembering is unshakable. Sadhanas are essential to dissolve our excess of invalid memories and to maintain a healthy and honest cognition. They are the gift the universe gave humans to cleanse themselves and to live gently upon the earth.

We experience creation through the two-pronged ahamkara: the experiential (individual) self and the cognitive (collective) self. Every being has an inherent memory refined from the beginning of time. When the fawn wobbles on its lanky legs minutes after birth, the memory of its species, from the very first fallow deer, is sustained. According to the Vedas, memory of all lives is remembered by the human embryo at the exact moment it leaves its watery domain and begins to emerge into the open world. After this passage, we gradually lose cognition of our magnificent inheritance and begin to function experientially.

Lymph, blood, muscle, fat, bone, marrow and nerves, and sperm and ovum—the seven vital tissues or *dhatus* of Ayurveda—carry the memories that shape the body and mind of each organism. Through these memories each life-form is able to adapt to the demands of its present environment and to function through all rebirths. The memory of each individual life, as well as the collective existence of the universe, is forever braided into the fabric of our being. These braided karmic imprints, which give us our singular identity, are referred to in Sanskrit as *samskaras.*

Every species is a form of remembering. The mountain goat has the memory of eons stamped in the structure of its feet, a structure that defies gravity. This creature was understood by the sages to be the living symbol of freedom—freedom from the cycle of rebirths. *Aja,* the Sanskrit term for goat, means "the one that has transcended birth." The original human tribes knew the memory of the universe because they observed the wild animals with whom they shared the earth. The early humans knew their own nature and sought to discover their cognitive memory by conquering wild animals. When they did so, they inherited that animal's power and what it symbolized. Essentially they sought to remember that which was forgotten in the brilliant flash of birth. We are given infinite clues and symbols in this universe to stir cognitive memory. The animals and plants are powerful guides, but every grain of sand can remove the fog surrounding remembrance when we learn to observe.

Sadhanas awaken the deeply embedded healing codes that are part of the emergent cognition of a timeless universe. There are many sadhanas that, when practiced with consistency, yield great inner fortitude and stir cognitive remembering. A simple walk through the forest, sitting in the river or ocean, riding a horse, walking barefoot on the early morning grass, digging into the soil, sowing seeds in a garden, sitting in the self, observing silence, prayer, chanting, practicing yoga asanas, dancing, doing t'ai chi, hiking in the mountains, swimming in a stream, smelling unplucked fruits in an orchard—these are just a few of the endless sadhanas that erase the invalid and give life to the primal, cognitive self.

*Be praised, my Lord,*
*For all your creatures,*
*And first for brother sun,*
*Who makes the day bright and luminous.*

*And he is beautiful and radiant*
*With great splendor,*
*He is the image of you, Most High.*

*Be praised, my Lord,*
*For sister moon and the stars,*
*In the sky you have made them brilliant*
*And precious and beautiful.*
*Be praised, my Lord, for brother wind*
*And for the air both cloudy and serene*
*And every kind of weather,*
*Through which you give nourishment*
*To your creatures.*

*Be praised, my Lord, for sister water,*
*who is very useful and humble*
*And precious and chaste.*

*Be praised, my Lord, for brother fire,*
*through whom you illuminate the night.*
*And he is beautiful and joyous*
*And robust and strong.*

*Be praised, my Lord,*
*For our sister, mother earth,*
*Who nourishes us and watches over us*
*And brings forth various fruits*
*With colored flowers and herbs.*

*St. Francis of Assisi*

## FOOD IS MEMORY

The Earth has been continuously refining herself from the beginning of time. Every species she contains contributes to the evolution of the universe. Each tree and mountain, cloud, and stream reflects the light of the universe. Cosmic memory is held and refined by the genetic code, the DNA, of all life-forms. For this reason, cosmic communion prevails among each of the Earth's inhabitants. When we walk, run, or climb, each cell recalls its cognition from the beginning of life. The land itself holds the cumulative cognizance of all ten million species. Our motions, our actions, set the stage for remembering. When we behold the beauty of a stream glittering in sunlight, or taste the nectar of a freshly ripened peach—even in passive moments, when our skin is brushed by the wind or our nostrils flooded by the fragrance of a flower, we are experiencing the elements—we are stirring cognitive memory.

Every food, every motion, every dream is memory of past and future. All vital memory is congealed within these three aspects of the whole. To realize that we are the inherent knowers of the elements is to remember from the beginning to the present. When we observe ourselves within the primacy of nature, we begin to thaw the frozen cognition of our being.

The five elements continuously transmute into each other to create atoms, molecules, minerals, foods, and life-forms. Food is the keeper of all five elements; in its transformation the body of life is formed. Our cognitive relationship to food can unravel the vast mystery of being in time and space. Food takes us through the complete cycle of being, from the original cosmic seed to the fragile sprout, to the flourishing plant and its fruits—our sustenance. Our need for food makes us dig into the land, feast on her bounty, and expel our bodily wastes back into her, so this Earth may continue to enrich herself. The food cycle is our complete memory. It is the constant remembering of our body. Food is memory. Memory is being. Eating is remembering. In our present spell of forgetfulness, we need "observing motion," conscious action, to warm the frozen cells of life.

We need to perceive this Earth as a referent of our being. We are all formed from the same ingredients as the tree and animal. The Earth is our physical body and Water is its fluid; Fire is the acids and enzymes of the body; Air is the prana and breath, and Space is the vibration of all vital systems together. The wholesome smell of Earth stirs fresh memory. Water allows us to taste and discern life. Fire enables us to digest the universe and transmute its cosmic intelligence; it gives us vision and sight. As well, Fire gives us the power to continually renew our observation—each moment contains a powerful potential for transformation. Air allows us to feel, to touch, to know. It is the gauge with which we measure our progress. The joy we feel pushes us forward into our cosmic nature; the pain we feel pushes us forward as well. Both happiness and sorrow allow us to review our growth. Space gives us the power to resonate within our observation and cognition. (We are ultimately taught the cosmic truth by sound and harmonic resonance.) The pull of Space is ever so subtle, the power ever so strong. The primal sound of being exists in this pull. Food, motion, and dream are all held within the stillness of Space. Our infinite nature as humans is born from the Water of life and resolved in the Space of God.

We hold the memory of the five elements in our physical body. The memory of Earth is kept in the heart; the memory of Water is stored in the kidneys; the memory of Fire is kept in the intestines; the memory of Air is held by the lungs; the memory of Space is stored in the brain.

Each of us contains a unique configuration of Earth, Water, Fire, Air, and Space within ourselves. In the human constitution, the five elements of nature are transmuted into the three doshas: Vata, Pitta, and Kapha. Known respectively as the Air, Fire, and Water principles, Vata has Space and Air as its dominant elements, Pitta has Fire as its dominant element, and the dominant elements of Kapha are Water and Earth.

In the section that follows we will examine how these five elements form the five bodies, the *panchakosha*, of the universe and of man. This doctrine of the five bodies, or sheaths, was first described in the Taittiriya Upanishad.

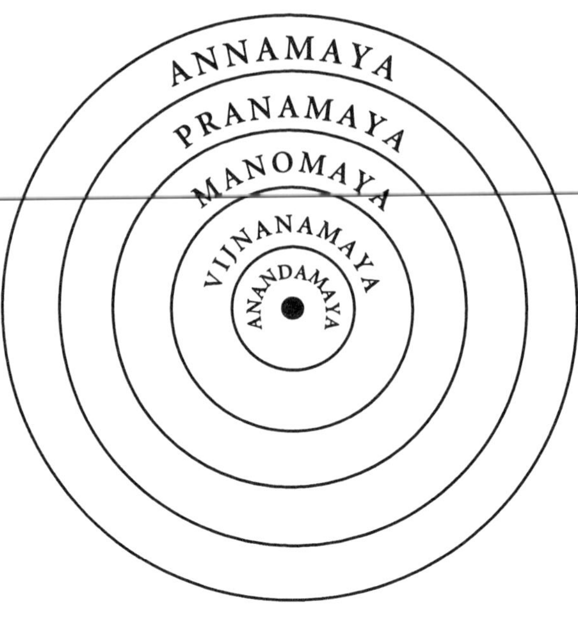


**Panchakosha:**
**The Five Sheaths Veiling the Absolute Nature of Man**

## THE FIVE BODIES

### *The Food Body: Earth and Water (Kapha)*

*I am food. I am the consumer of food.*
*I eat the consumer of foods, I consume the whole universe.*
*Taittiriya Upanishad (11.96)*

*Annamaya,* the first layer of the material self, is sustained by food. The earth and water of the universe are the counterparts, on a massive scale, of the earth and water elements in our own bodies. They make up the food body of humans and other life-forms.

The essential elements of life feed both our inner and outer nature. Essentially we are formed from soil, air, rain, and light that nourish the food we eat from the plant kingdom. It takes food for us to be sustained and grow; it then returns to feed the earth and springs up again in a new life. In the light of consciousness, this cycle continues until all obstacles to penetrating our true nature are resolved. In perceiving the external foods of earth as distant from our food body, we have embarked on a rapid cycle of self-demise. As a result of four hundred years of technological thinking, we have become densely self-absorbed. We are savagely raping the planet for food without recognizing that in fact we are violating ourselves.

From the more than ten million species that remain on the planet, we are losing one million every thirty years. Unless our earth can miraculously replenish herself, we will be extinct in three hundred years, the fastest extinction rate of any species. The Earth is losing her powers of continuance due to the ravages of technology, and to our removal from cognitive memory.

The food body of the universe and her species has been on a sharp decline for the past five hundred years. In its wake, the industrial and technological revolution has left us with a hoard of new and fatal diseases. The diseased planetary food body is also the diseased human food body—the planet and her life-forms suffer analogous afflictions at the same rate of deterioration. The idea of an inside-outside division is a myth. Similarly, if the patience and endurance of all life-forms were measured and added together, they would correspond directly to the endurance and patience of this amazing planet. Perhaps the species that has contributed least to the vast evolutionary score is the human.

Without a healthy food body, we cannot remember. Without a healthy food body, the planet too shall forget. Acorns will embed themselves in the soil and begin to sprout tomatoes, and we humans will probably applaud this abhorrent distortion. Cognitive memory is carried in the impulse and throb of everything that has existed through the passage of billions of years, from the beginning of time and space. Food is the most vital link to our entire history of cognition. The food body is the most tangible form connecting us to universal consciousness. Ironically, it is this very density of form that prevents easy access to the subtle and pervasive forces of awareness. Unless we are able to use our holy vision and see the matter-body as densely packed energy, we will not be able to shed our delusion of body/consciousness alienation.

We have turned upon ourselves. Through time, our cultural heritage and family traditions have dissipated and the values intrinsic to them have collapsed. We have gradually moved away from the core of intelligence and are held in the myopia of cosmic amnesia. The cords of balance have become invisible. Human food is defined in the Vedas as that which is rooted in the earth. Yet animals are being savagely and indiscriminately killed as fodder for humans. We are losing the vision of the ancient shamans and seers. They remembered the self-supporting principle of life. They knew the tree, water, sky, air, soil, light, animal, and human to bear the same immanence as the universe. As humans we have the power of self-reflection. This unique quality is felt through instinctual resonance by the whole cosmos except by the very species that possesses it. We incur the forces of separation and isolation through our vain egoity and false primacy over nature.

Food is our most vital link to cognitive rememberance. When the harvest is planted, reaped, and used in a salubrious way, the valid memory of all time will come to our aid. Unless we can remember, we cannot even begin to reflect on, much less contribute to, the continuance of a healthy planet. The old pine that stood before me for centuries remembers when to drop her cones and her needles. The oak knows when to let go of her leaves and when to bud again. Each tree knows its development to be gradual and gentle. It is in no hurry to leap into the sky. It has no separate awareness from the earth in which it is rooted. Every microorganism knows instinctively how to protect, flourish, or recede to balance the dignity of the earth. This instinctual knowing is the retention of memory deeply transmuted within the DNA of all life-forms. Because of the complexities of the human form, equipped as it is with will, choice, and self-reflection, we have greater burdens to master. As a highly developed species in the evolutionary prime of its extinction cycle, we are pressed to consider our excesses and lack of observation. As our powers of observation and inquiry replace our self-absorption we can hope to vibrate with more maturity.

An impaired food body indicates that the earth and water elements are dysfunctional. These elements make up the Kapha principle, the main structural support of creation. This Kapha principle, which is also in all living entities, lubricates the universe and holds her together. Diseases associated with the vitiation of Kapha proliferate at the present time. The sticky glutinous stuff that gels our cells together and glues us to the universe is beginning to erode. The earth is losing her magnetism and her ability to absorb. All degenerative diseases occur as a result of deterioration of this stuff that seals us together.

The spell that once compelled humans to observe nature is broken. The spell, which beckoned us to bask in the glow of the moon to transform and cool our energies, or to restore our solar body through the rays of the sun, is now an inertia into which we sink deeper with each day. The replenishing walk through the woods and the swim in the open stream or river are quickly becoming faint specks of yesteryear.

## Earth

As we continue to damage our external food body, our earth, we witness an enormous increase in Kapha disorders. Life-forms are becoming more liquid, denser, heavier, colder, cloying, and cloudy. This is reflected in lung congestion and its relative, grief. Tonsillitis and sinusitis, and their corresponding frustration and inertia, are on the increase. Extreme conditions, such as obesity, anorexia, and bulimia, predominate as never before, with their matching emotions of attachment and greed.

The stickiness of the universe helps heal our wounds. It fills the open spaces of earth with abundant foliage, flowers, fruits, and herbs. It supports memory retention. Kapha directs moisture and immunity to the nucleus of the universe, to buffer the natural forces of entropy that accompany her long existence. Kapha alone lubricates the circulatory and nervous systems of Earth and her life-forms, and so helps maintain a constant immunity.

When we inflict damage to the food body, we are breaking down a system that has been stoic and almost impenetrable. We are undermining Kapha's dignity. As Earth's magnetism loosens and her electrical impulses weaken, we drift farther away from the core of remembering. Kapha's patience is extensive and her forgiving expansive; she is the Mother Nature whom we applaud. She is the maternal protector and spirit of the universe. If we observe her even now, in the dismal hours, she will respond with vital resonance. For it is her nature that is deeply embedded in our Kapha nature.

### Water

The waters of the earth are the primal birthing element of all life. All elements are fathered by space and resolve into water. The greatest factor in memory is taste, and only the water element of Kapha can provide us with this faculty. Plants, and thus all food for humans, are totally dependent on water. The conch shell bears the memory of billions of years of ocean life, and through its form and sound we experience the primal circadian rhythm of timeless existence. The conch has kept its spatial memory intact because the sea has sheltered it. The cosmic sea and river shelter all life. They swallow the negative energies of the living and cleanse us. The Ganges has remained a holy and healing source of water despite the human waste, decay, and debris she has carried for hundreds of years. The Hudson River and the rocks of New York City also imbibe the pain of the human spirit and yet miraculously manage to hold all together.

The Water element is sweet and cool. She anoints and lubricates the smooth functioning of the body. She contains the cosmic memory of all taste. When we taste wholesome foods, we remember all time. Smell is created by the Earth. When we smell the Earth's natural fragrance, we remember all time. The Earth element is the magnetic energy that is perceived in the form of molecular configurations by the nose. Because Water and Earth, the electrical and magnetic forces of the universe, are inseparable, they are symbolized by the twin deities Ap and Prithivi in the Hindu scriptures.

## *The Prana Body: Air and Space (Vata)*

*Pranamaya,* the second layer of material self, is sustained by the breath. Wind and air are to the universe what the prana body is to humans, and all life-forms. The prana body is more subtle than the food body. This vital air is responsible for all bodily functions and urges. The ahamkara, which stores memory, is fed by prana. All remembrances expressed in human urges are activated by breath.

All of our past and future is held in the space of ahamkara. Our urges, such as the urge to write, paint, create music, sing, dance, use computers, procreate, have a relationship, love, hate, eat, or evacuate are rooted in the ahamkara. Through it, we are unconsciously predisposed to certain likes and dislikes, images of ourselves, quirks, compensatory behaviors, resistances, insecurities, emotional soft spots, and physiological and psychological tendencies of all kinds. When we are able to properly access the memory files through specific sadhanas, we no longer need to be victim to these tendencies; we are guided from moment to moment in our action and service to the cognitive self. The universe gave us sadhanas as a natural means of remembering. Hypnosis, regression therapy, and other similar forced techniques are unnatural ways of remembering cognitive details, the effects of which may be more harmful than helpful to our vital harmonic system.

Each layer of consciousness is interlaced with other layers. The prana dosha of the planet is the Vata dosha in the human. When the food body of the planet and its inhabitants is violated and plundered, the whole balance of prana is disrupted, both internally and externally. Outside, the inevitable harsh storms and killing winds begin, bringing with them the swift karmas of Vata diseases within our bodies. The natural shifting and decline of an aging planet does not fully account for the distortion of our seasons or other unnatural occurrences and diseases. These are propelled by humankind tampering with its own nature. Once the food body is diseased, the prana body suffers.* Memory function is the first to be vitiated. Forgetfulness, which is rampant in our world, is the direct symptom of pranic impairment. As a result, the cognitive self becomes less accessible. Prana is the breath of the universe. When the life force is impinged, hunger, thirst, and deprivation caused by indulgence prevail. Evidence of this abounds:

> Today a greater percentage of the human race is overweight than [at] any other time in history. Meanwhile, a greater percentage of the human race suffers from malnutrition than [at] any other time in recorded history.
>
> **John Robbins, *May All Be Fed***

Prana is the kinetic force of the universe. It causes the earth's movement around the sun. This heap of dirt called earth becomes a mobile dynamic entity, vibrating with complex life, because of prana. She is made alive, and in turn generates life for every organism that dwells on her, whether human or one-celled. Prana moves the air, water, nerves, and memory cells, and controls expansion and contraction of the earth's surface. The ebb and flow of the oceans and the moon's orbit around the earth are propelled by prana.

Air is the kinetic energy perceived by the skin; the sense of touch is born of prana. Space is registered by the saccule of the ear; our spatial orientation within our gravitational field and sound is produced by space.

Prana alone controls the breath of the planetary heart. The sharp rise of heart-related diseases is due wholly to the dysfunction of bodily prana, or the Vata dosha. When breath suffers, sadness prevails. This eternal breath moves the entire universe. Imagine the earth spinning in her galactic dance with other planets in the cosmos. What a gorgeous feat it is. The breath of the planet is the source of vitalization and renewal. When this layer of energy is sickened, the earth exudes fear, pain, tremors, and spasms. These are indications that her stalwart food layer has been pierced. Planetary deterioration is more readily visible in this dosha because prana is affected more easily than the food body, owing to its subtler nature. Likewise, the system of vibrations is the first to deteriorate within the prana body because of disharmonious noises and impulses. The vitiation of universal prana is directly responsible for the enormous increase of planetary insecurities.

Prana is directly descended from cosmic space. This is why we are able to dream and to reflect on her timeless and spatially limitless aspects. When prana resonates in nervousness, the very spirit of our being is pierced and pain permeates like endless rain. We are presently enduring this grief. During this time, we need to become vigilant and cherish our individual differences, while also knowing our true nature to be the One consciousness.

## *The Mind Body: Fire (Pitta)*

*Manomaya,* the third layer of the material self, is supported by the mind and its mental functions. Fire is to the universe what the mind is to humans. The mind is highly evolved and controls a variety of emotions. It is the basis of the will and the architect of desires. Manomaya, the transforming expression of consciousness, is the propitious power of universal transmutation and the fire force of all life-forms.

The Earth has a mind of her own and her self-constructing principle is fire. Fire makes the entire universe visible. That which we perceive in terms of ideas, vision, and imagination is but a speck of the mind's dynamism within the earth. Our ability to project the names and forms of creation, *nama rupa,* only hints at the earth's supremely intelligent principle.

Our potential for ordered intelligence is manifested in our galaxies and planets. As the earth metabolizes

* Although vitiation of the prana body is primarily caused by degeneration of the food body, occasionally disease can originate in the subtle body. This occurs when, at the time of death, the unresolved pain of the mind body is transported into the subtle body. Then at the time of rebirth, the impaired subtle body reawakens to its ambiance of pain, which in due course permeates the physical being.

oxygen and fuel into fire, so the Pitta function in the body metabolizes acids and enzymes to digest foods and thoughts. Her ability to balance and maintain the precise temperature within the immanent force of the cosmos is our ability to maintain bodily temperature. Her mind and intelligence are our emotions and thoughts.

The transmuting fire of the universe is the fire, or *agni,* of all living forms. As well as providing heat for proper digestion, it is kin to the waters of taste and appetite. Fire is perceived by sight, and is the power of all existing forms. The eye and the sense of sight are created by the element of fire. The simple art of cooking with fire transmutes food to make it suitable for the human system. Every life-form transmutes food in its own way. In most life-forms the power of transmutation resides entirely within the digestive system. Humans are the only species known to transmute foods with both external and internal fire.

This creation will never be defined or captured by words. Our capacity as humans to transcend thoughts and dwell in the oneness of the universal presence is due to the self-constructing prowess of earth's fire.

When the intelligence embodied and living in us loses its connection to the core of the earth's magnetism and dynamism, the thought process becomes distorted and the emotions random. Once the food and prana bodies are impaired, the more subtle body of the mind is dramatically altered. From this ominous transformation all destructive actions take birth. The abhorrent acts of fanaticism are the result of a distorted mind body. The savage turning of one human against another signifies the intense impairment of the mental fire.

The epidemic of self-obsession and self-absorption is an early symptom of a mind whose fire has leapt its bounds. Our innate ability to reflect, to choose, to construct so we may celebrate the dream is being consumed in the conflagration. Self-reflection is the most valuable asset granted to the human species. The power to transform and refine the blaze into cool flames, *tejas,* is our divination. The power of the mind has been greatly misunderstood. It was never meant to make us exclusive, superior beings. We have simply evolved by our own karmic actions. We are all One consciousness. But unless we can remember, the cognitive self will not prevail. Every human search for discovery of self is a good thing. But the process has to become clear and simple. Implementing a healthful lifestyle will not in itself be fruitful, as long as we continue to block memory.

> The guidance of our mind is of more importance than its progress.
>
> **Joubert, *Pensees***

The mind is our faculty for receiving. When the mind-body is impinged, we weaken knowledge with forgetfulness. We forget the art of graciousness, of being a guest in each others' presence. We rush to embroil ourselves in maya, as if believing that self-inquiry will seep through, by osmosis, into the blanket of fog and disregard. Drink from the well with grace. Maintain a distance, and inquiry will be fulfilled. When the universal fire is reflected as the cool flame of the mind, humankind is at its best. The virtues, or dharmas, of sharing, embracing, giving, and participating are all the brilliance, the tejas, reflecting from a happy planet. The Earth is awaiting our conscious evolution. She has endured epidemic proportions of our anger, jealousy, and hatred. The time has come to sustain our goodness and know that our minds are of one mind.

> *This we know. All things are connected*
> *Like the blood that unites us.*
> *We do not weave the webs of life.*
> *We are merely a strand in it.*
> *Whatever we do to the web, we do to ourselves.*
> *We love this earth as a newborn loves its mother's heartbeat.*
> *Hold in your mind the memory of the land*
> *As it is when you receive it.*
> *Receive the land and the air and the rivers*
> *For your children's children and love it as we have loved it.*
>
> ***Chief Seattle (1790-1866)***

## The Intelligence Body

*Even knowledge is the intellect's reflection of consciousness.*

***Taittiriya Upanishad (11.12)***

*Vijnanamaya,* the fourth layer of the manifest self, is sustained by universal intelligence. The intrinsic knowledge of every life-form refines itself as the planet sheds and produces because of the self-constructing intelligence of the universe. The palm tree does not need to perform any action to remember that it produces palms, nor does the horse doubt its young will be in its image instead of that of a geranium. Milk inside the mother is produced for feeding at the precise moment that the baby needs to be fed.

Intelligence is the natural order of all life. Genuine human response is a resonance of intelligence. When cognitive memory is functioning, thoughts are resolved in inquiry and observation.

Human activities are mostly based on self-absorption. We look at ideas and vision as issuing singularly from individuals. We believe that there is an independent "I" who does the thinking. We assume, because of our ignorance of our elemental nature, that the universe takes its cues from us. The concept of the "I" is generated by humankind out of great ignorance. And when ignorance is reinforced we become densely arrogant. To impugn nature, believing it to be a reflection of the elite human, is the most hopeless action our species can perform. Selfish action has no link to cognitive memory; it is an extension of a mental faculty that has forgotten its nature.

Vijnanamaya is the all-knowing presence of the human entity. The human is the only known species able to resolve thoughts within intelligence. But to reaccess this natural process of being, we need to remain alert to the harmony of all our bodies. The food body depends on the prana body, which in turn lives on the mind body. The mind body rests in its turn on the intelligence body. These four bodies resolve only in the consciousness body.

### *The Consciousness Body*

*The one who sees me in all beings, and all beings in me.*
*Lord Krishna, Bhagavad Gita (Ch. 6)*

*Anandamaya* is the complete fullness of being. It is the harmonic fullness of all living things within the universe. It is the sheath covering our boundless, infinite nature consciousness, since we are not aware of real nature. Pure consciousness has no attributes, no modification, and no differentiation. It is beyond the grasp even of intelligence. Because it is spatially limitless, all is dissolved into it, the source of all sources. The consciousness body is beyond the elements. This non-state is often referred to as "the abiding happiness and complete fullness." When the four bodies are in excellent health, they dissolve within this consciousness. Stillness, like a mountain standing in a cloudless blue sky, is the natural state of the conscious entity.

Purity and happiness exist at all times. We are too busy fluctuating between our joys and regrets to celebrate this truth, to celebrate nature. Living within our nature resolves all the obstacles. In time, when full cognition is gained, all the bodies dissolve within consciousness.

The five bodies we have just examined are the principle reflections of the universal structure. They are our cosmic anatomy. When we look at the creation, we see ourselves. Unfortunately since what we see is a mirror image, our foremost perception is of the densest body. Close your eyes and all your senses of perception. See the body without a mirror. See consciousness to be the primal source. See intelligence taking birth from consciousness, as the outermost layer. Next see the mind, and then prana, and finally, the food body. This is the natural order. To know this is to remember all time.

## THE POWER OF TRANSMUTATION

The intelligence of the universe is based on billions of years of memory and absorption. While each element has its own pure nature, it cannot assume form without also being absorbed in each other element. Each gross element, *mahabhuta,* is a synthesis of all others. This bonding of the elements is what makes the universe visible. For example, gross fire, from which the material universe emerges, has the character of heat and form, as well as the sound of space, the smell of earth, the feel of air, and the taste of water. Each element stores the eternal memory—our link with the universe and the secret food of every human source of wellness.

The physical body is formed by the transmutation of the five gross elements into doshas. Human intelligence, a power transmuted from the subtle elements, exists within the receptacle of mind. Ideas and visions are discerned from the glorious abundance of information and energy fluctuating in the memory bank of the universe, ripened by billions of years of radiance and absorption. These are all transformed within awareness. The infinitesimal magnitude of change evolves endlessly as we exchange our atoms and molecules with all the elements around us. While we bask in the sun, that solar energy becomes part of our being; when we walk through a forest, the trees and moisture and the god-filled black earth become part of our energy field. Our field of energy and that of the forest and the sun are identical.

Through the physiological blueprint of humankind, Ayurveda studies the macrocosm. It is simpler, in this way, to study what is immediately accessible first, and then intelligently observe other forms of life and the planet itself. The study of Ayurvedic physiognomy is not meant to further our self-obsession. Rather it is meant to reveal the trees and soil, rivers and light, galaxies and stars—the awesome playing field of creation through which we recognize our human potential. By reverence and observation, we can learn how to be human.

The Vedas create a cosmic map, which clearly delineates a network linking this planet and the whole universe. The doshas of Vata, Pitta, and Kapha in every life-form are the same energies of mobility, transmutation, and absorption as those in the universe. The seven body constituents, or dhatus, correspond in humans and other life-forms to such planetary constituents as oceans, land masses, skeletal deposits, and liquid fire. The main channels of the human body have their counterparts in the tracks and rivers, ducts and connective networks of the universe. Like the wastes of the body, or *malas*, the earth generates her own natural waste without the unnatural breakdowns and pollutants resulting from human actions.

Transmutation occurs with varying degrees of intensity throughout the earth, and within each life-form. From the earth's internal heat come the blood-red lakes of Africa, the hot springs under the glaciers of Iceland, the rock-melting infernos of the Andes. Transformation occurs on a colossal scale. On our planet, one land mass became six separate continents; one vast body of water became the seven seas. The continent of India moved northward over two hundred million years at the speed of fifteen feet every century until it collided with Asia, sending the land and sea sky-high to create the tallest mountain range on earth. Some six thousand feet above the sea, the fossilized limestone of prehistoric sea ammonites are embedded in the Himalayan peaks. The power of change occurs from the grand to the infinitesimal. All the while the coolness of the oxygenated atmosphere is maintained so that we may flourish as a life-form. The intelligence of the universe is based on roughly 120 billion years of intrinsic memory. This knowledge enables her to make very precise adjustments. Through our powers of observation and proper practice, we can access this same knowledge for our infinite transformation and refinement.

Both the creative and destructive forces depend upon transmutation for their respective prowess. The emergence process can be harmonious to the living and in keeping with the earth's cognitive memory, or it can be an abhorrent manifestation born from the action of human amnesiacs. One fulfills the destiny of a healthy universe and the other destroys its intrinsic harmony.

The entire intelligence of the cosmos functions through the same doshas and dhatus as those of the human body. When we identify the blueprint of personal functioning and learn how to access, guide, and encourage our real nature, we will begin to serve our specific destiny with true humanity and happiness.

## CHAPTER 2

# AYURVEDIC ANATOMY

## THE PHYSICAL BODY AND PRAKRITI

The ancient science of Ayurveda provides guidelines to help us identify our constitutional nature, enabling us to choose and live wisely on the earth. From the three doshas—Vata, Pitta, and Kapha—the seven body types are formed. Our body type, which is determined at birth by genetic and karmic memory, is our constitutional nature, or our prakriti. Once birth has made its elemental imprint, we cannot alter it to suit our needs. While we may be influenced positively or negatively by our culture, society, and environment, our basic nature at birth is established from the interlacing of the five cosmic elements. Being at the very core of our numinous nature, Vata, Pitta, and Kapha are essentially the motion, dream, and food of being. Patterned within the physical body, the doshas are the organizing forces that maintain health and eliminate bodily waste.

### *The Doshas*

Vata, Pitta, and Kapha are referred to as the dhatus of the body when they are in a balanced state. The doshas are basically waste products, and are thus considered supporters of the organism or dhatus, while performing their functions as they move out of the body. The mucus, which is a form of Kapha, protects the sensitive tissues, but it must be expelled regularly from the body by expectoration or defecation. If it accumulates, it will cause disease. Likewise with the bile, a form of Pitta which works properly only when it is excreted into the gut and expelled in the feces, and the Vata [air] which is released from the body as it causes other wastes to be released. The three doshas are forces, not physical manifestations, but when they accumulate, they cause the congregation of physical substances which they are associated with, and this leads to disequilibrium and disease.

Dr. Robert E. Svoboda, Lecture
Boulder, 1993

Ayurvedic anatomy is based on the doshas (bodily humors), the dhatus* (bodily tissues), and malas (bodily wastes). Formed from the elements, the doshas Vata, Pitta, and Kapha are referred to respectively as the air, fire, and water principles. Each dosha has a dominant element, which is contained within a secondary element. Vata's main element is air, and its container is space—as air is contained within the spaces and channels of the body. Pitta's main element is fire, and it is contained within the protective waters of the body. Kapha's main element is water, and it is contained by the mass bodily structure, or earth. Each dosha is generally defined by its main element.

Vata, the most dominant of the doshas, governs all movement of the body, the nervous system, and the life force. Pitta governs the enzymatic and hormonal activities of the body, and is responsible for digestion, pigmentation, body temperature, hunger, thirst, and sight. Pitta balances the kinetic energy of Vata and the potential energy of Kapha. Kapha governs the structure and stability of the body. It lubricates the joints, provides moisture to the skin, heals wounds, and regulates Vata and Pitta. In the cosmos, earth is the collective force of stability; water is the force of cohesion and absorption, fire is the force of transmutation and dynamism, air is the quality of exhilaration and mobility, and space is the field where all activities happen in dynamic containment.

Vata, Pitta, and Kapha pervade the entire body, but their primary domains, or centers of operation, are in the lower, middle, and upper body respectively. Kapha rules the upper body—the head, neck, thorax, chest, upper portion of the stomach, fat tissues, and all joints. Pitta dominates the chest, umbilical area, stomach, small intestines, sweat and lymph glands, blood, eyes, and skin. Vata rules the lower body—pelvic region, colon, bladder, urinary tract, thighs, legs, bones, ears, and nervous system.

In Ayurveda, the individual dosha is the fundamental consideration for diagnosis. Although there are numerous causes of disease, such as hereditary, congenital, external, and providential factors, the aggravation of the doshas exists either as the result of or the cause of ill health.

## The Five Airs of Vata

Each dosha manifests in five forms or divisions. Through these vehicles of systematic outreach, the doshas influence the entire bodily system. The five divisions of Vata, referred to as the five airs, are *prana, udana, samana, apana,* and *vyana.* Prana, which is the life breath and the first air, is situated in the heart, brain, face, and chest. Prana's action is to give life power to the body. It maintains inhalation and exhalation, and the swallowing of food. It sustains the heart, arteries, veins, and the nervous system, and controls the mind, senses, and intellect. Prana is the cosmic breath infused in the living universe by the creator. Psychologically, it inspires wisdom and knowledge of the inseparable nature of body, mind, and spirit. The second air, called udana, is situated in the throat. Prana and udana are somewhat analogous to the sympathetic and the parasympathetic nervous systems.

Udana is the time clock that ticks life away with every breath. Each person has a certain number of breaths inherent in life, and when the final breath is used, the body dies. Udana flows upward from the umbilicus through the lungs into the throat and to the nose. It gives vocal power, preserves the body's natural forces, and strengthens the mind, intellect, and memory. Loss of memory and impaired speech are caused by the vitiation of the udana. Psychologically, udana is the recorder of our cognitive memories. It inspires us to remember our journeys throughout time. The third air, known as samana, flows through the entire intestinal tract. This air fans the fires of digestion and aids assimilation and transport of nutrients to the various tissue elements. It further assists in the discharge of food waste to the colon.

* The term *dhatu* is used to define both the balanced state of the doshas (as in the preceding quote) and the seven bodily tissues. In this book the term refers to the bodily tissues.

Psychologically, samana—as the central air of Vata—fosters both mental and spiritual assimilation. When samana air is in balance, it inspires clarity, alertness, and spiritual equilibrium.The fourth air, called apana, is situated in the colon and in the organs of the pelvic region. Its action is to expel feces, urine, semen, and menstrual waste. Its downward pressure helps maintain the equilibrium of the fetus suspended in fluid and helps in its eventual birth. Apana, the most dominant of the five airs, is the primary location of Vata in the body. Psychologically, apana renews our sense of freedom and lightness.

The circulatory flow of vyana, the fifth air, is diffused throughout the body. Vyana's site is the heart. It functions with the circulatory channels, such as blood vessels, and transports nutritive juices and blood throughout the body. It is the carrier of sweat from the glands to the skin and it controls such movements as blinking and yawning. Vyana resonates psychologically as the accommodating, allowing, and compassionate nature of a person.

Vata is the main bodily principle: Sixty percent of diseases are caused by Vata derangement. Disturbances in the bladder, colon, anus, testicles, and heart and any impairments related to the five divisions are considered to be Vata disorders. Other common Vata symptoms are pain, stiffness, paralysis, hypertension, hoarseness, and defective assimilation, as well as certain malfunctions of the eyes, ears, nose, throat, and the airs of respiration.

## The Five Fires of Pitta

The five fires, or agnis, of Pitta are *pachaka, ranjaka, sadhaka, alochaka,* and *bhrajaka.* The first fire of pachaka, which is in the stomach, duodenum, and small intestine, has a digestive and dissolvent action. After digestion, pachaka separates the nutritive elements of food and discards the waste. It also supports the remaining agnis. Its psychological function is to fan the fires of proper mental assimilation and maintain a discriminating mind. The site of the second fire, ranjaka, is the liver, spleen, and stomach. Ranjaka, which is carmine red, controls blood formation. Its proper functioning relates to calmness and the general well-being of the body. The third fire, sadhaka, is located in the heart. It governs memory retention and the wellness of all mental functions. Psychologically, sadhaka assuages the mind and fosters humility. It is the central and most subtle of the five fires. The fourth fire, alochaka, resides in the pupil of the eyes. Animating the sense of sight, alochaka's fire inspires intuition, creative vision, clarity, alertness, and accommodation of others. The fifth fire, known as bhrajaka, exists in the skin. It governs the color and glow of the skin, and absorbs moisture and substances applied to the skin. Psychologically, the fire of bhrajaka sanctifies external beauty and cleanliness.

Thirty percent of diseases are caused by Pitta drangement. Disorders of the stomach and small intestines, fevers, indigestion, jaundice, pharyngitis, vitiation of sight, skin ailments, psychic disorders, and all vitiation related to the five divisions are considered to be impairments of Pitta.

## The Five Waters of Kapha

The five waters of Kapha are referred to as *kledaka, avalambaka, bodhaka, tarpaka,* and *sleshaka.* The first water, kledaka, originates in the stomach. It is the moist, foamy liquid that aids digestion. Kledaka nourishes the remaining four waters, coalesces the thinking faculties, inspires fluid interaction with the world, and pours gentility into human nature. The currents of the second water, avalambaka, flow in the heart, providing it with lubricating plasma and thus insulating it from heat. It makes the limbs limber. Avalambaka resonates psychologically as the protective, embracing, and maternal nature of a person. The third water, bodhaka, strings together the five waters of the body river. It wets the tongue and gives perception of taste. It channels the sensory perception that beckons the convivial juices before eating. Psychologically, bodhaka guards the impulse of quantitative intake to body, mind, and senses. The fourth water, tarpaka, flows in the head and calms the sense organs. It washes the senses of discretion and vitalizes the gates of memory. Proper functioning of tarpaka ensures clear memory and vital fulfillment of the senses. The fifth water, sleshaka, causes the joints to operate smoothly. By lubricating and solidifying them with its unctuous protective gel, it gives cohesion to body movements and fluidity to both mind and body.

The Kapha principle generally has the least malfunctions. Disorders such as impairment of taste and digestion, obesity, anorexia, bulimia, inertia, loss of memory, excess phlegm, water retention in joints, and certain respiratory conditions are considered Kapha disorders.

## *The Seven Dhatus*

In the Taittiriya Upanishad, the physical body is referred to as the food body, and food is referred to as medicine. The quality and quantity of our foods directly relate to the health of our bodily systems and thus our psychic mechanism. In Ayurveda, the physiological and psychological functions of the body are interwoven. Ayurveda proposes that matter does not exist without energy, and that matter essentially is energy.

The dhatus are the basic bodily tissue elements. Like the doshas, they too are formed from the five elements of space, air, fire, water, and earth. With the help of the digestive fire, the dhatus form the protective biological system of the body. They nourish, develop, and protect the body's immune mechanism. If one dhatu is defective, it affects each successive dhatu thus triggering a chain reaction of impairment throughout the entire system of dhatus. A dhatu enters the internal body structure in a concentric fashion.

The quality and energy of the foods that enter the body strongly affect the quality of the life-supporting nutrient plasma, or chyle. After the foods are digested, nourishment of the dhatus begins with the plasma dhatu, or *rasa.* Each dhatu is fed by the previous dhatu from the grossest, which is the chyle or nutrient plasma, to the most subtle, which is the sperm and ovum elements of the male and female.

The main element of the plasma dhatu is water. After this first dhatu is fed, nutrients are refined and transported to the blood dhatu, called *rakta.* The dominant element of the blood constituent is fire. After the hemoglobin of the blood is fed, the nutrients are further refined and proceed to the muscle tissue of the body, known as *mamsa.* The dominant element of this dhatu is earth. Once the bodily mass is nourished, a further refinement of the nutrients occurs and the dhatu of the fat tissue, or *meda,* is fed. The main elements of this dhatu are water and earth. Next in order of nourishment is the bone and cartilage dhatu, known as *asthi,* which is pervaded by the elements of air and space. The continuously refined nutrients are then transported to the red and white bone marrow, called *majja.* The main element of bone marrow is fire. Finally, the refined essential nutrient, which remains after all the dhatus have been fed, replenishes the ovum and sperm dhatus of the female and male, or *artava* and *shukra.* The quality and vitality of this subtle essence of nutrients directly depend on the quality and quantity of the foods ingested and their accompanying sadhanas.

Artava/shukra, the final dhatu, is the one that gives life and joy. This is the finest of the dhatus, and its dominant element is the subtle atom of water. Artava/shukra is also referred to as the "refined water," that which remains after all the bodily processes have been completed. The condition of this dhatu directly affects the health of the ovum and sperm, which are the raw materials for procreation. If the artava/shukra dhatu is polluted, this will impact on the very life formed from the union of that sperm and ovum.

## *The Three Malas*

Malas are the waste products of the body. They are also called *kittas,* which is the Sanskrit term for "that which must go away." The three principal malas are urine, feces, and sweat. These waste products, like the doshas and dhatus, are also composed of the five elements. The secondary malas include the fatty excretions of the intestines, earwax, hair (body, head, and beard), nails, tears, and menstrual discharge. Feces, the primary waste of the body, is the refuse of foods and substances excreted from the tissue cells that is meant to go back to the Earth and aid in her fertility. Two daily eliminations are vital to good health. Urine is the water waste of the body. Passing water five times daily is necessary for maintaining good health. Ample intake of pure water is vital to replenish the body fluids. Sweat expels waste from the skin tissues. The normal flow of the malas is obstructed when the doshas are increased or decreased beyond their natural state.

The Ayurvedic therapy of *panchakarma* refers to the "five-fold method" for eliminating excess doshas from the body. Once the primary forces of the doshas are brought into balance, the elimination of wastes becomes an incidental result. Vata, the main dosha implicated in the manifestation of disease, is responsible for the retention or ejection of feces, urine, bile, and other excretions from the body. When wastes such as mucus, bile, excess water, and gas remain in the body, Ayurveda urges the informed use of the five processes of cleansing. To balance Vata disorders, for example, herbal oils and decoctions are used as enemas. Pitta disorders are tended to by purgation therapy, and Kapha excess is reduced by emesis therapy. Frequently a variety of oils and aromas are used in massage therapy to balance, stimulate, or calm the doshas. These practices are essential to eliminate blockage, toxins, bile, mucus, and so on from the bodily systems.

## Ama

When the circulatory channels are blocked, bodily substances accumulate in them and the tissue metabolism is adversely affected. Stagnation is generally caused by unabsorbed foods, due to impaired digestive fire. This foul-odored stagnant substance, known as *ama,* clogs various channels of the body, such as the intestines and blood vessels. The prolonged presence of ama in the system generates toxins, which are transported through the blood to various viscera of the body. Ama settles in the lungs, heart, and in those organs encased within cavities, such as the cranium, thorax, abdomen, and pelvis, as well as in the joints. When doshic excess and ama ominously unite, they travel with great rapidity to a weakened site in the body and disease manifests.

Ama causes the deterioration of strength; it reduces rasa and induces lethargy and fatigue. Equally crippling to the system is mental ama, which is gathered as a result of misperceptions and disturbed thoughts. Emotions such as greed, selfishness, possessiveness, and anger convert into mental pollutants, or ama. When ama exists in the mind, it has a destructive influence on the digestive process and may even convert wholesome foods into the fetid bodily ama.

All internal diseases begin with ama's presence in the body, and all diseases caused by external factors eventually produce ama. An early sign of ama is a sticky coating on the tongue. Usually Kapha types will have a thick sweetish, whitish coating. Pitta types will have a sourish, yellowish coating, and Vata types will have a bitter, grayish coating. When these early symptoms of ama are noticed, they may be gotten rid of by fasting and a thorough cleansing of the bodily systems. The Ayurvedic panchakarma therapy is recommended for each body type, in accordance with the appropriate season.

## The Thirteen Channels of Circulation

The body contains numerous channels through which the dhatus, doshas, and malas circulate. Known as *srotas* in Ayurveda, these consist of both gross channels, such as the intestinal tract, lymphatic system, arteries, veins, and genitourinary tracts, and subtle channels, such as the capillaries and the *nadis.* The latter are analogous to the meridians in acupuncture, which are perceived as the central channels of the body's energy. All diseases in Ayurveda are diagnosed with consideration to which individual doshas are compromised and to which channels are obstructed.

An excess of any one dosha necessarily creates a blockage in the various channels of the body. Thus a disease originating from one vitiated dosha may travel through these channels to the site of another dosha. Ayurveda explores a complex system of diagnosis that traces the cause of the disease. The primary difference between the holistic approach of this ancient science and allopathic medicine is that Ayurveda provides cures based on the original cause of diseases, not symptoms.

Males have thirteen groups of channels, or srotas, and females have fifteen groups. Of the thirteen groups of channels common to both, the first three are governed by Vata, Pitta, and Kapha respectively. In essence, the first three srotas are conduits of breath, food, and water respectively.

### 1. Air Srotas

Air srotas, which originate in the heart and the alimentary tract, conduct pranic force and vitality through the respiratory and circulatory systems. These channels become impaired by the suppression of natural bodily urges, by ingestion of dry, unctuous food, and by physical exertion, as well as by fear, anxiety, and nervous tension. The symptoms of the vitiated air channels are shallow and restricted breathing.

### 2. Food Srotas

Food srotas, which originate in the stomach, are carriers of food through the digestive system. Vitiation of these channels is caused by untimely eating, indiscriminate eating, eating unhealthy foods, and low digestive fire, as well as by attachment and possessiveness. The symptoms of affliction are loss of appetite, indigestion, vomiting, and anorexia.

### 3. Water Srotas

Water srotas, which originate in the palate and pancreas, regulate the bodily fluids. Obstruction of these passages is caused by excessive exposure to heat, excessive use of alcohol or other addictive substances, and ingesting very dry foods, as well as by aggressiveness and selfishness. The symptoms of vitiation are excessive thirst, and dryness of lips, throat, tongue, and palate.

The following seven groups of channels service the seven dhatus of the body. Like the dhatus, these channels range from the gross to the subtle.

### 4. Plasma Srotas

Plasma srotas, which transport chyle, plasma, and lymphatic fluid to the plasma dhatu, begin in the heart and its ten blood vessels. Obstruction of these passages is caused by excessively cold and heavy foods, as well as by stress and grief. The symptoms of vitiation are anorexia, drowsiness, nausea, fainting, anemia, and impotence.

### 5. Blood Srotas

Blood srotas, which originate in the liver and spleen, transport blood, and especially hemoglobin, to the blood dhatus. This group is often referred to as the circulatory system. Vitiation of this system is caused by hot and oily foods, excessive exposure to the sun or fire, and exposure to radioactivity, as well as by anger, dullness, and stress. The symptoms of affliction are skin diseases and rashes, abscesses, excessive bleeding, and inflammation of the genital organs and the anus.

### 6. Muscular Srotas

Muscular srotas, which originate in the ligaments, tendons, and skin, supply nutrients to the muscle dhatus. Impairment of these channels is due to regular intake of heavy, greasy foods, excessive sleep, sleeping after meals, and a sedentary lifestyle, as well as to attachment and nervous tension. The symptoms of vitiation are usually benign tumors produced by the muscular system, tonsillitis, a swollen uvula, hemorrhoids, and swelling of the thyroid glands and adenoids.

### 7. Fat Srotas

Fat srotas, commonly known as the adipose system, supply ingredients of fat tissue to the fat dhatus. These channels originate in the kidneys and the fat tissue of the abdomen. Vitiation of this system is due to inertia, suppression of digestive activities, an excess of fatty foods, and an excess of alcohol or other additive substances, as well as greed, possessiveness, and indulgence. The symptoms of affliction are generally diabetes and urinary disorders.

### 8. Bone and Cartilage Srotas

Bone and cartilage srotas, commonly known as the skeletal system, supply nutritive ingredients to the bone and cartilage dhatus. This group begins in the hipbone. Affliction of these channels is generally caused by excessive activity, friction of the bones, and excessive intake of Vata-type foods, as well as by fear and deprivation. The symptoms of vitiation are generally dry, brittle nails, decaying teeth, painful joints, and dry and thinning hair.

### 9. Bone Marrow Srotas

The bone marrow srotas, commonly referred to as the nervous system, supply the marrow and nerve tissue nutrient to the bone marrow dhatus. In Ayurveda, marrow refers not only to the white and red matter inside the bone encasement, but also to the brain and spinal cord. Impairment of the bones and joints is usually caused by incompatible foods (for example, ingesting hot and cold at the same time) or incompatible activities (walking and eating). Eating foods incompatible with one's body types, such as Vata eating cold, dry foods, is also a factor. After impacting the bone and joints, these transgressions then have an effect on the bone marrow. Impairment can also be caused by isolation and fear. The symptoms of a vitiated nervous system are pain in the joints, fainting, dizziness, loss of memory, blackouts, and compounded abscesses.

### 10. Ovum and Sperm Srotas

The ovum and sperm srotas are the most subtle of all the nine preceding channel groups. They transport the semen and ovum to the reproductive tissues, or the shukra dhatus. Originating in the testes and ovaries, these channels are ordinarily referred to as the reproductive system. Afflictions of these passages are normally the result of excessive or suppressed sex, unnatural sex, sex at improper times, drug addictions, and abortions, as well as aggression, selfishness, and greed. The symptoms of vitiation are impotence, infertility, and defective pregnancy. These channels transport the essence of *ojas.*

The body's cycle of nutrition begins with rasa and culminates with ojas. Ojas allow tejas to project from the subtle body into the physical body, where it appears as the digestive fire. Ojas is the flow, the aura, the luster of the body when the ingested foods are wholesome, the mind is peaceful, and when the essence of nutrition is received. Every human is gifted with the potential of excellent ojas. A reflection of bodily and mental health, it permeates from the innermost self to beyond the physical body. It is said that Lord Krishna's ethereal blue aura projected for thousands of miles, and that all who came within that distance were blessed with tranquility. When ojas is plentiful, the body's natural immunity is impenetrable, and we may protect all that exists around us. Psychologically, ojas gives clarity and allows the cognitive self to flourish.

The remaining groups of channels common to both the male and the female are the three elimination systems of the body.

### 11. Urinary Srotas

The urinary srotas, which eject urine from the body, begin in the kidneys and the bladder. Impairment of these passages is caused by the suppression of urination, as well as fear and nervousness. The symptoms of vitiation are generally excessive, scant, or frequent urination.

### 12. Excretory Srotas

The excretory srotas, which evacuate feces from the body, are ordinarily referred to as the excretory system. They originate in the colon and rectum. Vitiation of this system is caused by weak digestive fire, eating before the previous meal is digested, suppression of defecation, and ingestion of disagreeable foods, as well as greed, attachment, and dullness. The symptoms of affliction are usually diarrhea, constipation, or excessively hard stools.

### 13. Sweat Srotas

The last of the excretory channels, which expel sweat from the body, is commonly known as the sebaceous system. These srotas originate in the fat tissues and hair follicles. Affliction of these channels is caused by excessive activity, heat, spicy foods, acidic foods, excessive alcohol or other addictive substances, as well as grief, fear, and anger. The symptoms of vitiation are excess perspiration or no perspiration, rough and dry skin, and burning sensation of the skin.

Two additional channels exist within the female body: the menstrual srotas, which expel menstruation from the body, and the breast milk srotas, which carry milk to the nursing mother's breasts. Both of these systems are part of the plasma srotas, which supply the plasma dhatus (see first item on this list).

# THE SUBTLE BODY

## The Fourteen Nadis

The *sushumna* nadi, along with *ida* and *pingala* nadis to her left and right respectively, are the three principal channels of the subtle body. These three branch into fourteen main nadis, which in turn divide into the many thousands of nadis which fill the entire system. Located within the central nadi, or sushumna, are subtle energy centers, or *chakras*. These chakras operate in close conjunction with the nadis.

The sushumna is the main subtle energy channel of the *pranavaha* nadi, which deals with physiological qualities. Related to the parasympathetic nervous system, the sushumna and three other pranavaha nadis are the carriers of the vital life force known as prana. The meridians in acupuncture are analogous to pranavaha nadis. The parasympathetic and sympathetic systems of the body would be rendered inoperable without the life currents of prana transmitted by the pranavaha nadis. The vehicle of the mind is prana, without which there is no impression of consciousness.

The ten *manovaha* nadis deal with psychological qualities and are related to the sympathetic nervous system. They are conduits of energies pertaining to the mind. While these two systems function inseparably, they are dealt with individually for the purpose of clarity. These two systems operate together since the mind is controlled by the air of prana.

### 1. Sushumna Nadi

The sushumna nadi, located within the spinal cord, begins at the pelvic plexus and ends in the space of the cerebrospinal axis between the two hemispheres of the brain. The seven chakras of the body are aligned along the sushumna nadi from the top of the head to the coccyx. Left of the sushumna is the ida nadi, and on the right the pingala nadi. Ida represents the feminine principle, which is the lunar energy; pingala depicts the masculine principle, which is the solar energy.

### 2. Ida Nadi

The ida nadi runs from the left testicle to the left nostril. All inhalation begins with the left nostril in yogic practices. The left breath stimulates the ida nadi and promotes creativity, visualization, and the nurturing of the emotions. It calms the nerves and silences the mind. The yogic sciences exhort the use of left nostril breathing during the day, when the body is vitalized by the sun's energy. This creates harmony and balance and is said to increase longevity. Ida is considered to be both a pranavaha and a manovaha nadi.

### 3. Pingala Nadi

The pingala nadi runs from the right testicle to the right nostril. It is activated by the breath of the right nostril. This stimulates the rational, practical self. Whereas both the breaths are cleansing, ida cleanses the mind and pingala revives the dynamic energy of the body. Right nostril breath promotes stamina, vigor, and vitality. It is wise to practice right nostril breathing during the night when the lunar energy is dominant. This activates a superior level of balance and vigor in the body, just as left nostril breathing during the day balances the aggression of the dominant solar energy. Pingala nadi is considered to be both a pranavaha and a manovaha nadi.

### 4–5. Gandhari and Hastajihva Nadis

The *gandhari* and *hastajihva* nadis are companion nadis to Ida. Gandhari originates from the lower corner of the left eye and ends at the big toe of the left foot. Hastajihva nadi begins on the lower corner of the right eye and ends at the big toe of the left foot. These nadis are used to ascend psychic energy from the lower body to the chakra between the eyebrows. The functions of both companion nadis relate to the main left channel of the ida nadi.

### 6–7. Yashasvini and Pusha Nadis

The *yashasvini* and *pusha* nadis are companion nadis to pingala. Yashasvini runs from the left ear to the big toe of the left foot; pusha nadi runs from the right ear to the big toe of the left foot. Their functions are related to the main right channel of pingala.

### 8. Alambusha Nadi

The *alambusha* nadi, which begins at the anus and ends in the mouth, provides prana for the assimilation and evacuation of food and liquid. This nadi is also responsible for the assimilation of ideas and thoughts.

### 9. Kuhu Nadi

The *kuhu* nadi begins in the throat and terminates in the genitals. Through tantric practices designed to give mastery over the senses, this nadi can be trained to induce the implosion and ascension of the seminal and vaginal fluids.

### 10. Shankhini Nadi

The *shankhini* nadi, which originates in the throat and ends in the anus, is located to the right of the sushumna nadi. It is activated by the cleansing of Vata from the colon and anus.

### 11. Saraswati Nadi

The *saraswati* nadi, named after the Hindu goddess of wisdom, begins in the tongue and ends in the vocal cord. It is responsible for speech and the dissemination of knowledge. Saraswati nadi is lunar in nature, and of the feminine principle. It is a companion channel to the sushumna nadi.

### 12. Payasvini Nadi

The *payasvini* nadi is located in the lobe of the right ear and connects to the cranial nerves. Traditionally, the point on the lobe was pierced with various precious metals to stimulate energy into the cranial nerves, thereby reducing stress and certain addictive behaviors.

### 13. Varuni Nadi

The *varuni* nadi, one of the four pranavaha nadis, aids in the purification of bodily wastes. This channel runs opposite and parallel to the alambusha nadi, and together they activate excretions of bodily waste. Varuni nadi originates between the throat and the left ear and ends at the anus. It works in concert with apana vayu, which circulates in the cavities of the large intestine. When this system is disturbed, stagnation of various bodily channels ensues and Vata disorders occur.

### 14. Vishvodara Nadi

The *vishvodara* nadi, last of the major fourteen channels, is located around the umbilical area or third chakra. It stimulates the adrenal glands and the pancreas, and also distributes prana throughout the body. Vishvodara nadi is the center energy stream of the body, often referred to as the *ki* or *chi*. All yoga and martial arts practices, especially t'ai chi, *quigong*, and *pranayama*, serve to strengthen this pivotal nadi.

## *The Seven Chakras*

The kundalini is the latent cosmic power within the human being. Lying coiled at the base of the spine like a serpent, when aroused she travels within the inner channel of the spinal cord known as the sushumna nadi. Very few yogis can properly arouse this coiled dormant power. The chakras, which are the most subtle manifestations of cosmic consciousness within the human body, symbolize our grandeur and the infinite spectrum of our nature.

As centers of consciousness within the individual, chakras do not work with the physiological or psychological functions of the body directly. However, all processes of the gross body have their basis in the vital force of the subtle body, and the chakras do interface with these subtle forces. Chakras operate with the spiraling rhythms of the elements within the body and mind. These energy centers influence and give insight into the absolute manifest potential of our psychospiritual nature.

In the classic tantric texts, each of the seven chakras is represented by a lotus with a specific number of petals, which reflect its intrinsic energy propagation. The list below outlines features of the seven chakras, starting with the first chakra.

### Muladhara

Known as the root chakra, the *muladhara* is located at the base of the spine. It is symbolized by a crimson lotus with four petals. Within the petals is a square, representing the element of earth.

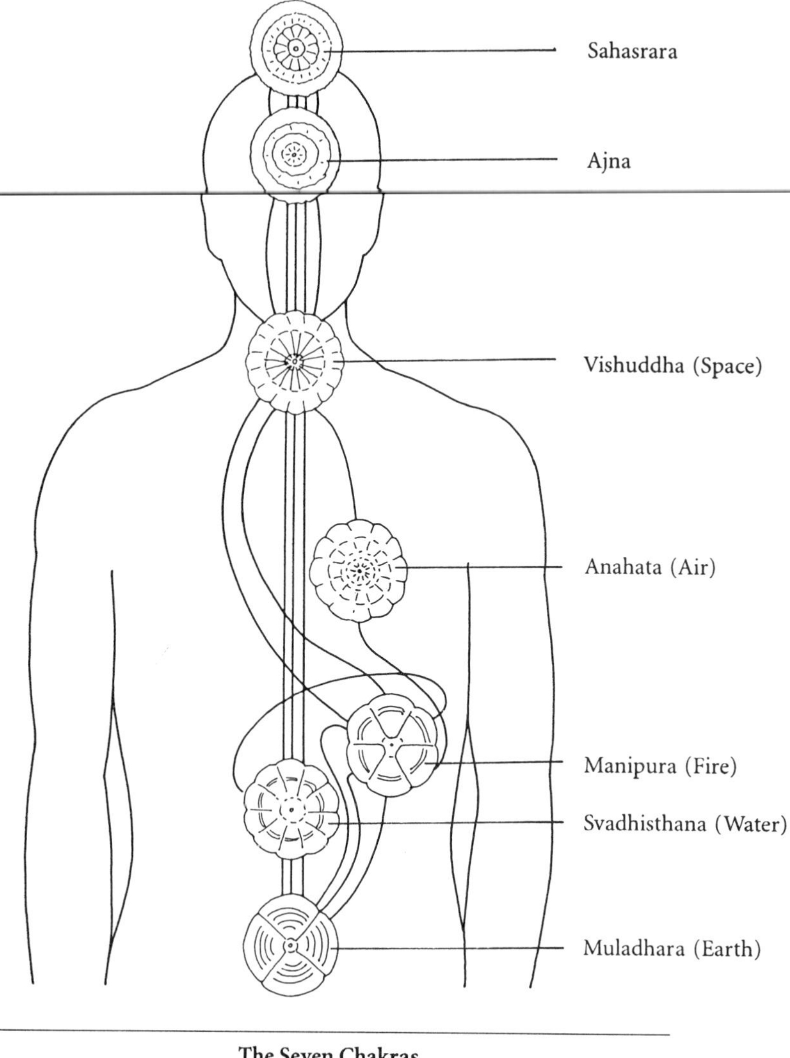


**The Seven Chakras**

## Svadhisthana

The second chakra, located in the region of the genitals, is symbolized by a carmine lotus with six petals. Within the petals is a crescent moon, representing the element of water.

## Manipura

The third chakra, which exists in the region of the navel, is represented by a lotus with ten petals the color of translucent smoke. It contains an inverted triangle, representing the element of fire.

## Anahata

The fourth chakra, which is located in the heart region, has twelve crimson petals. These petals hold a hexagram, representing the element of air.

## Vishuddha

The fifth chakra, which exists at the base of the throat, is represented by a smoky purple sixteen-petalled lotus. Within it is a circle, representing the element of space.

The Psychospiritual Nature of the Body Types (chapter 4) is presented against the tapestry of these five chakras.

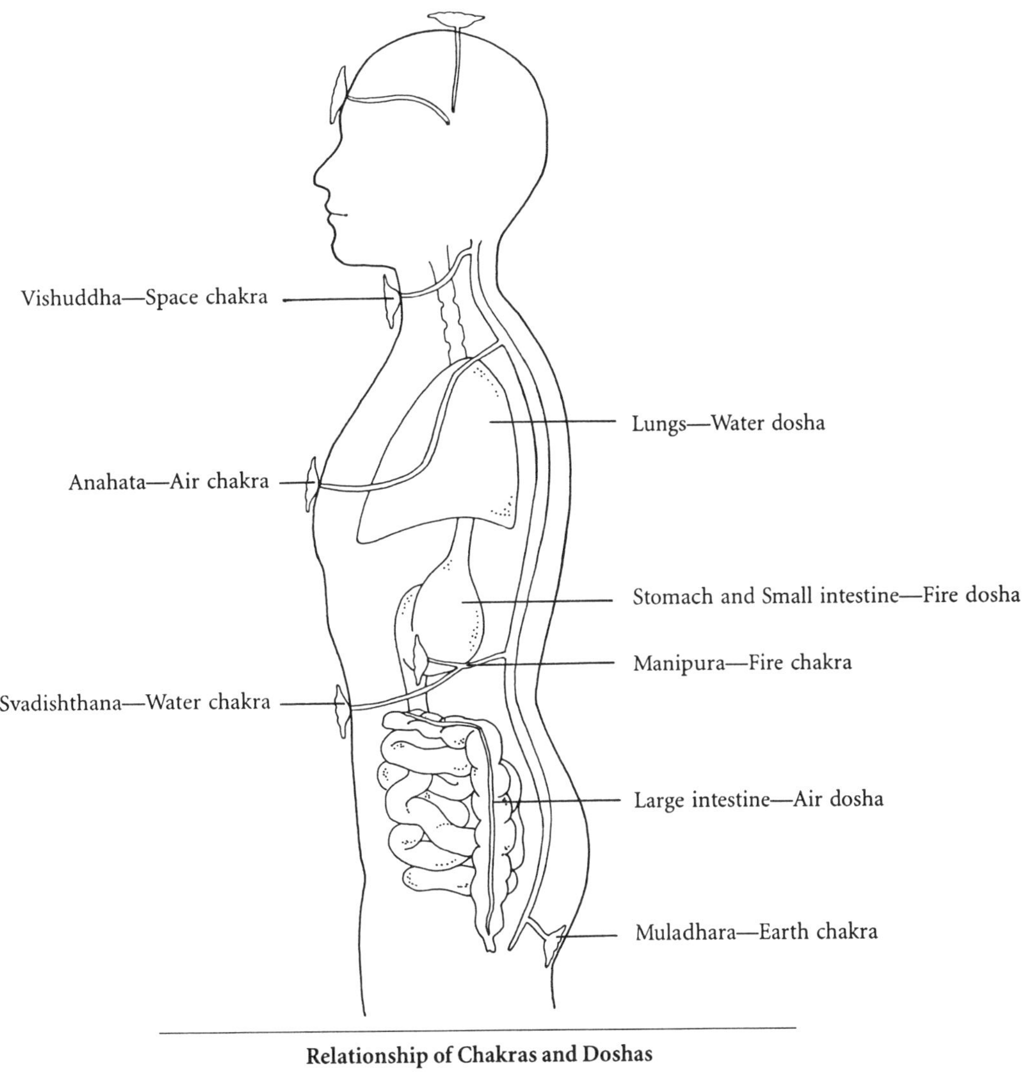


**Relationship of Chakras and Doshas**

## Ajna

The sixth chakra, located in the region of the third eye, has ninety-six white petals. At this site the gross elements of the individual dissolve into the pure elements of consciousness. It is known as the energy center of the Guru, the teacher of self-knowledge.

## Sahasrara

This final chakra is symbolized by a thousand-petalled lotus. It is said that before making her final ascension through the *sahasrara* chakra, the kundalini rests at an energy center known as the twelve-petalled soma chakra, which is located in the middle of the forehead directly above the ajna chakra. For those rare souls who have finished their cycles of rebirth, it is here that the kundalini rests before making her final ascension through the sahasrara chakra.

CHAPTER 3

# THE BODY TYPES

## ORIGIN OF THE BODY TYPES

*Earth, water, fire, air, space, manas (mind), buddhi (intellect), and ahamkara (ego)—*
*these are the eight-fold divisions of my manifestation.*

***Lord Krishna, Bhagavad Gita***

The cosmos and the human body are variants of the same energy principle. Air is located in the space of the universe just as prana exists within the spaces of the body. The waters of the universe are contained by the earth, as our fluids are held by the solid structure of our bodies. The cosmic elements are transmuted by fire in order to maintain harmony and existence of the universe. In like manner, the acid fire of the body transforms food into energy and balances the kinetic forces of Vata and the static forces of Kapha.

All truth is integrated with the knowledge of the conscious self. It is important to understand the individual self and its differences before we are able to serve the One consciousness. The fundamental aim of life is the eventual unison of the individual and the creator. When we begin to serve the individual self as the single bead on a rosary, and to know its idiosyncrasies and (apparent) differences from other individuals, we are better prepared to understand and serve all humans, all life-forms, and the planet.

In Ayurveda, when we identify ourselves as Vata, Pitta, or Kapha, we are relating to our body as a composition of the great elements of the universe. Once this correlation is made, there can be no

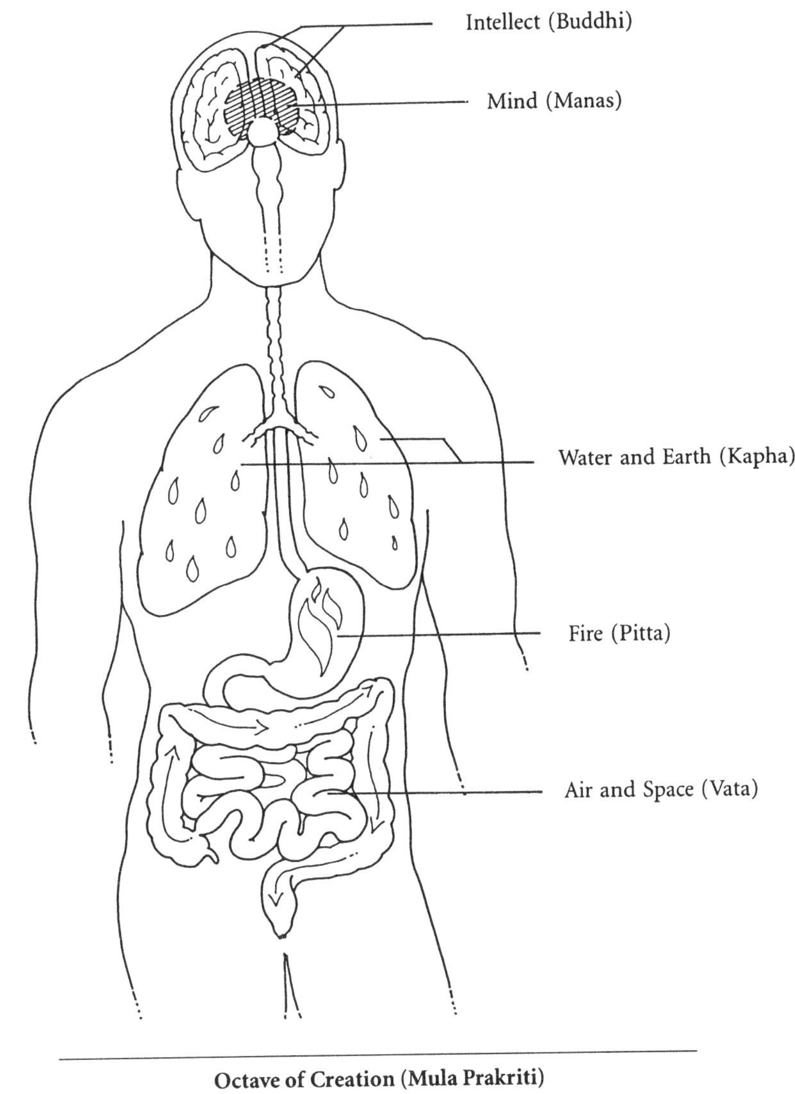


**Octave of Creation (Mula Prakriti)**

further separation from the environment: We witness the forces of the elements, inside and outside of us. As our regard for the elements of nature comes alive, we realize their majestic splendor within ourselves. In contrast, our disregard creates havoc and disease. We cannot hurt the external without affecting the internal and vice versa, nor can we separate one from the other. It is essential to know that we are incapable of helping our universe if we do not first nurture and respect our own health. All progress, all awareness, begins at home, and the body is our first home. It is the place within which we sit. It is the place within which we live, from the first breath to the last. As we clean our internal spaces, the external spaces will also become brisk and bright. By equipping ourselves with knowledge, all the vital forces will shimmer in harmony.

## *The Seven Body Types*

The human constitution, or prakriti, is comprised of all three doshas. Every individual contains the dynamic forces of Vata, Pitta, and Kapha. The difference is the degree to which the three doshas interact within each type. As we noted earlier, the constitution of each person as determined at birth by genetics remains constant throughout one's lifetime. Only our physio-psychological aspects change, in response to social, environmental, and cultural factors.

It is essential to understand the distinct differences of the doshas in order to grasp their whole, unified nature. The body types' ultimate reality is one of unison. If this is not grasped, the entire concept of the individual differences will be misunderstood. Essentially, the body type is merely adjectival to the endless list of an individual's attributes. However, the individual is not the body type. The doshas are an impressive example of apparent adversaries capable of functioning at a level of absolute equilibrium. It is worth remembering this in our relationships with each other.

The seven classic body types are defined in Ayurveda as Vata, Pitta, Kapha, Sama, Vata-Kapha, Vata-Pitta, and Pitta-Kapha. The first four types—in pure form—are rare; seldom is anyone influenced by one dosha alone. Rarer still is the Sama dosha, also called Tridosha, which is Vata, Pitta, and Kapha in equal proportions. The dual body types, referred to as dual prakritis, are the most common. There are considerable differences between the two components of a dual prakriti. A Vata-Pitta type contains more air energy, whereas a Pitta-Vata type contains more fire energy. For this reason, I have added three additional body types to the classic seven.

### *The Ten Body Types*

*Four Rare Classic Types*

- Vata — Air/Space
- Pitta — Fire/Water
- Kapha — Water/Earth
- Sama — Equal proportion of all three doshas

*Three Classic Dual Types*

- Vata-Pitta — Air/Space: main; Fire/Water: subordinate
- Vata-Kapha — Air/Space: main; Water/Earth: subordinate
- Pitta-Kapha — Fire/Water: main; Water/Earth: subordinate

*Three Additional Dual Types*

- Pitta-Vata — Fire/Water: main; Air/Space: subordinate
- Kapha-Vata — Water/Earth: main; Air/Space: subordinate
- Kapha-Pitta — Water/Earth: main; Fire/Water: subordinate

## ATTRIBUTES OF THE BODY TYPES

As the information below reveals, the physiological and psychological sites in both Vata and Kapha types are located in different parts of the body. For Pitta, however, the two sites are both located in the center of the torso.

### *Vata*

*Physical*

Its physical attributes are influenced by the shape of air.
Its force is kinetic.
It is the sense of touch.
Its organ is the skin.
Its shape is the hexagram.
Its vehicle is Anahata, the black antelope who dies for sound.
Its location is the heart.

*Mental*

Its mental attributes are influenced by the shape of space.
Its force is gravitational.
It is the source of sound.
Its organ is the ear.
Its shape is the circle.
Its vehicle is Gaja, the gray elephant who tames all the senses.
Its location is the thorax.

### *Pitta*

*Physical and Mental*

Its physical and mental attributes are influenced by the shape of fire.
Its force is radiational.
It is the sense of form and vision.
Its organ is the eyes.

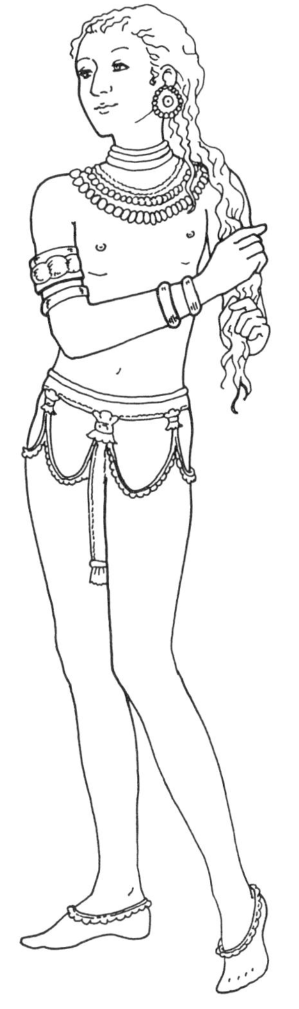

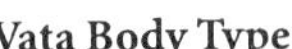

Vata Body Type

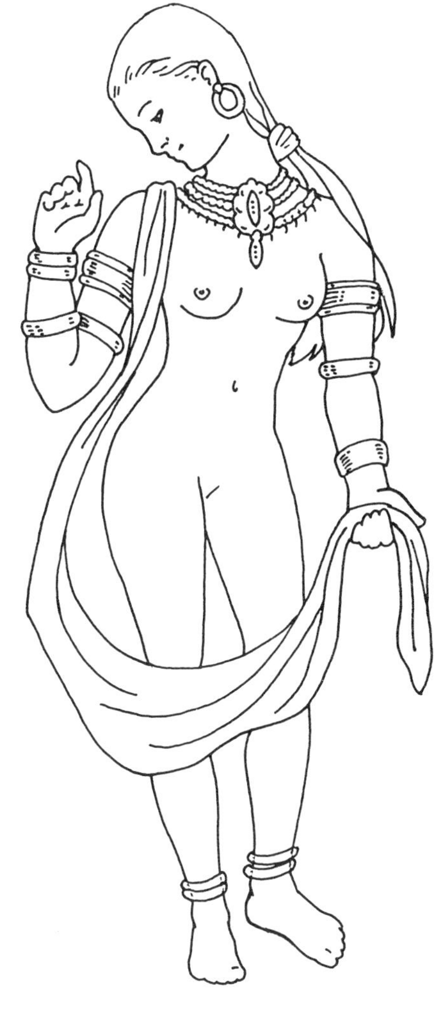

Pitta Body Type

Its shape is the inverted triangle.
Its vehicle is the Ram, the carrier of the fire god, Agni, who is the solar power.
Its location is the solar plexus.

## Kapha

*Physical*
Its physical attributes are influenced by the shape of earth.
Its force is magnetic
It is the sense of smell.
Its organ is the nose.
Its shape is the square.
Its vehicle is Airavata, the young four-trunked elephant who carries Indra, lord of the firmament.
Its location is the coccyx.

*Mental*
Its mental attributes are influenced by the shape of water.
Its force is electrical.
It is the source of taste.
Its organ is the tongue.
Its shape is the crescent.
Its vehicle is Makara, the crocodile.
Its location is the genitals.

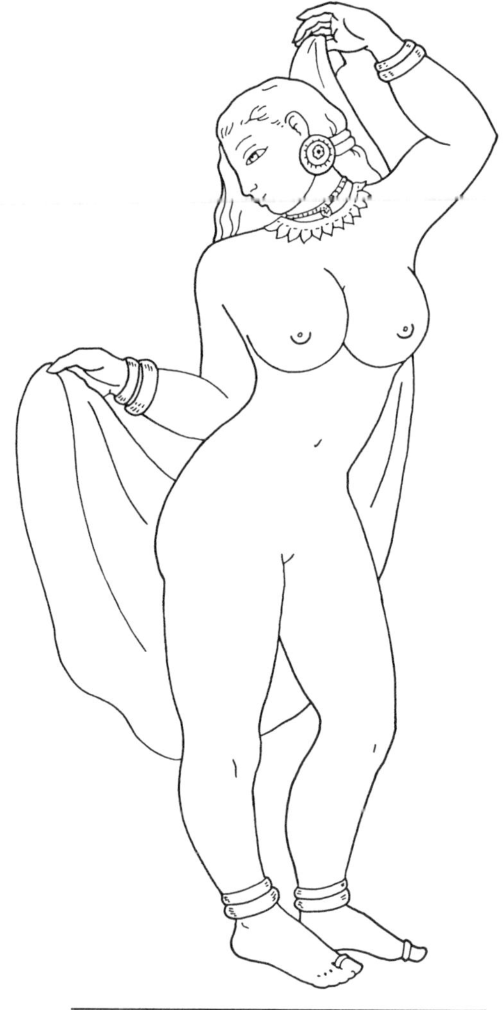

Kapha Body Type

## WHAT IS YOUR BODY TYPE?

### *Vata*

I am very tall (or very short), very thin, and underweight. My joints protrude, and my movements are generally discombobulated. My features are irregular and my nose bent.

My skin is generally gray, dry, dark, cold, callused, leathery, and rough.

I love heat. I am a sun worshiper.

My hair is generally dull, scant, wiry, and dry.

My eyes are narrow, itchy, and dull.

I have a raw nervous system. I am highly sensitive to sounds.

My mind is restless.

I am enthusiastic, vibrant, and quick to learn.

My memory retention is very poor.

I tend to sleep for four to six hours on my left side. I have great difficulty in falling asleep.

I find it difficult to have close relationships.

I tend to be fearful, anxious, and indecisive.

Under stress, I am an insomniac, paranoid, restless, and have a great deal of physical pain and anguish.

I tend to be constipated and cannot tolerate gaseous foods.

I have a spiritually perceptive and disciplined mind.

I am happiest amidst the wholesome beauty of nature.

I am an excellent counselor or teacher.

### *Pitta*

Generally, I have a toned athletic body of medium height.

I gain weight evenly.

My appetite is enormous, and under stress I crave spicy, hot, intoxicating foods and beverages.

My voice is sharp and penetrating.

My skin is yellowish or reddish, and prone to freckles, rashes, and sunburns.

I love cool temperatures and foods. Heat irritates me.

I am susceptible to premature graying or baldness. My hair is generally straight and reddish.

My eyes are green, hazel, or light brown. My sclera are sometimes yellow and bloodshot.

I am very competitive, success-oriented, and driven. I am quick to lose my temper.

I have a tendency to be hot, irritable, acidic, and arrogant.

I am blessed with great intelligence, alertness, precision, and brilliance. I am very organized and enjoy leadership.

I tend to sleep on my back for six to eight hours. My dreams can be violent.

I sweat profusely and have a strong, unpleasant body odor.

Under stress I can be gluttonous and promiscuous, and have a tendency toward ulcers, insomnia, diarrhea, and weight loss.

### *Kapha*

I am generally overweight.

My voice is soft and mellifluous and often blocked by mucus.

My body is strong, compact, wide. My thighs, buttocks, chest, and hips are big.

My skin is gleaming, pale, and cool.

I love heat. Cold, damp weather is bothersome.

My hair, which is blond or black, is abundant and wavy.

My eyes are large, clear, sensual pools of blue or black.

I am a complacent, calm, maternal, loving, and attached person. I love to gather and store possessions.

I prefer to be lazy, but I am hard working.

I am slow and methodical and have good endurance.

I sleep excessively (from eight to twelve hours), mostly on my stomach.

I have an excess of milky bodily secretions.

Under stress I overeat, oversleep, become greedy, stubborn, attached; I may even become anorexic.

## WHAT ARE THE QUALITIES OF MY BODY TYPE?

| VATA<br>*Like Wind* | PITTA<br>*Like Fire* | KAPHA<br>*Like Water* |
|---|---|---|
| dry | hot | oily |
| cold | oily | cool |
| light | light | heavy |
| mobile | intense | stable |
| erratic | fluid | dense |
| rough | fetid | smooth |
| bitter | sour | sweet |
| astringent | pungent | sour |
| pungent | salty | salty |

## WHAT ARE THE ELEMENTS, TASTES, AND ENERGIES OF MY BODY TYPE?

| VATA | VATA-KAPHA | KAPHA-VATA |
|---|---|---|
| Air and Space; bitter (cold) | Air and Earth; astringent (cold ) | Earth and Air; astringent (cold) |
| **PITTA** | **PITTA-VATA** | **VATA-PITTA** |
| Fire and Water; salty (hot) | Fire and Air; pungent (hot) | Air and Fire; pungent (hot) |
| **KAPHA** | **PITTA-KAPHA** | **KAPHA-PITTA** |
| Water and Earth; sweet (cold) | Fire and Earth; sour (hot) | Earth and Fire; sour (hot) |

## WHAT NURTURES MY BODY TYPE?

### VATA: *Nurtured by fire, water, and earth*

| | | |
|---|---|---|
| moist (lubricating) | hot | salty |
| heavy (solid) | sweet | sour |
| smooth (consistent) | | |

### PITTA: *Nurtured by water, air, space, and earth*

| | | |
|---|---|---|
| cool | calming | bitter |
| substantial | sweet | astringent |
| aromatic | | |

### KAPHA: *Nurtured by fire, air, and space*

| | | |
|---|---|---|
| dry | uncloying (moderate) | bitter |
| warm (stimulating) | pungent | astringent |
| light | | |

# THE AYURVEDIC BODY-TYPE QUIZ

It is important to approach the assessment of your body type with honesty. Keep in mind that your evaluation will be colored by the features of your present lifestyle. Six months after making the necessary changes in your activities and diet, assess yourself again. The results of your second assessment will be more in keeping with your true body type.

When completing the Body-Type Quiz Chart below, move vertically down each of the seven columns circling the attributes that most closely reflect you. Generally everyone bears characteristics from all three categories, with predominance in one or two of them. Double-check your answers and then place the total number of attributes within each body type in the last column. You may seek the help of those who know you well. Men are advised to seek the assistance of their mother or spouse, or a female friend.

## *Determining Your Score*

If your totals are, for example, Vata 18, Pitta 14, and Kapha 6, then your body type is Vata-Pitta.

## BODY-TYPE QUIZ CHART

### VATA

| SKIN | HAIR | EYES | NAILS | BODY FRAME | EMOTIONAL TEMPERAMENT | UNDER STRESS | TOTAL VATA ATTRIBUTES |
|---|---|---|---|---|---|---|---|
| Dry | Brown | Gray | Grayish | Very short or very tall | Raw nervous system | Loses weight | |
| Cold | Black | Brown | Brittle | Thin | Low tolerance to pain, noise, bright lights | Insomnia | |
| Rough | Dry | Unusual color | Dry | Narrow frame | Indecisive | Easily addicted to substances | |
| Leathery | Thin | Dull | Ridged | Big jointed | Fidgety | | |
| Tans easily | Tightly curled | Narrow | Tendency to bite nails | Flat-chested | Fearful/frigid | Paranoia | |
| Rarely burns | Frizzy | Small | | Sharp or bent nose | Introspective* | Restless | |
| Dark | Body hair: very fine or very coarse | Dry/itchy | | Gains weight in midriff | Perceptive* | Blurred mind | |
| Sallow | | | | | Disciplined* | Constipation | |
| Premature wrinkling | | | | | Spiritual/ austere* | Excess gas | |

* Your natural state when your doshas are in balance

## PITTA

| SKIN | HAIR | EYES | NAILS | BODY FRAME | EMOTIONAL TEMPERAMENT | UNDER STRESS | TOTAL PITTA ATTRIBUTES |
|---|---|---|---|---|---|---|---|
| Moderately oily | Strawberry-blonde | Light brown | Clear/pink | Medium build | Hot/arrogant | Violent dreams | |
| Soft | Auburn | Hazel | Reddish-yellowish | Well-shaped | Irritable | Excess sweat/ body odor | |
| Warm | Red | Green | Well-formed | Athletic | Self-centered | Promiscuous | |
| Freckled | Straight | Almond-shaped | Pliable | Toned | Alert/acidic | High stomach acid/ulcers | |
| Moles | Silver | Piercing | | Moderate weight | Adaptable* | Gluttony/ weight loss | |
| Yellowish/ reddish | Prematurely gray | Easily bloodshot | | Aquiline nose | Intelligent* | Insomnia | |
| Rashes | Prematurely bald | Yellow sclera | | Gains weight evenly | Bright* | Addiction to intoxicants, hot spices | |
| Pimples | | | | | Successful* | Diarrhea | |
| Tans moderately | | | | | | | |

## KAPHA

| SKIN | HAIR | EYES | NAILS | BODY FRAME | EMOTIONAL TEMPERAMENT | UNDER STRESS | TOTAL KAPHA ATTRIBUTES |
|---|---|---|---|---|---|---|---|
| Cool | Blonde | Black | Clear | Heavy | Stable/attached | Oversleeps | |
| Soft | Jet black | Blue | Pale | Strong | Narrow-minded | Overeats or loss of appetite | |
| Dense | Dark brown | Clear | Strong | Overweight | Stubborn | Inertia | |
| Oily | Oily | Big/bright | Square | Compact | Neglectful | Anorexia | |
| Smooth | Abundant | Sensual | Even | Wide, square frame | Forgiving* | | |
| Clear | Wavy | White sclera | | Well-lubricated joints | Calm/ complacent* | Water retentive | |
| Pale | Shiny | Thick lashes | | | Contemplative* | Greedy | |
| Fair with gleam | | | | | Nurturing* | | |
| Burns when over-exposed | | | | Gains weight in great mounds (buttocks, thighs, chest, arms) | Maternal* | Lazy | |

* Your natural state when your doshas are in balance

CHAPTER 4

# THE PSYCHOSPIRITUAL NATURE OF THE BODY TYPES

The doshas embody our karmic and genetic codes, which are irrevocably linked to and affected by the universal codes of the stars, planets, galaxies, and elements. Each dosha is further influenced by the subtle energy centers, or chakras, of the body. The doshas and chakras together serve as our essential connection to the universe. Understanding our physio-psychospiritual ties brings us closer to knowing the affairs of the self, the universe, and God. Through its knowledge of the body types, Ayurveda has systematized the codes for human behavior. While modern scientists are attempting to fathom the nature of DNA, Ayurveda has made use of its blueprints for more than five thousand years.

> The fate of every individual is written at birth in the genes. Our predispositions of character, our intelligence, the varying inclinations and strength throughout youth, maturity and old age, are all stamped there in indelible script. Not only our future physical strength and weaknesses are written there, but also the moment in the future when our body and its organs will begin to break down and dip towards feebleness and senility.
>
> **Biologists J. D. Watson, F. H. C. Crick, and M. H. F. Wilkins**
> **Nobel prize winners for Chemistry**

While our destiny is inscribed at birth, it is worthwhile to remember that we may alter fate through our choices, the power of our will, and self-reflection.

The five elements also pervade the seven chakras. The first five chakras are directly related to the elements. Earth (muladhara) and water (svadhisthana) are the physical plane of existence. Fire (manipura) is the mental and celestial plane, and air (anahata) is the plane of ultimate balance. Space (vishuddha), within which all four elements dissolve, is the plane of the unmanifest.

Although physiologically Vata occupies the lower cavities of the body, psychospiritually it is ruled by the region of the heart, the anahata chakra, which is presided over by the air element. It is also influenced by the region of the throat, the vishuddha chakra, which is ruled by the space element. Kapha physiologically occupies the upper parts of the body; psychospiritually it is presided over by the region of the genitals, the svadhisthana chakra, which is ruled by the water element. It is also influenced by the region of the base of the spine, the muladhara chakra, which is ruled by the earth element.

By contrast, both Pitta sites are in the center of the body. Physiologically Pitta is located in the small intestines and stomach, and psychospiritually it is in the solar plexus and the navel area, which is pervaded by the manipura chakra and ruled by the fire element. Pitta is strategically centered in the body to balance the energies of both Vata and Kapha.

The personality guidelines that follow unfold the salient characteristics of Vata, Pitta, and Kapha. It is worth remembering that we are all influenced to some degree by all three doshas and all seven chakras.

## THE VATA PERSONALITY

### Psychological Nature

*Swift as a deer, cold as ice. The coldness of the harsh winds against the variegated sands of the desert nights—such is the nature of Vata.*

Vata, the mobile force of the universe, is influenced by the air and space elements. Vata permeates the subtle body.

The Vata character is juxtaposed to the material notions of daily living. This type always appears to be on the precipice of isolation. Against the solidity of the earth type, Vata appears inconsistent and awkward. Much of Vata's innate worries and insecurities stand out by comparison against the canvas of Kapha's stoic endurance and Pitta's dramatic activities. In comparison with its partners, Vata appears to be the shifting oddity. But appearances are often deceiving.

Vata has the greatest potential among all three doshas for attaining a profound spiritual life. This dosha is ruled primarily by the subtle body and its elevated ethereal existence. The black antelope, called Anahata, is the symbol of the heart chakra and represents the innocence and purity of the fourth chakra person. The lotus of the fifth chakra, or vishuddha, is supported by the translucent gray elephant named Gaja. As the oldest of the surviving mammals, the elephant carries the past history of earth, herbs, and plants. Gaja represents the element of space, which is the most subtle of the elements; even in the process of manifestation—called grossification—it does not undergo transformation. (This is the reason space—*akasha*—is often likened to Brahman, or pure consciousness.) This chakra symbolizes the attainment of self-knowledge and the dissolution of the ego into total self-awareness. Vishuddha represents purity of cosmic sound.

Anahata and Gaja personify the essence of the Vata individual. The deer personifies the heart and the compassionate, reflective nature of the evolved person. There is an innate innocence in the conscious Vata personality. A delicate, sensitive, and aware nature reveals the graceful Vata component of any type. A person evolving from the fourth chakra has a very short karmic slack, as this energy center rules dharma. There is much physical and emotional pain attached to rubbing against the grain of right and proper actions. When Vata goes astray, the consequences are enormously painful.

Each chakra has a seed mantra, or *bija,* which is the memory sound that governs the manifested power of each element. The sound of anahata is YAM, the *m* being a nasal sound. This sound contains the divinity to be invoked during meditation upon that chakra.

The sound of vishuddha is HAM, the *m* being a nasal sound.

Each chakra has a presiding deity and a Shakti power, or feminine manifestation. From the heart to the middle of the eyebrows is said to be the region of air. Air is hexagonal in shape and black in color. Carrying the breath along the region of air and holding the syllable "Ya" in the mind, Vata types should meditate upon Isvara, the omniscient One who possesses faces on all sides and who is the presiding deity of the anahata chakra.

From the center of the eyebrows to the top of the head is said to be the region of space. Space is circular in shape and smoky in color. Raising the breath along the region of space and holding the syllable "Ha" in the mind, Vata types should also meditate upon Sadashiva, the dissolver of the universe and the presiding deity of vishuddha chakra. He is pure crystal and wears the rising crescent moon on his head. He has five faces representing the panchakoshas (the five bodies) and the panchabhutas (the five elements). He has three eyes representing the universal qualities or *gunas* (aspects of mainfestation) of *sattva, rajas,* and *tamas* (harmonic balance, necessary activity, and rest, respectively). He boasts ten hands, symbolizing the absolute authority and cause of all causes in the universe. Sadashiva is adorned with precious jewels, signifying His great splendor, and the cosmic weapons with which to slay ignorance. Vata types may meditate upon Him in the form of a *bindu,* a teardrop-shaped crystal that inspires wisdom and clarity.

Shakini, the Shakti potential of Sadashiva, has rose-colored skin and is adorned in a sky-blue sari with an emerald green bodice. She has five heads like the omniscient Sadashiva, and sits on a pink lotus. Her four hands hold the following objects: a skull, which symbolizes detachment from the experiential world of mind and sense perception; the staff of Gaja, the elephant symbol of vishuddha chakra, which represents the taming of the mind and the retrieval of humility from the intellect; the holy Vedic scriptures, which disseminate knowledge of the self; and the *mala* (rosary), symbolizing the art of meditation through the repetition of mantras.

Vata is heightened by this presiding Shakti. Meditation upon Shakini Shakti allows Vata to access its natural potential for cognitive remembering, as well as the instinct for wisdom.

Vata people have the luminous gift of being able to experience love and sensuality on a spiritual plane. Generally as the Vata person matures, physical desires subside and a profound cosmic love, which holds all of creation in embrace, begins to bloom. Vata types must allow their numinous nature to revel in the true spirit of universal sensuality. This is ultimately their most fulfilling sensual experience.

The sages gave elaborate descriptions of the gods and goddesses, or *devatas.* This was done so that we may visualize and properly invoke the energies necessary to attain a proper mental state during each meditation.

The upward energies of anahata and vishuddha, representing air and space, render Vata the potential high priestess of spirituality. Anahata is the energy center of the prana air, and vishuddha is the center of the udana air.

Vata people are the most misunderstood of all the types. They usually contrast the stalwart and dynamic nature of their lesser evolved partners, and seem to come up short and displaced. In the modern world we function on a simplistic level of existence. We are deeply rooted in judgmental conduct while the necessary strides toward self-reflective and conscious behavior are being stifled. Like the black antelope and the smoky elephant, the Vata person is the oldest of the surviving humans, and in many ways just as endangered by a mostly disoriented world. The most common mistake made by the Vata person is to attempt to meld into the routines created by Pitta and Kapha. Vata is analogous to mobility itself, which sweeps across austere terrains where Pitta and Kapha dare not go. When Vata attempts to keep in step with water and earth types, or with fire people, Vata will inevitably lose. The so-called norms are to be avoided by Vata types. While they need to ground themselves from time to time to satisfy daily family and work duties, their grounding principles differ in nature from those of Pitta and Kapha. It is imperative that Vata responds to its inherent mobility with rest periods from time to time.

Fortunately Vata will always be ahead of the game

of existence without actually forging forward. It is innate in the nature of Vata to be compelled by the pure cosmic sound of its own nature. Anahata, the antelope, dies for pure sound. Gaja, the elephant, is the energy of sound represented by space. The most vital insulation for the austere structure of Vata is fine and harmonious sound. It is essential for Vata to retire into the space of pure and natural sound after the jarring cacophonies of the day. The most healing sadhanas for these types are wholesome and contemplative activities, which resonate deeply with Vata's fine vibratory nature. The heart chakra, which is Vata's main link to the universe, is bathed and nurtured by fine sound. It is very difficult for every Vata to live by a babbling brook, chirping birds, a rustling forest, or within the environs of great music. But everyone is capable of retreating to a tiny space of natural sounds, or of closing off the senses and listening to the strumming of the inner sounds. Like the wind, Vata can be comfortable anywhere except in the modules designed by Pitta and Kapha. Vata is like the force of a windswept desert in the night. The easing of the wind within the vast and timeless space is Vata's natural lullaby.

Vata is also ruled by a heightened sense of touch, as air rules the organ of the skin. As natural sounds oil the arid minds of Vata, the gentle buffering touch of soft natural clothing is essential to Vata's physical well-being. It is difficult for these types to invest time nurturing the body. Soaking in a hot tub or succumbing to an oil massage are the farthest things from Vata's mind for fear that these activities would rob them of their time to worry, be fearful, and be generally bothersome to others. However, it is imperative that every Vata person reserve a few hours a day for exactly such nurturing activities.

These divine antelopes tend to shrink from being embraced, which is so necessary to calm their overwhelming antics and to keep ablaze the fire of their spiritual being. It takes great humility on the part of Vata types to accept that they need a relationship with the meandering Kapha type, grazing in the distance, or with the furious, tract-burning Pitta type.

When Vata types recognize their true role in this multi-faceted existence, it will become easier for them to initiate a physical and emotional embrace with their dynamic and potential counterparts. For Vata the bridge of self-acceptance is the longest and hardest to cross. In recognizing its potential self, it becomes easier for Vata to invite the evolving self. When the antelope person is able to do this, the sad becomes funny and the funny becomes sublime. It is not that the world does not accept Vata. It is only that Vata has not recognized its true ability and has not reconciled its awkward appearance with its sublime nature.

## *Sexuality*

Vata is ruled primarily by Venus and Jupiter. The lunar feminine principle of Venus influences the love of such things as art, culture, and social relationships. Vata has innate sensuality and appreciates the marvels of beauty more than any other type. With Vata, intimate relationships are processed and developed on a long cord. Vata needs to be careful not to extend this process indefinitely or allow the cord to become a treadmill. There is a time to allow the cord to run its course, and a time to make the necessary commitments.

Pure and romantic dating ideas are of more value to Vata than the malaise that accompanies modern sexuality. Traditional values are very important to these types, even though they may not readily recognize this fact. Sex in itself is not important to Vata, and those who are foolhardy enough to defy this fact usually achieve a devastating state of impotence. Sensuality is more likely to trigger their mind than their natural bodily reflexes. The Vata maiden or male, who may appear frigid by general standards, is a creature of poetic fantasies who blossoms into a sex god or goddess when the right partner arrives. For Vata it is the process of love that is love, not the results of love, as in sexual interplay.

The Vata type has an inborn sense of dharma and is generally quite faithful and honorable to a relationship once a commitment is made. Vata can go for long stretches without sexual interplay, but can also be a very fulfilling sexual partner.

It is imperative that Vata types choose the right partners in life. Their best partners are generally matured Kapha-Pitta, Pitta-Kapha, or Kapha-Vata types who have already conquered the crocodiles and tigers of excessive passion and sexuality.

## Career

Jupiter is known as the planet of the *guru*—that teacher who imparts the highest knowledge of Self, God, and universe. A true guru can lead one from ignorance to immortality. The austerity of Vata is naturally suited to aspire to this rare calling. Vata types make the best counselors for human plight as they ply compassion with objectivity. They are natural teachers of esoteric education. They are the champions of social dharma and are usually the best at enforcing laws. Psychologically they tend to be the most mature of all types, and they are suited to the natural role of fathering the universe. Usually it is very difficult for Vata to be an intimate family person. Since their vision and acuity are focused on the general and unbiased good of all, the family role tends to be the most difficult. Their natural nondiscriminating sense of justice is usually resented by close family members and friends. Vata has a direct conflict with granting partiality to the inner family. Vata has the natural ability to become a renunciate and live the monastic life with great happiness.

Those Vata types who have worked through their fears and addictions make the best guides. They naturally invite and relieve the misery of others. Vata types are natural teachers, philosophers, lecturers, musicians, law enforcers, international liaisons, foreign ministers, communicators, political consultants, religious ministers, monks, bankers, charity organizers, and union leaders, and counselors for the handicapped, abused, or addicted. Although Vata types themselves do not make dynamic leaders in the material arena, no leadership is successful without their support. They are unparalleled when it comes to providing the right-handed support behind the scenes. They are literally the heart and guts of an organization.

## Seasonal and Daily Activities

Fall is Vata season, and this is when most of their difficulties arise. It is essential that Vata prepare itself for a quiet and nurturing fall season each year. The times of days and nights when Vata energy is most active is between the hours of 2:00 and 6:00. In the early morning hours, Vata types are restless and lose sleep. Vata needs to maintain a regular schedule of pranayama and relaxation before bedtime. It is wise for Vata to retire early to insure proper sleep before the disturbed hours of early morning begin. If possible, Vata types should nap for a short while daily between 2 and 4 P.M., because during these hours their energies become scattered and dispersed. If napping is not possible, Vata should at least maintain a light schedule during the afternoon hours and minimize any intense activities. Due to the influences of anahata and vishuddha chakras, Vata types sleep an average of four to six hours nightly, mostly on the left side.

Vata types benefit from three full meals daily, beginning with an early breakfast at 7 A.M., lunch at 12 noon, a snack at 4 P.M., and a full dinner at 6 P.M. Ideal bedtime for Vata is around 10 P.M.

The most important sadhana for Vata types is to maintain a consistent daily schedule, one that allows a few hours for reflection, napping, and nurturing of the body and mind. Vata does not need intense exertion. Exercises should be tempered to gentle pursuits such as yoga asanas, do-in, t'ai chi, gentle walks, quigong, idle swimming, hot jacuzzi dips, occasional running, and golfing. (See Daily Routines in chapter 8; see *Diet for Natural Beauty* for the yoga asanas suited to Vata types.)

## Appearance

Vata types tend to be drawn to austerely tailored styles of clothing when they need the gentle buffering of soft, flowing clothes. With their lean, lithe antelope frames, these types may choose to adorn themselves from a wide spectrum of clothes and jewelry. Vata needs clothes for insulation as well as for confidence. There is no one more elegant than a Vata person draped in soft, exquisite clothes and adorned with the appropriate jewelry. These provide the fitting complement to the dry, lean, and hungry Vata look. Most high-fashion models exemplify the Vata look, although many may not be of the Vata constitution. Vata can afford the frills and fancies in clothing even though they are probably the last to visualize themselves with such frivolity.

While all types have simple, elegant clothes made from natural fibers in common, the colors, styling, kinds of fiber, and jewelry change from type to type. With a nature steeped in aesthetics, Vata is the natural clothes horse. The healing gems and metals for the Vata type are amethyst, sapphire, yellow garnet, white moonstone, red and yellow opal, silver, and gold.

The warm and soothing colors of the earth tones, reds, oranges, greens, and all combinations thereof, inspirit the confidence and assurance which Vata needs to project.

## THE PITTA PERSONALITY

### Psychological Nature

*The brilliance of a raging fire dragon in the city of sparkling gems—such is the nature of Pitta.*

Pitta is influenced by the fire element, which is the dynamic dream force of the universe. Pitta permeates the mental body.

The ram, vehicle of the fire god which thrusts forward with great energy, represents the dynamic and cosmic powers of the sun. Pitta is blessed with a powerful solar energy that is reflected in its lofty intellect and noble presence. As with other types, the evolving Pitta personality gradually unfolds toward its true character, and as such has varying degrees of self-awareness.

Pitta demands the lion's share and usually gets it. These raging fire dragons leave long stretches of burnt tracks behind them as they forge forward with their ram power. Pitta's fire energy is represented by the third chakra, or manipura. This Sanskrit term, which translates as "the glittering abode of precious gems," is an ideal description of Pitta energies. Pitta is unique in that both its physiological and psychological centers are located in the central region, or solar plexus, of the body.

Energy, ambition, and aggression are the primary qualities of Pitta. Born of the radiating energy of the universe, Pitta transforms ideas into reality. Ultimately, our potential for cosmic love and dream is made possible by the numinous fire of the universe. Fire energy is perceived by the sense of sight and forms the ability for great vision. This fire is tejas, that which shines and is the moving energy within the billions of atoms in the universe.

The inverted triangle seated within the ten-petalled lotus of the manipura chakra indicates the downward flow of fire energy. When Pitta is balanced through conscious living, this fire energy moves upward in its natural direction. The seed mantra, which holds the energy memory of the third chakra, is the sound RAM, the *m* being a nasal sound. The carrier of the seed mantra is the ram, who is the vehicle of Agni, the fire god.

Fire is triangular in shape and a vivid red in color. The region from the anus to the heart is said to be the region of fire. Carrying the breath along this region, while holding the syllable "Ra" mentally, Pitta types should meditate upon Rudra, Lord of the South. As presiding deity of the manipura chakra, Rudra is destroyer of evil forces in the universe. Picture mentally his crystal blue body daubed with holy ash and sitting on a tiger skin. Visualize his smiling countenance and his three eyes ready to grant you your deepest wishes. Rudra is the one who controls the fiery tigers of the mind.

Pitta is the catalytic force that keeps both Vata and Kapha in check. The Pitta types naturally enjoy absolute control over all situations. Ram-powered for success, they are brilliant and able to focus single-mindedly on whatever task is at hand. Driven by solar force, Pitta types are spectacular in their accomplishments. As with the other types, each person's level of accomplishment varies. For every superbly fine-tuned ram, there is a sheep lurking in the bushes. The Pitta type has its existence on the celestial plane, which signifies mental balance.

Pitta types lose control with great rapidity. It takes a great deal of awareness for them to remember that other humans—namely Vata and Kapha—inhabit the planet. Tempering the Pitta will is tantamount to controlling a forest fire. Yet this very will is responsible for humanity's giant leaps in the area of science and technology. (The backlash, of course, is the immense glutting of planetary industries.) Ambition and power are the trademarks of the Pitta type. While Vata best take note of some of this ego strength, Pitta necessarily needs to underplay its rule of "I-ness." Remember, Pitta types, you do not have to prove yourself as the central and synergistic force in the interaction among types. Pitta is manipura—the central axis of manifestation. This role was defined by the creator; everyone bears the mark of his or her karmic contributions—it's not necessary to redefine the brilliant plans of the super Architect. This is the most essential lesson for Pitta types to learn. Manipura rules the stage of young adulthood. It is natural for the Pitta to be red-headed, irascible, and untamed at the starting line. But somewhere along the marathon trail, Pitta must slow down and take note of its counterparts. The central axis cannot exist alone. It needs a front and a back, respectively Vata and Kapha, in order to fulfil its own noble destiny.

Consideration for others is the main issue Pitta types must keep foremost in their minds. This may slow down the fire dragon from time to time, but it will give Pitta time to reflect.

Pitta's deeper nature is the path of karma. The Bhagavad Gita teaches that karma cannot be performed without dharma. These third chakra types serve the highest potential of all living beings. Their brilliant intellect is capable of grasping the most profound knowledge of the self when they are able to discipline their excesses, indulgence, and arrogance. They have the greatest capacity for a sattvic mind—a mind that is free from the fetters of living, a mind that is in harmony with the universe, a mind that achieves balance. It is a common mistake for the dynamic Pitta type to feel that material conquests are the pinnacle of success. Under this blazing fire is a hidden gem cooled by its own brilliant radiance. When Pitta knocks down the obstacle of its own self-centered ego, Pitta will begin to discover the real pursuit.

## Sexuality

Pitta is ruled primarily by the Sun. This masculine brilliance is stamped indelibly on all of Pitta's activities. The sun power influences fame, purpose, and individuality. Much like this peak of brilliance at the center of the planetary system, Pitta types occupy center stage. Fueled by the primal forces of the rambutting power, Pitta charges to the front lines in the worldly areas of life and love. The fire element of manipura is represented by the inverted triangle, which shows the flow of Pitta's energy propagating downward. When Pitta's fire of intelligence interacts with the waters of deceit (symbolized by the crocodile, Makara), difficulties may ensue. For example, Pitta's overwhelming passion for winning may reign supreme and leave very little room for wholesome interplay.

It is typical for Pitta to be compelled forward with passion, only to burn out before the finish line. Sexually, Pitta types visualize themselves as great lovers, but in reality they often lack the patience and psychological humility necessary to comingle with another. In short, they can be the most passionate lovers if they do not have to depend upon someone else to participate. These types often sabotage their gentler nature due to their overwhelming achievements and their gift of intelligence. Potentially the Pitta types can command great happiness within intimate relationships without compromising their powerful profiles.

The profound brilliance of the Pitta masculine planet is balanced by the eternal powers of Lakini, the Shakti potential. She has three heads, which symbolize the resolve or merging of the physical, astral, and celestial planes of existence. In one of her four hands she carries the *vajra*, a thunderbolt that symbolizes the radiational energy of manipura. A second hand holds the arrow, representing the arrest of desire from Kama, the Lord of sex in the second chakra. This arrow symbolizes the upward turn of Pitta's potential sexual energy. For Pitta types sexuality cannot be simply fulfilling the basic functions of procreation, or the lustful acts of desire. They will always short their fuse when their sensuality is motivated by these ends. Because they are blessed with great intelligence, Pitta's sexual interactions must be conducted at a noble and caring level. The only way Pitta can sustain its juices without burning out is to redirect its emotions to flow through the heart rather than through the genitals. The sexual frustrations of the Pitta type are due to going against their natural (upward flowing) energy and to the modern approaches to sexuality. They are often besieged by impotence—through frustration, insufficient semen, or premature ejaculation—and often suffer from the inability to conceive. It is important for this type to know how to direct the flow of their natural virility. It is paradoxical that the most potent of types needs the most patience to benefit from their own prowess. The lack of knowledge of our true potential nature creates many unwholesome inclinations. With Pitta types this manifests as a need to be sexually indulgent and fanatical, with deleterious results.

In her third hand, Lakini holds fire which only she can control. With her fourth hand she demonstrates the final resolve of the manipura chakra by means of the *mudra,* or hand gesture, that dispells the fear created by duality.

Once Pitta's energy is directed toward the heart, which is a boundless well of compassion, patience, and nurturing, the Pitta type will truly excel with splendiferous virility. If the fire continues to burn hot, it will invariably turn on itself and wipe out even its master. Those Pitta types who have channeled their energies in the right direction are blessed with the most sublime relationship with their spouse, and have great numbers of offsprings.

The most suitable partners for Pitta are Kapha, Kapha-Pitta, and Pitta-Kapha types. These beings are the salve that heals the multitude of burns Pitta sustains. It is important that a partner to the Pitta type also relish physical activities and have a passion for nature's beauty.

## *Career*

The domain of material gain is Pitta's most comfortable seat of existence. There are truly no obstacles in the operational universe that the ram cannot pierce with its radiant lasers. When all else fails, Pitta will charge and butt against the impossible with awesome results.

The fire people are truly a marvel. They deserve our applause and gratitude for pioneering work that no other type is capable of. They were born to the center stage of life, and we need to maintain them there with due respect. When this acknowledgment is given, Pitta can wholeheartedly proceed with the fire dragon tasks ahead, or else they will stubbornly sear the very spots on which they stand and demand recognition.

The solar power of the Pitta type illuminates the world of activities—it is maya's lamp of rajas, or progressive activities (on the material plane). Whereas Kapha naturally meets the earthy and maternal needs of our universe and Vata champions the right actions of fortitude and knowledge, Pitta's place is in activities that foster progress on the planet. They are the administrators, directors, and pioneering forces of our planet. Stand in their way and you will be cauterized to oblivion. Holding such a lofty and visible spotlight amidst the quietude and flightiness of their counterparts, Pitta types have the most difficult of routine challenges. They are equipped for the Hundred Year's War each day, generally prepared with their sharp wielding swords. Pitta's arrogance does not come from being ignored or envied by others, but from Pitta's own ignorance of its nature. Pitta's real power is sharpened by accommodation, in the form of patience and respect for others. Pitta types will only continue to scorch endlessly unless they learn the elementary lesson of regard. It is important that Pitta pace itself with those sadhanas that ignite compassion and reduce judgment toward others.

It is vital for all types to know that the importance of another's existence is not a matter for contention. Every existing life is equally important. Only each purpose and each stage of individual evolution differs. Karma is the gift that brings us here, but dharma is the blessing that determines our real scores. Fire people have a karma that is rajasic, the nature of universal activity. When this type stubbornly digs its heels into the ground, it regresses into the terrain of tamas, the stagnant, inert principle. Pitta must not look downward, as their lessons are held forward in the guna of sattva. Sattva is a state of balance, the harmony of all three gunas. This is the highest state mortals can attain. Sattva is our ability to cognize the stupendous love of cosmic intent. It is here that the rash, young, blazing fire is tamed into cool radiance. Pitta has the greatest potential for becoming sattvic, harmonious, and gentle in nature, if it is willing to work tirelessly on the ego.

The professions most suited to the Pitta types are presidencies or directorships within governments and organizations. They generally make excellent designers, architects, engineers, and scientists. Their acute vision lends itself to all pursuits that require pioneering and foresight. Pitta types excel in fields involving high technology, such as the space programs and the military.

Pitta's sense of vision is superior to its partners. The ram person is capable of producing significant progressive work in the areas of visual arts and design. As a leader Pitta is without a second, and in courage, persistence, and energy, this fireball is unparalleled.

## Seasonal and Daily Activities

Summer is Pitta season, and this is when most of its difficulties arise. Pitta's natural heat is reinforced by the scorching of the sun. It is important that this type prepare for a cool and reticent summer season, in contrast with the rest of the year's activities. Summer is ideal for frolicking with family and friends, and splashing about in cool streams and lakes. The ocean is not the best choice for summer outings, as the hot and caustic fire types burn too easily. Late afternoon strolls and jogging on the beach are the best use of the salty sea terrain, if Pitta has to be there.

Fire people are natural athletes. While running, swimming, tennis, boating, and all high-energy sports are excelled in by these types, it is important that Pitta chooses the cool of the day to engage in them. Pitta types burn off excess energy through sports, but they need to remain alert to themselves and not practice sports for the "metabolic high." When the fire energy is fueled by anger, it becomes detrimental to Pitta's health. Remember, you fierce and fast rams, that you deplete the container of your strength and life force, the *hara,* when you allow anger to run your activities. It is much better to calm yourself when feeling stressed than push to the limit. Pitta's calm is attained through pleasant visual activities, such as painting or observing a green meadow or field of flowers, or a glistening stream. Cool, quiet, comtemplative activities and bathing in the moonlight—these are also excellent sadhanas for Pitta types.

The universe is most likened to Pitta between the morning and evening hours of 10:00 to 2:00. Pitta must be careful not to indulge in rash, hot-tempered conflicts during these times. These types are famous for their eruptions during the midday meal and after the evening meal. Gentle foods and beverages are helpful to Pitta's raging appetite. Pitta needs to avoid spicy foods and intoxicants. These measures will reduce Pitta's need to be temperamental.

The Pitta digestive system peaks at noon and midnight. Pittas are allowed large and filling meals during the day, to meet their metabolic needs. Wholesome foods play the most vital role in fire people's life—it is the medicine that soothes and calms their eruptive nature and aids in the remembrance of their cognitive self. These types cannot afford to indulge in careless and unconscious eating habits.

Evening meditations are enormously important to quiet the overactive Pitta mind. Pitta types need to tone down their activities after 6 P.M. Visualizations are good aids for Pitta meditations—soothing images of cool streams, white sands and snows, green forests, and animals and birds of grace and color are all instrumental in calming these volatile minds.

While the midnight hours bring another spurt of creative energy, the wise Pitta forgoes the temptation of staying up all night, only to crash at dawn. These types normally sleep from six to eight hours squarely on their backs. They can afford to sleep in later than their counterparts to replenish the enormous energy they expended during daytime hours.

Pitta's optimum meal times begin with breakfast at 7 A.M., lunch at noon, a snack at 3 P.M., and dinner at 6 P.M.

At day's end, it is recommended that Pitta leave its worldly conquests outside the home. Pitta needs to surrender to the nurturing of Kapha and the wisdom of Vata so as to regenerate its virile power for the next day. Pitta has much to learn of life's gentle graces from its air and water partners.

Pitta's spare time is best spent with various community charities. Time away from the power treadmill is vital for Pitta. Humanitarian work inspirits the much needed lesson of compassion. When Pitta does work within these dharmic boundaries, a low profile needs to be maintained. It is a difficult testing ground for Pitta, but with practice this shining gem can develop the subtle qualities necessary to invoke its own graceful and dynamic nature. (See also Daily Routines in chapter 8; for the yoga asanas suited to Pitta types, see *Diet for Natural Beauty.*)

### *Appearance*

Pitta is usually best dressed for success. The fire person conforms to the appropriate codes of dress and is careful not to be too obvious. If one looks closely enough, Pitta will always have something different, which is rearing to bloom into a spark of eccentricity. Fire people have enormous power appeal. They love to hang expensive clothes on their athletic and virile bodies.

Subtlety is the best trademark for Pitta. Style and subtlety of presentation are unbeatable combinations for power. Natural fibers are best for all types. Pitta's most complimentary colors are white, blue, lavender, purple, mauve, green, pastels, and all combinations thereof. Pitta is the original preppy, without fitting into any mold. Always two steps ahead of the current trend, Pitta can always be identified by that one offbeat insignia.

## THE KAPHA PERSONALITY

### *Psychological Nature*

*Solid as a rock, cool as a glimmering stream in the white moonlight; such is the essence of Kapha.*

Kapha is influenced by the water and earth elements, which are the energies of attraction and fascination in the universe. Kapha pervades the food body, and has its base in the upper thoracic cavity of the body.

The energies of Kapha's earth principle are symbolized by Airavata, the translucent elephant with four trunks displaying the rainbow. He is the vehicle of Lord Indra, ruler of the firmament. Airavata is the symbol of the foundation chakra, or muladhara. Earth dissolves into the water element of the second chakra, or svadhisthana, and translates as the abode of the self.

The element of earth has the figuration of a square and is yellow in color. The seed mantra that holds the energy memory of the muladhara chakra is LAM, the *m* being a nasal sound. This sound contains the divinity to be invoked during meditation upon that chakra. The element of water bears the sign of the crescent and is white in color. The sound of svadhis-thana is VAM, the *m* being a nasal sound.

Svadhisthana is the dominant energy pervading Kapha. It is ruled by Mercury, which is feminine and lunar in nature. This primal feminine force of procreation is contained by the masculine solar energy of muladhara. The vivacious water person is ruled by both the masculine principle of muladhara and the feminine principle of svadhisthana. Together these energies form the basis of the creation as a whole.

Kapha's spiritual nature is influenced by the first and second chakras, which permeate the pelvic plexus and the genital areas of the body. Its physiological and psychological sites are the exact reverse of Vata, which is also balanced by the upper and lower bodies: Vata's psyche is in Kapha's physiological terrain and Kapha's psyche is in Vata's physiological area. In essence, Vata and Kapha are the two opposite extremes, which are regulated by Pitta. At the cosmic level, Kapha is the food force, Vata the mobile force, and Pitta the dynamic force of dream.

The principles of the planet earth were perfectly defined for Kapha. Of all the body types, Kapha types are the most attuned to the pace of earthly survival. They wrote the social and familial dharmas for humans. Compared to Kapha, Vata flightiness and Pitta fury stand out in sharp contrast. Kapha's basic energy sustains everything. She is the principal foundation upon which all the blocks of existence are built. Kapha is the archetypal Mother Earth.

From svadhisthana she procreates and maintains the universal cycles of life. The apana air, which circu-

lates through her chakras, flows downward to give birth to life. She is the late winter and early spring of all living things. Kapha washes away the blood and mud of daily existence, to reveal vital freshness. She is the basic and continuous routine of life and without her, there is no home, no children, no family. Being the maternal bosom of the planet, both Pitta and Vata types go to her for replenishing. She is like the calm, beautiful cow grazing contentedly with her calves on lush and fragrant fields of buttercups and grass. The primordial elephant who carries the pains and burdens of earth is her mascot. Her symbols, the square and the crescent, represent our foundation, and the maternal, feminine nature of both male and female life. The Kapha person is the classic synthesis of stoical grace, calm, and sensuality. This buoyant life-form provides stability to insure the freedom of Vata and Pitta. Kapha insures the present for her partners.

The Kapha type exists on the physical and astral planes. Kapha, in the form of earth and water on the planet, dominates more than fifty percent of our total existence in space and time. These elements also pervade over sixty percent of the dhatus and approximately eighty percent of the total body weight. As a result Kapha types tend to be frightfully attached to the material world. Their predominant senses—taste and smell—get them into deep trouble with excessive rich foods and possessions.

Just as pure sound is imperative to Vata, clear and unobstructed spaces are essential to Kapha's well-being. Their ability to breathe while performing herculean tasks is aided by brisk conditions. Their terrain may be filled with prolific energy, but it may not be cluttered. The environment of the home should be comfortable but practical. The greatest sadhana for Kapha types is to generously detach themselves from unnecessary hoarding. The difficulty for Kapha is to determine what is necessary. It is usually one quarter of everything this type deems essential.

These solid, gleaming people have a strong tendency to lose their progressive incentives and to head straight for the murky waters. Excessive and unconscious intake of foods, visuals, sounds, and fragrances render them lethargic. During the vulnerable seasonal and daily times, Kapha types need to remain especially observant of their desire to turn inward so as not to add to their inertia and bodily weight. When these magnificent elephant people slip, they often dive deeply into the vortex of the waiting crocodile. True to their implacable nature, Kapha can break free from the clutches of these behaviors, though it may require years of tedious effort.

Kapha's primal nature is dominated by the svadhisthana chakra. The element of this chakra is water, and its symbol is the crocodile, known as Makara. When Kapha tampers with the clarity of her waters, she begins to slip to the bottom of the dark whirlpool where the crocodile of every Kapha personality lurks. It is here that Kapha types attempt to trick and deceive others by inaccurate representations of themselves. Whereas Vata will commit a non-dharmic, or adharmic, action from fear, Kapha will do likewise from delusion. Depression and melancholia are the vibrations that fill these dark waters. When Kapha types descend to these depths, they switch from the role of a universal builder to that of an active destroyer. This is the space from which many malignant cancers are created.

The water type needs to maintain a strict schedule of things to do throughout the day. It is necessary that Kapha people remain current with their emotional self by keeping abreast of inner conflicts. Water people cannot afford to store antagonism and unrest within their absorbent boundaries. Like the streams and rivers, Kapha must remain constantly awash and moving.

## *Sexuality*

Kapha is ruled by both Mars and Mercury and is gifted by a profound equilibrium. Mars, which is solar and masculine in nature, gives robust strength and endurance to the hard working Kapha types. Mercury graces those types with profuse femininity and sexual prowess. The vital synchrony of endurance and sensuality make Kapha people the most formidable carriers of life, procreation, and sexuality on earth.

All the Kapha female has to do is think of sex and she generally becomes pregnant. Both sexes are blessed with abundant fertility and great stamina in love-making. It is one of the few exerting activities that these adept ceiling-viewers take great pleasure in. Kapha's juices of life are always streaming forth with great rapidity. The great classical portraits of Vedic times depict the gods and goddesses with voluptuous bodies that connote the essence of Kapha's sensuality.

The presiding deity of the svadhisthana chakra is Vishnu, the Lord of preservation. With skin the color of pure crystal, he is adorned in orange cloth, symbolizing immortality. While carrying the breath along the region of water, which extends from the knees to the anus, and holding the syllable "Va" in the mind, Kapha types should meditate upon Vishnu in his form as Narayana, the preserver of the universe. He is always ready to grant wishes for fertility, procreation, and wealth.

The Shakti power of the svadhisthana chakra is Rakini. Her skin is pale pink in color and she is adorned in a brilliant red sari and exquisite precious stones. Her four hands hold the following objects: an arrow, shot from the bow of Kama, the Lord of love, which symbolizes the sensual prowess as well as the piercing pain of love-related emotions; a skull, which symbolizes being emotionally indiscriminate—a condition that accompanies the lovelorn and emotionally attached; a drum, which represents the birth of universal music, art, and rhythm; and an axe, which represents both a labor-intensive existence and the implaccable stamina that cuts through all obstacles.

The Kapha female has the rare gift of being both lover and mother to her spouse. The Kapha male shares an equally exceptional position as great lover and nurturing father. Meditation upon Rakini Shakti allows Kapha to access its maternal and yet erotic nature, as well as its instinct for work (symbolized by the axe), perseverance, and the protection of the human family.

Brahma, the presiding deity of the muladhara chakra, is exquisitely golden in color and boasts four heads, which represent the four directions of the universe. In the Vedic trilogy, Brahma is considered the creator. Kapha may meditate upon Brahma and visualize His firm golden body and four heads. He is the one who inspires the stoic and dharmic nature of action. Dakini, the Shakti potential of Brahma, has pink skin and is adorned in either yellow-peach or vermillion. Her eyes are bright red. While she is often depicted as fearsome, she should be visualized in her beneficent aspect. In one of her two left hands she holds a trident, symbolizing her triune nature as creator, preserver, and destroyer. In her other left hand she holds a skull indicating detachment from fear of death. In her upper right hand she holds a sword, symbolizing the overcoming of difficulties and the destruction of ignorance. Her other right hand holds a shield as protection against problems.

Kapha people are the sole heirs of sensuality. Whereas sensuality is a mental exercise for Vata and a desired condition for Pitta, it is the natural state of Kapha's existence. These types will innocently flirt with everyone and everything. They are inherently fresh and unobstructed in their primal flow of sexual energy. They are the procreators of karma and the beneficiaries of kama, sensual desire.

Like all of Kapha's engulfing tendencies, their quest for love may imprison others if they do not develop an alertness to the nature of those they embrace. They are, after all, the wide bosoms of maternal and material consolations.

Generally Kapha types make wonderful partners for all the types. A Kapha is considered the prime catch for a good marriage. A suitable partner for Kapha must be strong and have vital sexual prowess as well as a need for many offspring.

### *Career*

The balance of the solar energy of Mars and the lunar energy of Mercury, which respectively belong to the muladhara and the svadhisthana chakras, make Kapha people the most suited to familial responsibilities. They are the natural providers of the nurturing and sustaining home. These people are often called the salt of the earth; true to that phrase, they guard and protect their loved ones through thick and thin. But they need to be careful not to transgress their limits and allow their mothering to turn into smothering.

Attachments are necessary for the task of nurturing, but water people must remain alert to their impulse of holding on too tightly and too long. Their natural tendency to forage and provide must be tempered with discretion. Kapha becomes attached to material possessions simply for the insatiable need to store. It is natural to plan ahead for the winter years, but Kapha's need to accumulate arises from a strong psychological urge to conserve, and this need quickly expands to mountainous hoarding. It is a typical syndrome for Kapha types to prepare food for twenty people when six are expected for dinner. Their need to give is often accompanied by a wasteful generosity. Overcompensation is Kapha's trademark.

Kapha works best in situations that demand stamina and nurturing. They are natural teachers and parents. They excel as healers and chefs. They are great task force workers for organizations, as well as accountants, technicians, and production facilitators. They have the sublime gift of being able to combine their earthy qualities with the fine arts of dance, poetry, and music. True to their nature of *bhuvar loka,* the earthly plane, they are lofty people with both feet firmly planted on the ground.

## Seasonal and Daily Activities

If it were possible, Kapha would find a way to have all the activities of life come to them. Kapha deliberates every move before it is executed, for fear that too much energy will be expended. Their most cherished activities are finely tuned basic patterns, such as journeying from the bed to the refrigerator, and moving, slowly and with precision, the hand from plate to mouth, while in a luxurious reclining pose. Often these activities are in stark contrast to their amazing ability to outlast all others in arduous work, should circumstances demand. They are truly motivated by the earnest need to help and embrace others. Unlike their Pitta counterparts, they do not operate from well-planned ulterior motives, nor do they look for great gains from their actions. However, a lack of acknowledgment or a graceless attitude in exchange for work well done will greatly displease them.

Late winter and early spring is Kapha season, and this is when most of its difficulties arise. During this time, when nature is about to break free from the earth's bondage, the Kapha person feels thunderously lethargic. It is imperative to set up the year so that this time of upheaval becomes nurturing. Kapha needs to make a firm commitment to maintaining a nonsedentary life. Activities such as gardening, sports, spring and fall cleaning, and redecorating are all suited to the Kapha temperament. Kapha types need to see valid and immediate results for their work, and thus going to formalized programs such as the gym or exercise classes do not work for them.

From 6:00 to 10:00 mornings and evenings, when the universe is most likened to the Kapha personality, a dramatic increase of Kapha tendencies occurs. Their energy becomes intense, heavy, and rooted. These types need to define clear-cut schedules and will themselves into maintaining consistency. The most harmonious day for Kapha begins with an early morning shower, meditation, and yoga or a physical workout. Breakfast should consist of suitable teas, with a light, crisp meal, if any. Kapha's main repast should be a large and healthy lunch followed by a brief walk. Upon returning to their normal work schedule, an even pace should be maintained until day's end. A light supper should be taken. If the meal is too heavy or eaten too late, Kapha will naturally submit to the sluggish slumbering energy prevalent during that time. The most certain way to transcend these danger times is for Kapha types to have a committed schedule of classes, workshops, and so on, to either attend or initiate themselves.

Early to bed and early to rise is the best maxim for Kapha. If Kapha types remain in bed after 6:00 A.M., they become trapped in Kapha-time and sabotage all hopes of being properly motivated for the day. Even though these types need more sleep than others before feeling refreshed, an excellent sadhana to improve the will is to maintain a rest schedule of no more than seven hours nightly.

Kapha's optimum meal times begin with breakfast at 8 to 9 A.M., lunch at 1 P.M., a snack at 4 P.M., and dinner at 6 P.M.

Due to the influences of the muladhara and the svadhisthana chakras, Kapha types normally sleep an average of eight to twelve hours nightly on the stomach or in the fetal position. (See also Daily Routines in chapter 8; for the yoga asanas suited to Kapha types, see *Diet for Natural Beauty.*)

### *Appearance*

Kapha is truly empowered by colorful and flowing clothes. Water types prefer to maintain uniformity in style and could wear the same styles for many years. Once they find a favorite style, they have a tendency to buy duplicates and triplicates of the same thing. There is great beauty in simplicity, but Kapha should not sell itself short. These buoyant people may wear an enormous variety of colors. However, the style should be simply draped and without frills. Kapha types do not need excessive jewelry or frivolous accessories. Nor do they need strictly tailored clothing. If the Kapha body is in excellent condition, simple and softly tailored clothing is the best. However, if there is excess body weight, they should wear loose, flowing clothing with classic styling. The most important gems for Kapha types are agate, red diamond, red and yellow garnet, red and yellow opal, ruby, and topaz. The important metals are copper and gold. Kapha can wear all the colors of the rainbow, and the muted shades thereof.

Kapha's style should be minimal but sensual, practical but soft, and never overt and obvious. The single fine gold chain, the tiny delicate earrings, the classically elegant and understated shoes with a delicate bow or jewel, the yoked and gently flowing shirt, the soft and loose blouse—these are all the adornment these extravagant, sensual creatures need. As much as possible, they should maintain natural fibers in all clothing, and natural metals and gem stones in all jewelry.

CHAPTER 5

# THE NATURE AND TASTES OF EACH DOSHA

The attributes of each dosha strongly influence the body types. A person who is a predominantly Vata type will bear more attributes of Vata, one who is predominantly Pitta will have more attributes of Pitta, and so also with Kapha.

The ancients define each type as follows. Vata, like the wind, is dry, cold, light, mobile, erratic, and rough. Vata is also composed of the tastes produced by her ruling elements of space and air, which are bitter, astringent, and pungent.

Pitta, like fire, is oily, hot, light, intense, malodorous, and fluid. It is composed of the three tastes inherent in fire, which are sour, salty, and pungent.

Kapha, like water, is oily, dense, cool, heavy, stable, and smooth. The tastes of its ruling elements of water and earth are sweet, sour, and salty, and these are the inherent tastes of Kapha.

Ayurveda is rooted in the principle of balance. To approach this balance, we must *decrease* the use of foods with qualities most like our body type. For example, if a Vata type ate dried, cold, rough, and bitter foods, Vata would be very disturbed. If a Pitta type used hot, spicy, and sour foods, Pitta would be aggravated. Similarly, Kapha would become immensely lethargic if the sweet, sour, and salty tastes were used to excess.

The nature of the universe was patterned from the five elements and their six original tastes. Each body type is nurtured by three of these tastes: the three that are not of its own nature.

Kapha types do best with pungent, bitter, astringent tastes, and warm and dry qualities, to counteract their nature of cool and cloying sweetness. This is not to suggest that Kapha types cannot use grains and fruits, which are mostly sweet. However, they need to be alert to the quality and quantity of sweet they use.

Pitta types are nourished by sweet, bitter, and astringent tastes, and cool and fresh qualities, to balance their hot, pungent, sour, and aggressive nature.

Vata types fare well with moist, smooth, warm, and sturdy qualities and sweet, salty, and sour foods. These qualities offset the arid, cold, deprived, bitter, and insecure composition of Vata.

In the doshas, the principle of like increases like applies. The inherent tastes of each dosha will be reinforced if that dosha is fed its own tastes. For instance, Kapha will greatly increase with the sweet taste, and moderately increase with the sour and salty tastes. Vata will be most increased by the bitter taste, and to some extent by astringent and pungent. Pitta will be most increased by sour taste, and then somewhat by pungent and salty tastes.

This does not mean that each type eats only foods with the specific tastes best for their body types. Since all three doshas operate in everyone, a combination of all six tastes is necessary in every person's diet. The proportions of these tastes are the determining factor in good health.

Think of the relationship of the doshas as analogous to the body, mind, and spirit. The harmony of these three diverse aspects is key to our happiness. The doshas are like three streams flowing into the one river of universal intelligence. That river is ourself.

## PROCESS OF MATERIALIZATION

| VATA<br>*Space and Air* | PITTA<br>*Fire and Water* | KAPHA<br>*Water and Earth* |
|---|---|---|
| Bodily air | Digestive acids and enzymes and fats | Body mass, structure, and fluids |
| Spatial cavities of the body | Protective fluids | |

The three doshas are formed from the five elements, which are the basis of the body types. Each element is transmuted into the body with its corresponding functions, thus producing the original six tastes. Further, each type benefits from the tastes other than its own.

## THE DOSHAS AND THEIR NATURAL TASTES

| VATA | PITTA | KAPHA |
|---|---|---|
| Bitter | Sour | Sweet |
| Astringent | Salty | Salty |
| Pungent | Pungent | Sour |

## BENEFICIAL TASTES FOR EACH DOSHA

| VATA | PITTA | KAPHA |
|---|---|---|
| Salty | Bitter | Pungent |
| Sour | Astringent | Bitter |
| Sweet | Sweet | Astringent |

## THE SIX TASTES

### The Sweet Taste

The sweet taste increases bodily tissues, nourishes and comforts the body, and relieves hunger. This taste is necessary for each body type, but the Pitta and Vata types can use more sweet foods than the Kapha types. Water and earth produce the sweet taste, which includes all carbohydrates, sugars, fats, and amino acids. Most grains and fruits are sweet. The primary element of life, which is water, is sweet. Milk is sweet. Almost all foods contain some degree of sweetness. This is the most dominant taste of all our forms of sustenance.

### The Sour Taste

The sour taste is used in small quantities by everyone, but it is most beneficial for the Vata types. Small amounts may be used by Kapha, and minute amounts by Pitta. It aids in digestion and the elimination of wastes from the body. Sour is formed from the earth and fire elements. All organic acids are considered sour. Many fruits—such as lemons, limes, grapefruit, soursop, and strawberries—are considered sour with some sweetness. All fermented foods—such as miso, soy sauce, yogurt, and pickles—are sour foods.

### The Pungent Taste

The pungent taste is most beneficial for the Kapha type. It is to be used in small amounts for Vata, and very sparsely by Pitta. The pungent taste stimulates appetite, and maintains the metabolism and balance of secretions in the body. This taste is formed from the elements of air and fire. Spices, such as garlic, ginger, asafoetida, peppers, and all volatile oils are considered pungent.

### The Salty Taste

The salty taste is used in small quantities by all types, but it is mostly beneficial to Vata. This taste cleanses bodily tissues, makes the system limber, and activates digestion. The salty taste is formed from water and fire, and exists in all salts and seaweeds. Most watery vegetables—such as zucchini, cucumber, and tomatoes—are naturally high in saline.

### The Bitter Taste

The bitter taste is good for everyone in medicinal quantities. It detoxifies the body, tones the organs, cleanses the liver, and controls skin ailments. It is of most importance to Pitta, moderate importance to Kapha, and of very little use to Vata. This taste is formed from air and space, and exists in all bitter foods—such as turmeric, aloe vera, neem leaves, endives, and lettuce—and in alkaloids and glycosides.

### The Astringent Taste

As with bitter, the astringent taste is to be used medicinally. Very small quantities can be used by each type. Pitta and Kapha can use more astringent foods than Vata. Astringency heals the body by its constrictive nature. It reduces secretion and is the most stark of the six tastes. It is formed from the elements of air and earth. Examples of astringent foods are those high in tannin, such as the teas made from the barks of trees. Most legumes contain the astringent taste along with the sweet taste. Most medicines are astringent in nature.

## RASA: THE TASTES OF NATURE

*Rasa* has many meanings in Sanskrit. In the book *Diet for Natural Beauty,* I have defined rasa as the culmination of maturity—the beauty which is earned. It is the achievement of a calm and resolved being. In Ayurveda, rasa is the vital lymph fluid or plasma that nurtures the cells of the body.

The term *rasa* in Ayurveda also refers to the complex chain of reactions that occur from the initial registration of a perception by a sense organ to the stimulation of the brain cells that excite the appetite. Appetite is not simply the initial hunger for food—it is the total intelligence of the body acting in harmony with the external environment. The correct response to the prompting of appetite begins with making informed choices from an array of healthy foods. Similarly, rasa is not merely the taste of foods. Taste is a tiny aspect of the prodigious spectrum within which rasa operates. Food is desired, ingested, digested, and its waste ejected. Rasa is present through all stages of this vital process.

The most important aspect of rasa is discrimination. Rasa is an intelligence to be learned, not the irresponsible throwing together of foods that appeal simply to the sense of sight and taste irrespective of ingestion and digestion. The proper "foreplay" of eating arises from (1) a knowledge of nature, its environs, and of the body; (2) a regard for the universe and the bounty of its grains and greens; and (3) the selection of seasonal and reparatory produce. The delicious taste that ensues from foods knowledgeably and cleanly prepared is only one of the many graces of rasa.

As food enters the system, it signals an immediate heating or cooling response. This factor, which is the active potency of food, is called *virya.* All pungent, sour, and salty foods lend a heating virya, the most heat being produced by those that are pungent. Bitter, astringent, and sweet foods yield a cooling virya, the coldest effect being produced by those that are bitter.

In addition to taste (rasa) and the heating or cooling energies of food (virya), each food has certain qualities or gunas. Each of the three basic doshas *is nourished by* foods having the following seven features:

Vata: moist/lubricating (guna)
heavy/solid (guna)
smooth/consistent (guna)
hot (virya)
sweet (rasa)
salty (rasa)
sour (rasa)

Pitta: substantial (guna)
aromatic (guna)
calming (guna)
cool (virya)
sweet (rasa)
bitter (rasa)
astringent (rasa)

Kapha: dry (guna)
light (guna)
uncloying/moderate (guna)
warm/stimulating (virya)
pungent (rasa)
bitter (rasa)
astringent (rasa)

By tracing the continuum of bliss that foods naturally afford us, the Vedic seers were able to define the properties and effects of food on the human system, and the causes of disease. This ancient science can be revived by the alertness of those who revel in nature. Food is known in Ayurveda as *ausadam,* that which is medicine. When food ceases to be medicine, medicine becomes impotent.

Once food has been digested, the action of rasa continues. The post-digestive effect of foods is called *vipaka.* Here the six tastes are synergized into three final tastes. Sweet remains sweet, in its vipaka state; salty becomes sweet; pungent, bitter, and astringent leave a pungent vipaka; sour remains sour. In essence, the sweet, pungent, and sour tastes are the three unchanging tastes from the beginning to the end of the process of rasa.

Occasionally certain foods or medicines do not follow these three stages predictably. When foods deviate from the established virya or vipaka, they are referred to by the Ayurvedic scholar Charaka as *prabhava,* the exceptions to the rule. Prabhava is most important in Ayurvedic pharmacology, since most ingredients with prabhava qualities are used to deliberately *increase* a specific dosha. In the Vedic diet, we generally attempt only to decrease the aggravated dosha. Certain foods, such as honey, lemons, bananas, and onions, are classified as prabhava foods. Honey, for example, has more of a pungent and volatile nature, even though it is considered sweet; for this reason, it has a hot virya instead of cold, like most sweets. Lemons are classified as sour, but have a cold virya instead of a heating energy. Bananas are considered sweet, but their subtle overriding nature is sour and thus their vipaka is also sour. Onions are classified as pungent, but have a sweet taste after they are cooked. I have discovered that many foods that are classified as prabhava display much more of their subtle tastes when subjected to heat. Most foods with dubious prabhava, such as honey, lemon, tamari, and bananas, should not be cooked.

Ayurveda considers certain foods to be contradictory in nature and cautions us on combining them. The following foods should not be combined:

- Dairy products and salts or salted foods
- Dairy products and animal foods (especially fish)
- Fruits and any other foods
- Hot and cold foods
- Ghee and honey in equal quantity

Ayurveda also enjoins us not to ingest alkaline foods over a long period of time, and not to take honey with warm foods or liquids.

## OJAS

> The excellent essence of the dhatus beginning from plasma and ending in sukra is called ojas. Ojas is also known as *bala* in the context of medical science. This strength provides stability, and nourishment of the muscle tissue, and the individual remains undeterred in all efforts. He is endowed with excellence of voice and complexion. His internal organs and external senses are capable of performing their will to their full abilities.
>
> **Vaidya Bhagwan Dash**

In review, the Ayurvedic concept of taste is observed in these three stages: the sensory stimulation and initial taste of the tongue (rasa); the heating or cooling energy that occurs during digestion (virya); and the post-digestive taste (vipaka), which reduces the six original tastes into three residual tastes of sweet, sour, and pungent. These three final tastes are transported within the nutritive plasma to the various organs and tissues of the body. After digestion and assimilation are completed, the singular essence known as ojas remains in the body. When the energies of the foods or the mental attitudes are impaired, or the seasonal influences are not observed, ojas is greatly diminished.Without this residual essence of ojas in the body, the autoimmune system becomes vulnerable to disease.

When the doshas are all in balance, the health of the dhatus is excellent. When the dhatus are healthy, the male and female sperm and ovum dhatus (shukra and artava) are aglow with brilliance. When the doshas and dhatus are unhealthy, the shukra and artava are polluted and the aura is impaired. The sperm shukra is the food of fertility for the ovum artava. The shining health of a child depends entirely on the shukra and artava condition of the parents. The union between male and female is fundamental to the feeding of the female artava. Sexual union takes place for the replenishment of the artava, the nurturing of the female hunger, in order to procreate. When the conditions of the shukra and artava are weak and without nutrition, the female loses her fertility and the male his potency. The male can no longer feed the female, and even though children continue to be born, the basic intelligence and health of their nature is dramatically diminished because of the depleted shukra and artava.

## DETERMINING THE TASTE AND ENERGETICS OF FOODS

> Air, fire, and water are the three fundamental bases of life.
>
> **Sushruta**

Each minute grain of sand has its own distinguishing feature, which makes it unique within creation. In observing nature, we are able to determine the inherent energy of each human, animal, vegetable, grain, bean, fruit, and seed.

Shape, size, color, scent, taste, temperature and season, as well as texture—these are the primary indicators used to determine a space, air, fire, water, or earth food. Like humans, most foods are a combination of

## THE ANATOMY OF THE SIX TASTES

| RASA | ELEMENTS | QUALITIES | VIRYA |
|---|---|---|---|
| Sweet | Earth/Water | Oily, cold, heavy | Cold |
| Sour | Earth/Fire | Oily, hot, heavy | Hot |
| Salty | Water/Fire | Oily, hot, heavy | Hot |
| Pungent | Fire/Air | Rough, hot, light | Hot |
| Bitter | Air/Space | Rough, cold, light | Cold |
| Astringent | Air/Earth | Rough, cold, light | Cold |

| RASA (Initial taste) | VIPAKA (Post-digestive taste) | EFFECT | | MAIN FUNCTION |
|---|---|---|---|---|
| Sweet | Sweet | increases K | decreases V, P | Increases body tissues |
| Sour | Sour | increases K, P | decreases V | Increases appetite |
| Salty | Sweet | increases K, P | decreasesV | Makes body limber and cleanses body tissues |
| Pungent | Pungent | increases P, V | decreases K | Reduces fluid in tissues |
| Bitter | Pungent | increases V | decreases P, K | Purifies organs and controls skin ailments |
| Astringent | Pungent | increasesV | decreases P, K | Purifies and constricts body |

## THE THREE STAGES OF TASTE

| RASA (Initial taste) | VIRYA (Energy of Food) | VIPAKA (Post-digestive taste) |
|---|---|---|
| Sweet | Cold | Sweet |
| Sour | Hot | Sour |
| Salty | Hot | Sweet |
| Pungent | Hot | Pungent |
| Bitter | Cold | Pungent |
| Astringent | Cold | Pungent |

## SUMMARY OF THE TRANSFORMATION OF THE SIX TASTES

Sweet remains sweet

Sour remains sour

Pungent remains pungent

Salty becomes sweet

Bitter becomes pungent

Astringent becomes pungent

two dominant elements. By observation, we are able to distinguish and use foods that are different from our own nature, and thus maintain a dynamic stasis within our organism.

All plants and other life-forms are derived from the water element. Through the process of transmutation, the other four elements also exist in varying degrees. Water gives taste to life, and earth gives scent to it. Fire transforms the shape and visual characteristics of food. Air creates the skin, feel, and texture of the food. Space gives the food sound, hollowness, and resonance.

When we learn to plant seeds in our own garden and observe the growth of our grains, vegetables, beans, fruits, and herbs, we become attuned to the nature of each plant. We instinctively become alert to its distinguishing features. A wholesome life is sustained by the excellent marriage of each life-form to its proper food.

Food speaks to us. All we need to do is listen... to be still and observe the grandeur of nature in every blade of grass. Every food has its innate markings, color, vibration, and taste. The ripe peach shimmers on a tree. It is golden and red. Human lips are caressed by its fine fur before its sweet pulp is released. A red, round, firm apple crackles under our bite. It may be sweet and juicy or tart and firm. A banana turns into mush and lubricates the digestive system. The chili pepper, which bites by sight and scent, consumes the tongue and stomach with fire long after it is eaten. All foods speak to us—some loudly, others delicately. Be still and observe.

It is best to eat the foods that are in season and that grow either locally or in a similar climate. Occasionally, foods that grow in other climates and terrains may be used for variety and the celebration of our universal spirit.

## ELEMENTAL FEATURES OF ALL FOODS

| SPACE | AIR | FIRE | WATER | EARTH |
|---|---|---|---|---|
| Hollow | Mobile | Intense | Cool | Solid |
| Resonant | Rough | Hot | Dense | Dense |
| Translucent | Hard | Medium-size | Heavy | Heavy |
| Blue | Dry | Sharp | Large | Large |
| Cold | Variable | Light | Moist | Oily |
| Astringent | Fresh | Fluid | Smooth | Sour |
| Pungent | Wiry | Oily | Cloudy | Sweet |
| | Light | Fetid | Sticky | |
| | Compact | Red | White | |
| | Dark (gray/green) | Orange | Clear | |
| | Bitter | Pungent | Sweet | |
| | Astringent | Salty | Salty | |

### ENERGETICS OF EACH FOOD ARE DETERMINED BY

| | | | |
|---|---|---|---|
| Shape | Color | Taste | Texture |
| Size (density/weight/buoyancy) | Scent | Temperature/season | |

### FIRE FOODS

| | | |
|---|---|---|
| All hot spices | All pickles, vinegars, and salts | All heating grains |
| All oily foods | All acidic foods /medicines | All nuts |
| All sour /pungent fruits and vegetables | All animal foods | All red foods |

### AIR/SPACE FOODS

| | | |
|---|---|---|
| Most leafy greens and lettuces | All hollow vegetables with tiny seeds* | All dry, rough, stale foods |
| All cabbage families | Most nightshade foods | |
| All bitter vegetables | Most dry, compact legumes | |

*Except for peppers, which are fire/air/space foods

### EARTH/WATER FOODS

| | | |
|---|---|---|
| All sweet, juicy fruits | All cool, milky foods | All sticky, cold foods |
| All salty and sweet watery vegetables | | All sweets |

The following examples are given so you may begin to use your own powers of observation and learn about the foods that are transformed into your body. Remember that in order to approach balance accord ing to Ayurvedic principles you must select foods with energetic qualities different from those of your basic constitutional type. If you are predominantly a space/air type (Vata), the foods most suited to you would be *other than* these energies. If you are a water/earth type (Kapha), your foods would be mostly of fire, air, and space. Once you learn the cosmic rule, you'll be intuitively deciphering the energies of all things with practice.

## EXAMPLES OF TASTES ACCORDING TO THE ELEMENTS

### **LETTUCE:** AIR/WATER FOOD

| | | |
|---|---|---|
| Primary element: air | Color: green | Texture: airy, wiry |
| Secondary element: water | Scent: fresh | Good for Kapha and Pitta types; occasionally for Vata types (with dressing) |
| Shape: variable | Taste: bitter | |
| Size: thin, light | Temperature: cool, moist | |

### **RED CHILI PEPPER:** FIRE/AIR/SPACE FOOD

| | | |
|---|---|---|
| Primary element: fire | Size: small, medium, light (with compact seeds) | Taste: pungent, salty |
| Secondary elements: space/air | Color: red | Temperature: hot |
| Shape: triangular, hollow (space) and variable | Scent: sharp and penetrating | Texture: smooth, oily |
| | | Good for Kapha types; occasionally for Vata types |

## **CROOKNECK SQUASH:** WATER/EARTH FOOD

Primary element: water
Secondary element: earth
Shape: crescent
Size: medium, buoyant

Color: yellow; white flesh
Scent: sweet
Taste: sweet, astringent
Temperature: cool

Texture: smooth, oily
Good for Vata and Pitta types; occasionally for Kapha types

## **COCONUT:** WATER/EARTH/SPACE FOOD

Primary element: water
Secondary elements: earth/space
Shape: round
Size: medium, hollow, resonant

Color: brown shell; white flesh
Scent: sweet, milky
Taste: sweet
Temperature: cool

Texture: variable, dry
Good for Pitta and Vata types

## **ACORN SQUASH:** EARTH/WATER FOOD

Primary element: earth
Secondary element: water
Shape: multi-crescent
Size: medium, large; solid

Color: cloudy orange
Scent: sweet, nutty
Taste: sweet
Temperature: cool

Texture: smooth, dense
Good for Vata and Pitta types

## **GREEN BELL PEPPER:** AIR/SPACE/FIRE FOOD

Primary elements: air and space
Secondary element: fire
Shape: triangular and variable, hollow (space)

Size: medium, small, light (with compact seeds)
Color: green
Scent: sharp, pungent

Taste: pungent, salty
Temperature: hot
Texture: smooth, oily
Good for Kapha types; occasional for Pitta types

## A REMINDER

***Tastes (Rasa) and Energy (Virya) suitable (in order of preference) for each dosha:***

Good for Vata: salty, sour, sweet; heating
Good for Pitta: sweet, bitter, astringent; cooling
Good for Kapha: pungent, bitter, astringent; heating

The following list categorizes foods according to their tastes. When a food has only *one* of the two tastes indicated, and/or has *an additional taste*, that information is in parentheses. Occasionally, certain additional charactericstics or gunas (see page 60) appear in italics after a food; these qualities can render an otherwise unallowable food permissible for a particular body type.

## TASTE (RASA) AND ENERGY (VIRYA) OF EACH FOOD

### VEGETABLES

#### *Sweet/Astringent; Cooling*

Asparagus
Broccoli
Cabbage (pungent)
Cassava
Cauliflower (astringent)
Celery (astringent)
Cucumbers
Gourd squash
Green beans
Jerusalem artichoke (astringent, bitter)
Lettuce (astringent)
Okra
Parsnip
Peas (pungent)
Potatoes, white (salty)
Spinach (astringent, pungent)
Sprouts (astringent, pungent)
Sweet potatoes
Taro potatoes (salty)
Winter squash: acorn, buttercup, butternut, spaghetti
Zucchini (pungent)

#### *Bitter/Astringent; Cooling*

Arugula (bitter)
Collards (bitter)
Dandelion greens
Endive (bitter)
Kale (bitter)
Karela (bitter)
Sprouts (astringent)

#### *Sweet/Pungent; Heating*

Artichoke (sweet, astringent)
Beets
Beet greens
Bell peppers (pungent)
Brussels sprouts(pungent, astringent)
Burdock root (astringent, bitter)
Carrots (pungent, astringent)
Corn, fresh (sweet, astringent)
Daikon (pungent)
Eggplant (astringent, bitter)
Garlic (pungent)
Horseradish (pungent)
Landcress (pungent)
Leeks
Mushrooms (sweet, astringent)
Olives, black
Onions
Parsley (pungent)
Peppers (pungent)
Plantain (pungent, astringent)
Radish (pungent)
Tomatoes (sour)
Turnips (pungent, astringent)
Turnip greens (pungent, astringent)
Watercress

### FRUITS

#### *Sweet/Astringent;Cooling*

Apples
Avocado
Berries
Coconut (sweet)
Dates (sweet)
Figs, ripe
Grapes, purple
Melon (sweet)
Pears
Prunes (sweet)
Raisins
Watermelon

***Sour; Cooling***

Lemons
Limes (bitter)
Mango, green
Pomegranate (sweet, astringent)
Quince (sour, sweet)
Strawberries (sour, sweet)
Tamarind

***Sweet/Sour; Heating***

Cantaloupe (sweet)
Grapes, green
Oranges
Papaya
Pineapple
Soursop

***Sweet/Astringent; Heating***

Apricots
Bananas (sweet, sour)
Cherries (sweet, sour)
Cranberries(sour)
Mango, ripe (sweet)
Peaches
Persimmon
Plums
Rhubarb

***Sweet/Sour; Cooling***

Rhubarb
Strawberries

## GRAINS

***Sweet/Astringent; Cooling***

Barley
Basmati rice (sweet)
Cereals (sweet)
Wheat (sweet)
Wheat bran (sweet)
White rice (sweet)

***Sweet/Astringent; Heating***

Brown rice (sweet)
Buckwheat
Cornmeal (sweet; *dry*)
Corn (sweet; *dry*)
Millet (sweet; *dry*)
Oat bran (sweet; *dry*)
Oats (sweet; *dry*)
Rye
Triticale

***Pungent/Sweet; Heating***

Amaranth
Quinoa (pungent)

## BEANS, LEGUMES, AND PEAS

***Sweet/Astringent; Cooling***

Aduki beans
Black beans
Black-eyed peas
Chickpeas
Lima beans
Mung dhal
Pinto beans
Soybeans
Split peas
Tofu
White beans

***Sweet/Astringent; Heating***

Kidney beans
Lentils, brown and red
Navy beans
Toor dhal (sweet)
Urad dhal

***Pungent/Astringent; Heating***

Tempeh

## SPICES, HERBS, CONDIMENTS, AND SEAWEEDS

### *Pungent/Heating*

- Allspice
- Ajwan
- Anise
- Asafoetida
- Basil
- Bayleaf
- Black pepper
- Caraway
- Cayenne
- Celery seed
- Cloves (*aromatic*)
- Curry powder (bitter)
- Ginger (sweet)
- Horseradish
- Marjoram
- Mustard seeds
- Nutmeg
- Oregano
- Paprika
- Parsley
- Pippali
- Rosemary (bitter)
- Sage (bitter, astringent)
- Savory
- Star anise
- Tarragon (bitter)
- Thyme
- Turmeric (bitter)

### *Pungent/Sweet; Heating*

- Cardamom
- Cinnamon (astringent)
- Fenugreek leaves (bitter)
- Garam masala (bitter)
- Mace
- Onion
- Orange peel (pungent, bitter, *aromatic*)

### *Bitter/Astringent; Heating*

- Fenugreek seed

### *Salty; Heating*

- Black salt
- Rock salt
- Sea salt

### *Pungent/Salty; Heating*

- Most seaweeds

### *Bitter/Pungent; Cooling*

- Black cumin
- Coriander
- Cumin
- Dill leaves and seeds
- Peppermint (pungent)
- Neem leaves (bitter)
- Mint leaves (pungent)
- Spearmint (pungent)
- Wintergreen (pungent)

### *Sweet/Pungent; Cooling*

- Fennel
- Saffron (astringent, bitter)
- Vanilla (pungent, astringent)

### *Sweet; Cooling*

- Kudzu
- Rose water

## SWEETENERS

### *Sweet;Cooling*

- Barley malt (astringent)
- Brown rice syrup
- Brown sugar (unrefined)
- Dates
- Fructose
- Fruit juice concentrates (astringent)
- Maple syrup (bitter)
- Sucanat
- Sugarcane juice
- White sugar

### *Sweet; Heating*

| | | |
|---|---|---|
| Amasake | Jaggery | Molasses (pungent) |
| Honey (astringent) | | |

## OILS

### *Sweet; Heating*

| | | |
|---|---|---|
| Almond oil | Safflower oil (astringent) | Vegetable oil, mixed |
| Apricot oil | Sesame oil (bitter, astringent) | Walnut oil (astringent) |
| Corn oil | | |

### *Sweet; Cooling*

| | | |
|---|---|---|
| Avocado oil | Coconut oil | Sunflower oil |
| Canola oil | Soy oil | |

### *Pungent; Heating*

| | | |
|---|---|---|
| Mustard oil | Olive oil | |

### *Sweet/Bitter/Pungent; Heating*

Castor oil

## DAIRY

### *Sweet; Cooling*

| | | |
|---|---|---|
| Butter, unsalted (astringent) | Cow's milk | Goat's milk (pungent) |
| Cheese, unsalted (sour) | Ghee | Mother's milk |

### *Sour/Astringent; Heating*

| | | |
|---|---|---|
| Buttermilk | Sour cream | Yogurt |
| Cheese, salted (pungent) | | |

## NUTS

### *Sweet/Astringent; Heating*

| | | |
|---|---|---|
| Almonds (sweet) | Macadamia (sweet) | Pine nuts |
| Cashews (sweet) | Peanuts | Pistachios |
| Filberts | Pecans | Walnuts, black or English |

## SEEDS

### *Pungent/Sweet; Heating*

| | | |
|---|---|---|
| Chia seeds | Poppy seeds (astringent) | Sesame seeds (sweet) |
| Flax seeds (sweet; astringent) | Pumpkin seeds (sweet, bitter, astringent) | |

### *Sweet/Astringent; Cooling*

| | | |
|---|---|---|
| Psyllium seeds | Sunflower seeds | |

## TEAS

| | | |
|---|---|---|
| | ***Sweet/Astringent; Cooling*** | |
| Alfalfa | Borage | Oat straw (sweet) |
| Barley (sweet) | Lotus | Raspberry |
| Blackberry (astringent) | Nettle (astringent) | Strawberry |
| | ***Bitter/Pungent; Cooling*** | |
| Chamomile | Lavender (pungent) | Peruvian bark (pungent) |
| Chicory (bitter) | Lemon grass | Spearmint (pungent) |
| Elder flower | Passionflower (bitter) | Violet |
| Hops | Pau d'arco (bitter) | Wintergreen (pungent) |
| Jasmine | Peppermint (pungent) | Yarrow (astringent) |
| | ***Pungent; Heating*** | |
| Ajwan | Eucalyptus | Mugwort (bitter) |
| Basil | Fenugreek (bitter, sweet) | Orange peel |
| Calamus (bitter) | Ginger, dried or fresh (sweet) | Osha (bitter) |
| Cardamom (sweet) | Ginseng (bitter, sweet) | Pennyroyal |
| Cinnamon (sweet, astringent) | Hyssop (bitter) | Wild ginger |
| Clove | Juniper berries (bitter, sweet) | |
| | ***Astringent/Sweet; Heating*** | |
| Burdock (astringent, bitter) | Hawthrone (sweet, sour) | Hibiscus |
| | ***Bitter/Sweet; Cooling*** | |
| Chrysanthemum | Marshmallow (sweet) | Sarsaparilla |
| Dandelion | Red clover | |
| Licorice | Sandalwood (astringent) | |
| | ***Sweet/Pungent; Cooling*** | |
| Corn silk | Lemon balm | Saffron (bitter) |
| Fennel | Rose flowers (bitter, astringent) | |

# PART TWO

# The Practice of Ayurveda

CHAPTER 6

# EATING ACCORDING TO YOUR BODY TYPE— THE FOOD CHARTS

All produce, grains, beans, and breads start out as fresh and alive with energy. Energy is the life force of a food from its inception as a fertile seed, which receives energy through fertile soil and agreeable climate, through the final stages of sowing and reaping. The source of this energy is referred to as *tanmatras,* the subtle aspect of the five elements. The longer a food is uprooted from the earth, the less energy it holds. Certain foods, such as grains and beans, can be stored successfully under specific conditions. But the extent to which these foods are then processed is proportionate to the depletion of their life-force. The energy of a food is determined by the natural or unnatural conditions under which it is farmed. Whether that energy is fully transmitted into our body is determined by the season in which it is picked and eaten, and by whether or not it is complementary to our body type. Since we no longer depend upon our own efforts of farming, and since the prices of organic foods can be high, continuous effort and commitment are required on our part to eat wholesomely. We must strive to regain and protect our natural farmlands and invest the time to create and harvest small gardens or communal plots. When we redistribute our purchasing power toward healthier choices, we will actually save money. Whole grains, for example, are less expensive than the conveniently processed grains and breads.

Foods are not inert. The depth and density of their energy invariably correspond to the level of our internal energy. Foods that are grown naturally, without the use of chemicals and without undue processing, are the optimum choice. Fresh produce, available at farmer's markets and supermarkets, is the second choice. Canned, frozen, or chemically-processed foods, and fast foods, are noxious to our health. They are dead foods, devoid of any innate energy.

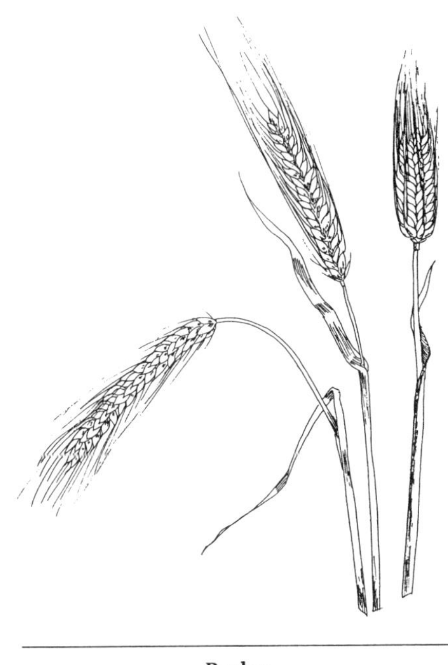

Barley

The vital energy in foods is what invigorates the various organs, tissues, fluids, and spaces of the body. When we consume dead food, food that barely yields the minimum energy needed for survival, we ensure the slow and dangerous demise of our internal environment.

The food charts that constitute the bulk of this chapter outline a large variety of foods suitable for each body type. The foods in the Major category are for everyday use, and those in the Minor category are for occasional use. The Regressive category contains the most negative foods for each type.

These food recommendations should be approached slowly and with consistency, especially by those just beginning a natural lifestyle.

Many of the foods listed in these charts can be found in ancient Ayurvedic texts, while some have only recently been evaluated and categorized. As research on the energetics of foods flourishes, more information is continually becoming available. These charts are designed only as guidelines. While you may use them to learn which foods are best suited to your body type, the ultimate determination about what is appropriate for you must come from your own conscious reactions.

The classic Ayurvedic texts enumerate seven body types. They are Vata, Pitta, Kapha; Vata-Pitta, Pitta-Kapha, Vata-Kapha; and Vata-Pitta-Kapha. However, each of the three dual types contains notable differences depending on which of the two doshas is dominant. Vata-Pitta may express itself as Vata-Pitta or as Pitta-Vata. For this reason I have added Pitta-Vata, Kapha-Pitta, and Kapha-Vata, to give a total of ten body types for the Food Charts.

In the Food Charts that follow, the foods in the Major category will generally exhibit two or more qualities suitable to your dosha. Thc foods in the Minor category will have at least one quality suitable to your dosha. The Regressive category lists foods that can negatively affect your dosha. This category includes all foods that are old, insect-eaten, frozen, dried, or canned. All body types should use fresh and seasonal foods.

Dairy references always refer to organic products. Unrefined brown sugar refers to jaggery, gur, Sucanat, or noncommercial turbinado.

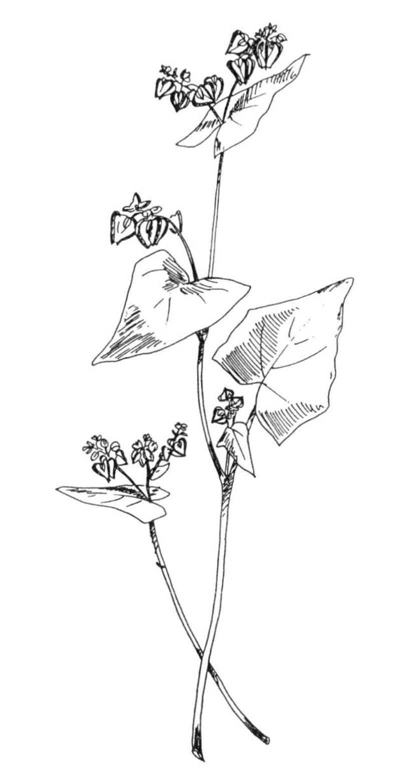

Buckwheat

## STAGES FOR INTRODUCING PROPER FOODS

*First Six Months (21 Meals per Week)*

| *Major* | *Minor* | *Regressive* |
|---|---|---|
| 10 out of 21 meals | 8 out of 21 meals | 3 out of 21 meals |

*Second Six Months (21 Meals per Week)*

| *Major* | *Minor* | *Regressive* |
|---|---|---|
| 12 out of 21 meals | 8 out of 21 meals | 1 out of 21 meals |

*After One Year (21 Meals per Week)*

| *Major* | *Minor* | *Regressive* |
|---|---|---|
| 17 out of 21 meals | 4 out of 21 meals | None/once in a very long while |

## THE FOOD CHARTS

### VATA

#### VEGETABLES

*Use fresh and seasonal vegetables.*

*Major*

Artichoke
Asparagus
Bok choy
Carrots
Daikon
Green beans
Landcress
Leeks, cooked
Onion, cooked
Pumpkin
Sweet potatoes
Summer squash (yellow crookneck, zucchini)
Watercress
Winter squash (acorn, buttercup, butternut)

*Minor*

Broccoli
Burdock root, cooked moist
Cassava
Collards
Corn, fresh
Cucumber, seedless
Gourd squash
Jerusalem artichoke
Jicama
Kale, well cooked
Karela
Lettuce
Mustard greens
Parsnips
Plantain
Radishes
Spinach
Sprouts
Taro root
Turnip greens
Winter squash (spaghetti)

### *Regressive*

| | | |
|---|---|---|
| Beet greens | Eggplant | Pokeroot |
| Bell peppers | Endive | Potatoes, white |
| Brussels sprouts | Kohlrabi | Rutabaga |
| Cabbage | Mushrooms | Swiss chard |
| Cauliflower | Onion, raw | Tomatoes |
| Celery | Peas | Turnips |

## FRUITS

*Use fresh and seasonal fruits.*

### *Major*

| | | |
|---|---|---|
| Apricots | Grapefruit | Peaches |
| Avocado | Kiwi | Pineapple |
| Bananas | Lemons | Plums |
| Berries | Limes | Rhubarb |
| Cherries | Mango | Soursop |
| Coconut | Melons | Tamarind |
| Dates | Oranges | Tangerines |
| Figs, fresh | Papaya | |

### *Minor*

| | | |
|---|---|---|
| Apples | Pears | Quince |
| Cranberries | Pomegranate | Raisins, cooked |
| Dried fruits, cooked | | |

### *Regressive*

| | | |
|---|---|---|
| Persimmon | Prunes | Watermelon |

## GRAINS (ALL YEAR)

*V types should avoid a mono-diet of brown rice.*

### *Major*

| | | |
|---|---|---|
| Basmati rice, brown or white | Oats, whole cooked | Wheat berries |
| Brown rice, all grains or sweet | Sushi rice, white | |

### *Minor*

| | | |
|---|---|---|
| Amaranth | Barley | Quinoa |

### *Regressive*

| | | |
|---|---|---|
| Buckwheat | Corn | Oats, dry |
| Cereals, dried | Millet | Rye |

## PROCESSED GRAINS (ALL YEAR)

### *Minor*

| | | |
|---|---|---|
| Bulgur | Oats, rolled or steel-cut, cooked | Udon noodles |
| Couscous | Pasta, whole wheat | Unbleached white flour |
| Mochi (pounded sweet rice) | Rice flour | Whole wheat flour |

## LEGUMES, BEANS, PEAS, AND SOYBEAN DERIVATIVES

### *Major*

| | | |
|---|---|---|
| Aduki beans | Tofu, cooked | Toor dhal |
| Mung dhal, split or whole | | |

### *Minor*

| | | |
|---|---|---|
| Black chickpeas | Muth beans | Urad dhal |

### *Regressive*

| | | |
|---|---|---|
| Black beans | Kidney beans | Soybeans |
| Black-eyed peas | Lima beans | Split peas, green or yellow |
| Chickpeas | Navy beans | Tempeh |
| Lentils, brown or red | Pinto beans | White beans |

## NUTS AND SEEDS

### *Minor*

| | | |
|---|---|---|
| Almonds | Macadamia | Pumpkin seeds |
| Brazil nuts | Peanuts | Sesame seeds, roasted |
| Cashews | Pecans | Sunflower seeds |
| Chestnuts | Pine nuts | Walnuts |
| Filberts | Pistachios | |

## DAIRY

### *Major*

| | | |
|---|---|---|
| Buttermilk | Cow's milk, certified raw | Yogurt |
| Cottage cheese | Ghee | |

### *Minor*

| | | |
|---|---|---|
| Cheeses, hard or soft | Ice cream, homemade | Sour cream |
| Goat's milk | | |

### *Regressive*

Dairy products, commercial or powdered

## OILS/FATS

### *Major*

Almond
Canola
Sesame, dark or light
Sunflower

### *Minor*

Coconut
Mustard
Olive
Safflower
Soy
Walnut

### *Regressive*

Animal fats
Corn
Vegetable, mixed

## SWEETENERS

### *Major*

Amasake (rice milk)
Brown rice syrup
Brown sugar, unrefined
Dates
Fruit juice concentrates
Honey, raw and uncooked
Maple syrup
Sucanat
Sugarcane juice

### *Minor*

Barley malt
Dried fruits, cooked (apricots, bananas, papaya, peaches, pineapples, raisins)
Molasses

### *Regressive*

Honey, cooked
Sugar substitutes (saccharin, Sweet 'n Low, NutraSweet)
White sugar

## HERBS, SPICES, AND FLAVORINGS

### *Major*

Almond extract
Anise
Asafoetida
Basil
Bay leaf
Black cumin
Black pepper
Caraway
Cardamom
Chili pepper
Cinnamon
Cloves
Coriander
Cumin
Curry powder
Dill, leaves or seed
Fennel
Garam masala
Ginger, dried or fresh
Kudzu
Mango powder
Mustard seeds
Nutmeg
Oregano
Paprika
Peppermint
Pippali
Rosemary
Saffron
Sage
Savory
Spearmint
Tamarind
Tarragon
Thyme
Turmeric
Vanilla

### Minor

Cayenne
Cilantro
Curry leaves
Fenugreek
Garlic
Horseradish
Mint
Parsley

### Regressive

Garlic, raw
Extremely bitter and astringent herbs and spices

## CONDIMENTS

### Major

Chutney, coconut or mango
Daikon, grated
Gomasio
Horseradish
Mayonnaise, noncommercial
Mirin
Mustard, noncommercial
Olives, black or green
Pickles, ginger or lime or general
Rock salt
Sea salt
Tamarind
Umeboshi plum
Vinegar, brown rice or herbal or umeboshi
Yogurt, spiced

### Minor

Cilantro
Chili pepper
Coconut, grated
Coconut milk
Rose water
Tamari

### Regressive

Garlic, raw
Ketchup
Mayonnaise, commercial
Mustard, commercial
Onion, raw
Preservatives and additives, chemical
Salt, iodized

## SEAWEEDS

*Soak and rinse thoroughly before use.*

### Major

Arame
Hijiki
Kombu
Wakame

### Minor

Agar-agar
Blue-green algae
Dulse
Kelp
Seaware

## BREWS AND BEVERAGES

***Drinks should not be cold, and most fruit juices should be diluted with water or milk for V types.***

### *Major*

Almond milk
Aloe vera drinks or juice
Apricot juice
Berry juice
Carrot juice
Cherry juice
Chicory blends
Coconut milk
Date shake
Grapefruit juice
Grape juice
Lemonade
Mango juice
Orange juice
Papaya juice
Peach juice
Pineapple juice
Salted drinks
Sour drinks

### *Minor*

Carob drinks
Carob-banana shake
Lassi (sweet yogurt drink)
Milk shakes
Mixed vegetable juices

### *Regressive*

Alcohol
Apple juice
Caffeinated drinks
Carbonated drinks
Cold drinks
Cranberry juice
Pear juice
Prune juice
Pungent drinks
Tomato juice

## TEAS

***Do not use chamomile if you are allergic to ragweed.***

### *Major*

Ajwan
Bancha (twig)
Basil
Chamomile
Chicory
Cinnamon
Cloves
Comfrey
Elder flowers
Eucalyptus
Fennel
Ginger
Hyssop
Lavender
Lemon balm
Licorice
Lotus
Marshmallow
Orange peel
Pennyroyal
Peppermint
Peruvian bark
Rose flowers
Rosehips
Saffron
Sage
Sarsaparilla
Sassafras
Spearmint

### *Minor*

Alfalfa
Barley (grain tea)
Chrysanthemum
Ginseng
Hibiscus
Hops
Jasmine
Nettle
Passionflower
Raspberry
Red clover
Strawberry
Violet

### *Regressive*

Blackberry
Borage
Burdock
Corn silk
Dandelion
Mormon tea
Yarrow

# VATA-PITTA

## VEGETABLES

***Use fresh and seasonal vegetables, mostly cooked. All vegetables with seeds should be well cooked with appropriate Vata spices to minimize aggravation of V-P types. Small amounts of bitter vegetables may be used.***

### *Major*

Artichoke
Asparagus
Bok choy
Carrots
Collards
Green beans
Jerusalem artichoke
Landcress
Mustard greens
Okra
Parsnips
Pumpkin
Rutabaga
Summer squash (yellow crookneck, zucchini)
Sweet potatoes
Winter squash (acorn, buttercup, butternut, spaghetti)

### *Minor*

Arugula
Beets
Bell peppers
Broccoli
Broccoli rabe
Burdock root
Cabbage
Cauliflower
Celery
Corn, fresh
Cucumber
Dandelion greens
Endive
Gourd squash
Jicama
Kale
Karela
Kohlrabi
Lambsquarter
Lettuce
Lotus root
Onion, cooked
Papaya, green
Peas
Plantain
Potatoes, white
Radicchio
Radishes, cooked
Shiitake mushrooms
Spinach
Sprouts
Watercress

### *Regressive*

Brussels sprouts
Eggplant
Mushrooms
Onions, raw
Pungent vegetables, in excess
Swiss chard
Taro root
Tomatoes
Turnips
Turnip greens

## FRUITS

***Use mostly sweet fruits with a small amount of sour ones.***

### *Major*

| | | |
|---|---|---|
| Apricot | Grapes | Pineapple, sweet |
| Avocado | Lemons | Plums, sweet |
| Coconut | Limes | Quince, sweet |
| Dates | Mango | Tamarind |
| Figs, fresh | Oranges, sweet | Tangerines, sweet |

### *Minor*

| | | |
|---|---|---|
| Apples | Kiwi | Prunes |
| Bananas | Papaya | Raisins |
| Berries, sweet | Peaches | Soursop |
| Cherries, sweet | Pears | Strawberries |
| Grapefruit, sweet | Pomegranate | Watermelon |

### *Regressive*

| | | |
|---|---|---|
| Cranberries | Persimmon | Sour fruits, in excess |

## GRAINS

***Since most dry goods are available throughout the year, grains are categorized by season for the dual body types.***

***V-P types should avoid a mono-diet of brown rice.***

### *Winter/Spring (December to end of April)*

| *Major* | *Minor* | *Regressive* |
|---|---|---|
| Barley | Brown rice, long-grain or sweet | Amaranth |
| Basmati rice, brown or white | Quinoa | Buckwheat |
| Oats, whole cooked | Wild rice | Corn |
| Wheat | | Millet |
| | | Oat bran |
| | | Rye |

### *Spring/Summer (May to end of August)*

| *Major* | *Minor* | *Regressive* |
|---|---|---|
| Barley | Brown rice, all grains or sweet | Amaranth |
| Basmati rice, brown or white | Wild rice | Buckwheat |
| Oats, whole cooked | | Corn |
| Wheat | | Millet |
| | | Quinoa |
| | | Rye |

*Fall (September to end of November)*

| *Major* | *Minor* | *Regressive* |
|---|---|---|
| Brown rice, medium- or short-grain or sweet | Barley | Amaranth |
| Oats, whole cooked | Basmati rice, brown or white | Buckwheat |
| Wheat | Brown rice, long-grain | Corn |
| | Quinoa | Millet |
| | | Rye |

## PROCESSED GRAINS (ALL YEAR)

*Major*

Bulgur
Couscous
Mochi (pounded sweet rice)
Oats, rolled or steel-cut, cooked
Pasta, whole wheat
Rice flour
Udon noodles
Unbleached white flour
Whole wheat flour

## LEGUMES, BEANS, PEAS, AND SOYBEAN DERIVATIVES

*Major*

Aduki beans
Mung dhal, split or whole
Urad dhal

*Minor*

Black beans
Chickpeas, black or yellow
Kidney beans
Lentils, brown or red
Muth beans
Soybeans
Tempeh
Tofu
Toor dhal

*Regressive*

Black-eyed peas
Lima beans
Navy beans
Pinto beans
Split peas, green or yellow
White beans

## NUTS AND SEEDS

*Minor*

Coconut
Pumpkin seeds, roasted
Sesame seeds, white
Sunflower seeds, roasted

*Regressive*

All nuts. Small amounts of almonds, cashews, pecans, pistachios, poppy seeds, and walnuts are permitted in the fall (September to end of November).

## DAIRY

*Major*

Butter, unsalted
Cottage cheese
Cow's milk, certified raw
Goat's milk
Ghee
Yogurt

### *Minor*

| | | |
|---|---|---|
| Butter, salted | Buttermilk | Cheeses, mild and salted |
| | | Sour cream |

### *Regressive*

| | | |
|---|---|---|
| Dairy products, commercial or powdered | Ice cream, homemade | |

## OILS

### *Major*

| | | |
|---|---|---|
| Canola | Safflower | Sunflower |
| Coconut | Sesame, dark or light | |

### *Minor*

| | | |
|---|---|---|
| Almond | Corn | Soy |
| Avocado | Olive | Walnut |

### *Regressive*

| | | |
|---|---|---|
| Animal oils or lard | Corn | Vegetable, mixed |

## SWEETENERS

### *Major*

| | | |
|---|---|---|
| Amasake (rice milk) | Dates | Sucanat |
| Barley malt | Fruit juice concentrates | Sugarcane juice |
| Brown rice syrup | Maple syrup | Sweet fruits |
| Brown sugar, unrefined | | |

### *Minor*

| | | |
|---|---|---|
| Fructose | Honey, raw and uncooked | |

### *Regressive*

| | | |
|---|---|---|
| Honey, cooked | Sugar substitutes (saccharin, Sweet 'n Low, NutraSweet) | White sugar |
| Molasses | | |

## HERBS, SPICES, AND FLAVORINGS

### *Major*

| | | |
|---|---|---|
| Basil, fresh | Dill | Saffron |
| Black cumin | Fennel | Sandalwood chips |
| Black pepper | Garam masala | Spearmint |
| Caraway | Kudzu | Tamarind |
| Cardamom | Mint | Turmeric |
| Coriander | Orange peel | Vanilla |
| Cumin | Peppermint | Wintergreen |

### *Minor*

Ajwan
Almond extract
Bay leaf
Cayenne
Chili peppers, mild
Cinnamon
Cloves
Curry powder, mild
Dill leaves or seed
Garlic, cooked
Ginger, dried or fresh
Licorice
Mango powder
Mustard seeds
Neem leaves
Nutmeg
Onions, dried
Orange extract
Oregano
Paprika
Parsley
Rosemary
Sage
Savory
Tarragon
Thyme

### *Regressive*

Asafoetida
Chili peppers, hot
Fenugreek
Garlic, raw
Mace
Marjoram
Onions, raw

## CONDIMENTS

### *Minor*

Cilantro
Coconut, roasted
Coconut milk
Daikon, grated
Gomasio
Horseradish
Lemon juice
Lime juice
Mayonnaise, noncommercial
Olives
Pickles, ginger or lime
Pumpkin seeds
Rock salt
Rose water
Sea salt
Sesame seeds, white
Sunflower seeds
Tamari
Vinegar, brown rice or herbal
Wasabi
Yogurt, spiced

### *Regressive*

Ketchup
Mayonnaise, commercial
Miso
Mustard, commercial
Preservatives and additives, chemical
Salt, iodized
Vinegar, commercial

## SEAWEEDS

***Seaweeds should be used mostly in the fall (September to end of November). Soak and rinse thoroughly before use.***

### *Minor*

Arame
Dulse
Hijiki
Kelp
Kombu
Seaware
Wakame

## BREWS AND BEVERAGES

***Fruit juices may be diluted with water or milk for V-P types.***

### *Major*

Apricot juice
Chicory blends
Coconut milk
Cow's milk or drinks, sweet
Date and fig shakes
Lassi (sweet yogurt drink)
Sweet fruit juices (berry, cherry, grape, mango, peach, pomegranate, sweet orange, pineapple)

### *Minor*

Aloe vera juice or drink
Apple juice
Carob drinks
Carrot juice
Cow's milk or drinks, hot spiced
Grapefruit juice
Mildly salted or sour brews
Mixed vegetable juice
Papaya juice
Pear juice
Prune juice

### *Regressive*

Alcohol
Caffeinated drinks
Carbonated drinks
Chocolate drinks
Pungent beverages
Tomato juice

## TEAS

*Do not use chamomile if you are allergic to ragweed.*

### *Major*

Bancha (twig)
Cardamom
Chamomile
Elder flower
Fennel
Hops
Lavender
Lemon balm
Lemon grass
Peppermint
Rose flowers
Rosehips
Spearmint

### *Minor*

Ajwan
Barley (grain tea)
Blackberry
Borage
Chrysanthemum
Cinnamon
Cloves
Comfrey
Eucalyptus
Ginger
Hibiscus
Jasmine
Mexican bark
Passionflower
Red clover
Strawberry

# VATA-KAPHA

## VEGETABLES

***Use fresh and seasonal vegetables. Vegetables with seeds should be well cooked with the appropriate Vata spices to minimize aggravation of V-K types.***

### *Major*

Artichokes
Asparagus
Beets
Green beans
Landcress
Lotus root
Mustard greens
Okra
Onion, cooked
Parsnips
Radishes, cooked
Summer squash (yellow crookneck)
Winter squash (acorn, buttercup, butternut, spaghetti)
Watercress

### *Minor*

Arugula
Bamboo shoots
Bell peppers
Bok choy
Broccoli
Broccoli rabe
Burdock root
Cabbage
Carrots
Cassava
Cauliflower
Celery
Corn, fresh
Cucumber, seedless
Daikon
Eggplant
Endive
Escarole
Gourd squash
Jerusalem artichokes
Jicama
Kale
Karela, well cooked
Kohlrabi
Lambsquarter
Mushrooms
Papaya, green
Parsnips
Peas
Peppers
Plantain
Pokeroot
Potatoes, white
Pumpkin
Radicchio
Shiitake mushrooms
Snow peas
Spinach
Sprouts
Sweet potatoes
Turnip greens
Zucchini

### *Regressive*

Brussels sprouts
Onions, raw
Swiss chard
Taro root
Tomatoes
Turnips
Vegetables, raw

## FRUITS

***Use fresh and seasonal fruits.***

***Major***

| | | |
|---|---|---|
| Apricots | Lemon | Peaches |
| Berries | Lime | Raisins, moist |
| Cherries | Mango | Rhubarb |
| Coconut | Melon | Strawberries |
| Dates | Papaya | Tamarind |
| Figs, fresh | | |

***Minor***

| | | |
|---|---|---|
| Apples | Kiwi | Pineapple |
| Avocado | Oranges | Plums |
| Bananas | Pears | Pomegranate |
| Dried fruits | Persimmon | Soursop |
| Grapes | | |

***Regressive***

| | | |
|---|---|---|
| Cranberries | Prunes | Quince |
| Dried, sour, or sweet fruits, in excess | | |

## GRAINS

***Since most dry goods are available throughout the year, grains are categorized by season for the dual body types.***

***V-K types should avoid a mono-diet of brown rice.***

***Winter/Spring (December to end of April)***

| ***Major*** | ***Minor*** | ***Regressive*** |
|---|---|---|
| Barley | Amaranth | Buckwheat |
| Millet | Basmati rice, brown or white | Oats, whole cooked |
| Quinoa | Brown rice, long- or short-grain | Wheat |
| | Rye | |

***Spring/Summer (May to end of August)***

| ***Major*** | ***Minor*** | ***Regressive*** |
|---|---|---|
| Brown rice, long-grain | Barley | Amaranth |
| Wheat | Brown rice, short- or medium-grain | Buckwheat |
| | Millet | Corn |
| | Oats, whole cooked | Quinoa |
| | Wild rice | Rye |

### *Fall (September to end of November)*

| *Major* | *Minor* | *Regressive* |
|---|---|---|
| Basmati rice, brown | Basmati rice, white | Amaranth |
| Brown rice, long-grain | Brown rice, medium-grain | Buckwheat |
| Oats, whole cooked | Millet | Corn |
| | Quinoa | Rye |
| | Wheat | |
| | Wild rice | |

## PROCESSED GRAINS (ALL YEAR)

### *Minor*

| | | |
|---|---|---|
| Bulgur | Oats, steel-cut | Udon noodles |
| Couscous | Pasta, whole wheat | Unbleached white flour |
| Mochi (pounded sweet rice) | Rice flour | Whole wheat flour |

### *Regressive*

| | | |
|---|---|---|
| Cereals, commercial or dried | Corn meal | Rye flakes |
| Corn grits | Oat bran | Wheat bran |
| | Oats, rolled | |

## LEGUMES, BEANS, PEAS, AND SOYBEAN DERIVATIVES

### *Major*

| | | |
|---|---|---|
| Aduki beans | Mung dhal, split or whole | Toor dhal |
| Lentils, brown or red | | |

### *Minor*

| | | |
|---|---|---|
| Black beans | Muth beans | Urad dhal |
| Chickpeas, black or yellow | Tofu | |

### *Regressive*

| | | |
|---|---|---|
| Black-eyed peas | Pinto beans | Split peas |
| Kidney beans | Soybeans | Tempeh |
| Lima beans | Soy by-products, except tofu | White beans |
| Navy beans | | |

## NUTS AND SEEDS

### *Minor*

| | | |
|---|---|---|
| Coconut | Pumpkin seeds, roasted | Sunflower seeds, roasted |
| Poppy seeds | Sesame seeds, roasted | |

### *Regressive*

All nuts. Small amounts of almonds, cashews, pecans, pistachios, and walnuts are permitted in the fall (September to end of November).

## DAIRY

### *Major*

Cottage cheese
Ghee
Goat's milk

### *Minor*

Butter, unsalted
Cow's milk, certified raw
Yogurt

### *Regressive*

***Small amounts of cheeses and sour cream may be used in the fall (September to end of November).***

Buttermilk
Butter, salted
Cheeses, salted
Dairy products, commercial or powdered
Ice cream, homemade
Sour cream

## OILS

### *Major*

Canola
Sunflower

### *Minor*

Almond
Apricot
Avocado
Coconut
Corn
Mustard
Olive
Safflower
Sesame, dark or light
Soy
Walnut

### *Regressive*

Animal oils or lard
Vegetable, mixed

## SWEETENERS

### *Major*

Amasake (rice milk)
Dates
Fruit juice, mixed
Honey, raw and uncooked
Sweet fruits

### *Minor*

Barley malt
Brown rice syrup
Brown sugar, unrefined
Fruit juice concentrates
Maple syrup
Sucanat
Sugarcane juice

### *Regressive*

Fructose
Honey, cooked
Molasses
Sugar substitutes (saccharin, Sweet 'n Low, NutraSweet)
White sugar

## HERBS, SPICES, AND FLAVORINGS

### *Major*

Allspice
Anise
Asafoetida
Basil
Bay leaf
Black cumin
Black pepper
Caraway
Cardamom
Cinnamon
Cloves
Coriander
Cumin
Curry powder
Dill leaves
Eucalyptus
Fennel
Garam masala
Garlic, cooked
Ginger, dried
Mace
Marjoram
Mint
Mustard seeds
Nutmeg
Onion, dried
Orange peel
Oregano
Paprika
Parsley
Peppermint
Poppy seeds
Rosemary
Saffron
Sage
Savory
Spearmint
Star anise
Tamarind
Tarragon
Thyme
Turmeric
Vanilla

### *Minor*

Almond extract
Cayenne
Dill seed
Fenugreek
Ginger, fresh
Horseradish
Kudzu
Mango powder
Mugwort
Neem leaves
Orange extract

### *Regressive*

Garlic, raw

## CONDIMENTS

### *Minor*

Cilantro
Chutney, coconut or sweet mango
Daikon, grated
Gomasio, mild
Horseradish
Lemon juice
Mayonnaise, noncommercial
Mint leaves
Mustard, noncommercial
Olives, black
Pickles, cucumber or ginger or lime or mango
Rose water
Rock salt
Sea salt
Sprouts
Vinegar, brown rice or herbal or umeboshi
Wasabi
Yogurt, spiced

### *Regressive*

Mayonnaise, commercial
Miso
Mustard, commercial
Preservatives and additives, chemical
Salt, iodized
Vinegar, commercial

## SEAWEEDS

***Use moderately during the fall (September to end of November). Soak and rinse seaweeds thoroughly before use.***

### *Minor*

Agar-agar
Arame
Blue-green algae
Dulse
Hijiki
Kelp
Kombu
Riverweeds
Seaware
Wakame

## BREWS AND BEVERAGES

### *Major*

Apricot juice
Berry juice
Carrot juice
Carrot-ginger drink
Cherry juice
Chicory blends
Grape juice
Mango juice, unsweetened
Peach juice
Soy milk, warm spiced

### *Minor*

Apple juice
Banana drink
Carrot-vegetable juice
Coffee
Mildly salted or sour brews
Orange juice
Pear juice
Pineapple juice
Pungent brews

### *Regressive*

Alcohol
Aloe vera juice or drinks
Caffeinated teas
Carbonated drinks
Chocolate drinks
Cold drinks
Fruit juices, sweetened
Goat's milk, warm spiced
Pomegranate juice
Tomato juice

## TEAS

*Do not use chamomile if you are allergic to ragweed.*

### *Major*

Bancha (twig)
Basil
Chamomile
Chicory
Cinnamon
Cloves
Elder flowers
Eucalyptus
Fennel
Ginger, dried
Lavender
Lemon balm
Lemon grass
Lotus
Mexican bark tea
Orange peel
Osha
Peppermint
Raspberry
Rose flowers
Saffron
Sage

### *Minor*

Ajwan
Alfalfa
Barley (grain tea)
Chrysanthemum
Comfrey
Dandelion
Ginger, fresh
Ginseng
Hibiscus
Hops
Hyssop
Jasmine
Licorice
Nettle
Pennyroyal
Red clover
Sarsaparilla
Spearmint
Violet

# PITTA

## VEGETABLES

### *Major*

Artichokes
Arugula
Asparagus
Bell pepper
Broccoli
Brussels sprouts
Cabbage
Cauliflower
Collards
Cucumber
Dandelion greens
Endive
Green beans
Jerusalem artichoke
Jicama
Kale
Karela
Lambsquarter
Landcress
Lettuce
Mushrooms
Okra
Parsnips
Peas
Potatoes, white
Radicchio
Sprouts
Winter squash (acorn, buttercup, butternut, spaghetti)
Watercress

### *Minor*

Bamboo shoots
Burdock root
Carrots
Carrot tops
Cassava
Celery
Corn, fresh
Daikon radish
Escarole
Kohlrabi
Leeks, cooked
Mustard greens
Parsley
Plantain
Pokeroot
Pumpkin
Rutabaga
Spinach
Turnip greens

### *Regressive*

Beets
Beet greens
Eggplant
Horseradish
Hot chili peppers
Onion, raw
Radishes
Swiss chard
Taro root
Tomatoes
Turnips

## FRUITS

### *Major*

Apples
Apricots
Berries
Coconut
Dates
Figs, fresh
Grapes
Mango
Melons
Oranges, sweet
Pears
Pineapple
Plums
Pomegranate
Raisins
Watermelon

### *Minor*

Avocado
Dried fruits, sweet
Kiwi
Lemons
Limes
Quince, sweet
Strawberries, sweet
Tamarind

### *Regressive*

Bananas
Berries, sour
Grapefruit
Papaya
Peaches
Persimmon
Rhubarb
Soursop

## GRAINS (ALL YEAR)

### *Major*

Barley
Basmati rice, brown or white
Brown rice, sweet
Oats, whole
Wheat

### *Minor*

Sushi rice, white
Brown rice, long- or medium-grain

### *Regressive*

Amaranth
Buckwheat
Corn
Millet
Quinoa
Rice, in excess
Rye

## PROCESSED GRAINS (ALL YEAR)

### *Minor*

Barley flour
Bulgur
Cereals, barley or wheat
Couscous
Mochi (pounded sweet rice)
Oats, rolled or steel-cut
Pasta, whole wheat
Udon noodles
Unbleached white flour
Wheat bran
Whole wheat flour

## LEGUMES, BEANS, PEAS, AND SOYBEAN DERIVATIVES

### *Major*

Aduki beans
Black beans
Black-eyed peas
Chickpeas, black or yellow
Lentils, brown
Lima beans
Mung dhal, split or whole
Muth beans
Navy beans
Pinto beans
Soybeans
Split peas, green or yellow

### *Minor*

Tempeh
Tofu, cooked
Urad dhal

### *Regressive*

Lentils, red
Toor dhal

## NUTS AND SEEDS

### *Minor*

Coconut
Poppy seeds
Pumpkin seeds, roasted
Sunflower seeds, roasted
Water chestnuts, cooked

### *Regressive*

All nuts
Sesame seeds, black or white

## DAIRY

### *Major*

Butter, unsalted
Cottage cheese
Cow's milk, certified raw

### *Minor*

Cheeses, mild or soft
Goat's milk
Ice cream, homemade
Yogurt, sweetened

### *Regressive*

| | | |
|---|---|---|
| Buttermilk | Dairy products, commercial or powdered | Goat's cheese |
| Cheeses, hard | | Sour cream |

## OILS

### *Major*

| | | |
|---|---|---|
| Canola | Soy | Sunflower |
| Coconut | | |

### *Minor*

| | | |
|---|---|---|
| Avocado | Safflower | Walnut |
| Olive | | |

### *Regressive*

| | | |
|---|---|---|
| Almond | Corn | Sesame, dark |
| Animal fats or lard | Mustard | Vegetable, mixed |
| Apricot | | |

## SWEETENERS

### *Major*

| | | |
|---|---|---|
| Barley malt | Fruit juice concentrates (apple, pear, mango, fig, apricot, grape) | Sucanat |
| Brown sugar, unrefined | Maple syrup | Sugarcane juice |
| Dates | | Sweet fruits |
| Fructose | | |

### *Minor*

| | |
|---|---|
| Amasake (rice milk) | Brown rice syrup |

### *Regressive*

| | | |
|---|---|---|
| Honey | Sugar substitutes (saccharin, Sweet 'n Low, NutraSweet) | White sugar |
| Molasses | | |

## HERBS, SPICES, AND FLAVORINGS

### *Major*

| | | |
|---|---|---|
| Black cumin | Dill leaves | Saffron |
| Cilantro | Fennel | Spearmint |
| Coriander | Kudzu | Turmeric |
| Cumin | Mint | Wintergreen |
| Curry leaves | Peppermint | |

### *Minor*

| | | |
|---|---|---|
| Almond extract | Cloves | Nutmeg |
| Basil, fresh | Curry powder | Orange peel |
| Black pepper | Dill seed | Parsley |
| Caraway | Garam masala | Tamarind |
| Cardamom | Ginger | Vanilla |
| Cinnamon | Mace | |

### *Regressive*

| | | |
|---|---|---|
| Ajwan | Fenugreek | Oregano |
| Allspice | Garlic | Paprika |
| Anise | Horseradish | Pippali |
| Asafoetida | Mango powder | Rosemary |
| Basil | Marjoram | Sage |
| Bay leaf | Mustard seeds | Thyme |
| Cayenne | Onion, raw | |

## CONDIMENTS

### *Major*

| | | |
|---|---|---|
| Chutney, coconut or mango | Coconut milk | Mint leaves |
| Cilantro | Daikon, grated | Rose water |
| Coconut, grated or roasted | | |

### *Minor*

| | | |
|---|---|---|
| Black pepper | Orange peel | Tamari |
| Gomasio, mild | Pickle, sweet ginger | Vinegar, brown rice or mild herbal |
| Mirin | Rock salt | Yogurt, sweetened or spiced |
| Olives, black | Sea salt | |

### *Regressive*

| | | |
|---|---|---|
| Chili peppers, hot | Miso | Pickles, sour |
| Garlic | Mustard, commercial | Salt, iodized |
| Gomasio | Preservatives and additives, chemical | Soy sauce |
| Ketchup | | |
| Mayonnaise, commercial | | |

## SEAWEEDS

*Use seaweeds sparingly. Soak and rinse thoroughly before use.*

### *Minor*

| | | |
|---|---|---|
| Agar-agar | Hijiki | Riverweeds |
| Arame | Kelp | Seaware |
| Dulse | Kombu | Wakame |

## BREWS AND BEVERAGES

### *Major*

Aloe vera juice or drinks
Amasake (rice milk)
Apple juice
Apricot juice
Berry juice, sweet
Carob drinks
Coconut milk
Coconut shakes
Cow's milk or drinks, cool
Date shake
Grape juice
Mango juice
Peach juice
Pear juice

### *Minor*

Almond milk
Carrot-vegetable juice
Chicory blends
Orange juice
Lassi (sweet yogurt drink)
Soy milk, spiced

### *Regressive*

Alcohol
Banana shake
Caffeinated drinks
Carbonated drinks
Chocolate drinks
Cranberry juice
Frozen drinks
Grapefruit juice
Papaya juice
Salted drinks
Sour fruit juice
Tomato juice

## TEAS

***Do not use chamomile if you are allergic to ragweed.***

### *Major*

Bancha (twig)
Barley (grain tea)
Birch
Blackberry
Catnip
Chamomile
Chicory
Chrysanthemum
Comfrey
Dandelion
Elder flowers
Fennel
Hops
Jasmine
Lavender
Lemon balm
Lotus
Marshmallow
Passionflower
Peppermint
Raspberry leaves
Rose flower
Saffron
Spearmint
Violet
Wild cherry bark
Wintergreen

### *Minor*

Alfalfa
Borage
Burdock
Cardamom
Cinnamon
Grain tea
Hibiscus
Rosehips
Strawberry

### *Regressive*

Ajwan
Cloves
Corn silk
Eucalyptus
Ginger, dried or fresh
Ginseng
Hawthorne
Hyssop
Mormon tea
Osha
Pennyroyal
Sage
Sassafras

# PITTA-VATA

## VEGETABLES

***Use mostly cooked vegetables. Use bitter vegetables in small amounts.***

### *Major*

Artichoke
Arugula
Asparagus
Bell peppers
Bok choy
Broccoli
Broccoli rabe
Carrot
Celery
Collards
Cucumber, seedless
Dandelion greens
Endive
Green beans
Jerusalem artichoke
Karela
Landcress
Lettuce
Mustard greens
Okra
Parsnips
Pumpkin
Radicchio
Rutabaga
Sprouts
Winter squash (acorn, butternut, buttercup, spaghetti)
Summer squash (yellow crookneck, zucchini)
Sweet potatoes
Watercress

### *Minor*

Beets
Burdock root
Cabbage
Cauliflower
Corn, fresh
Dandelion greens
Gourd squash
Jicama
Kale
Mushrooms
Onion, cooked
Papaya, green
Peas
Plantain
Potatoes, white
Radishes, cooked
Spinach

### *Regressive*

Brussels sprouts
Eggplant
Onion, raw
Pungent vegetables, in excess
Swiss chard
Tomatoes
Turnips
Turnip greens

## FRUITS

***Use mostly sweet fruits with a small amount of sour ones.***

### *Major*

Apricot
Coconut
Dates
Figs, fresh
Grapes, dark
Lemons
Limes
Mango
Oranges, sweet
Pears
Pineapple, sweet
Plums, sweet
Pomegranate
Prunes
Quince, sweet
Raisins
Tangerines, sweet

### *Minor*

| | | |
|---|---|---|
| Apples, sweet | Cherries, sweet | Papaya |
| Avocado | Dried fruits | Peaches |
| Bananas | Grapefruit, sweet | Strawberries |
| Berries, sweet | Kiwi | Tamarind |

### *Regressive*

| | | |
|---|---|---|
| Cranberries | Rhubarb | Sour fruits, in excess |
| Persimmon | Soursop | Watermelon |

## GRAINS

***Since most dry goods are available throughout the year, grains are categorized by season for the dual types.***

### *Winter/Spring (December to end of April)*

| *Major* | *Minor* | *Regressive* |
|---|---|---|
| Barley | Brown rice, long-grain or sweet | Amaranth |
| Basmati rice, brown or white | Quinoa | Buckwheat |
| Oats, whole cooked | Wild rice | Corn |
| Wheat | | Millet |
| | | Oat bran |
| | | Rye |

### *Spring/Summer (May to end of August)*

| *Major* | *Minor* | *Regressive* |
|---|---|---|
| Barley | Brown rice, long-grain or sweet | Amaranth |
| Basmati rice, brown or white | Wild rice | Brown rice, medium- or short-grain or sweet |
| Oats, whole cooked | | Buckwheat |
| Wheat | | Corn |
| | | Millet |
| | | Quinoa |
| | | Rye |

### *Fall (September to end of November)*

| *Major* | *Minor* | *Regressive* |
|---|---|---|
| Basmati rice, brown | Barley | Amaranth |
| Brown rice, long-grain or sweet | Basmati rice, white | Buckwheat |
| Oats, whole cooked | Brown rice, medium- or short-grain | Corn |
| Wheat | Quinoa | Millet |
| | | Rye |

## PROCESSED GRAINS (ALL YEAR)

### *Minor*

Barley cereals
Barley flour
Bulgur
Couscous
Oats, rolled or steel-cut, cooked
Rice cereals
Rice flour
Udon noodles
Pasta, whole wheat
Whole wheat flour

## LEGUMES, BEANS, SEEDS, AND SOYBEAN DERIVATIVES

### *Major*

Aduki beans
Mung dhal, split or whole
Urad dhal

### *Minor*

Black beans
Black chickpeas
Chick peas
Kidney beans
Lentils, brown or red
Muth beans
Soybeans
Tempeh
Tofu

### *Regressive*

Black-eyed peas
Lima beans
Navy beans
Pinto beans
Split peas, green or yellow
Toor dhal
White beans

## NUTS AND SEEDS

### *Minor*

Coconut
Poppy seeds
Pumpkin seeds, roasted
Sunflower seeds, roasted
Water chestnuts, cooked

### *Regressive*

All nuts may be used occasionally for cooking

## DAIRY

***Dairy products should not be taken with salted or sour foods, or with animal foods.***

### *Major*

Butter, unsalted
Cottage cheese
Cow's milk, certified raw
Ghee
Yogurt

### *Minor*

Butter, salted
Cheeses, mild
Ice cream, homemade

### *Regressive*

Buttermilk
Cheeses, salted
Goat's milk
Dairy products, commercial or powdered
Sour cream

## OILS

### *Major*

Canola
Coconut
Safflower
Soy
Sunflower

### *Minor*

Almond
Avocado
Sesame, light
Olive, sparingly

### *Regressive*

Animal oils or lard
Corn
Mustard
Vegetable oil, mixed

## SWEETENERS

### *Major*

Amasake (rice milk)
Barley malt
Brown rice syrup
Brown sugar, unrefined
Dates
Fruit juice concentrates
Maple syrup
Sucanat
Sugarcane juice
Sweet fruits

### *Minor*

Fructose
Honey, raw and uncooked

### *Regressive*

Honey, cooked
Molasses
Sugar substitutes (saccharin, Sweet 'n Low, Nutrasweet)
White sugar

## HERBS, SPICES, AND FLAVORINGS

### *Major*

Basil, fresh
Black cumin
Black pepper
Caraway
Cardamom
Coriander
Cumin
Dill leaves
Fennel
Garam masala
Kudzu
Mint
Orange peel
Peppermint
Saffron
Spearmint
Tarragon
Turmeric
Vanilla
Wintergreen

### *Minor*

Ajwan
Almond extract
Bay leaf
Cayenne
Cinnamon
Cloves
Curry powder, mild
Dill seed
Garlic, cooked
Ginger
Licorice
Mango powder
Mustard seeds
Neem leaves
Nutmeg
Onion, dried
Orange extract
Oregano
Paprika
Parsley
Rosemary
Sage
Savory
Tamarind
Thyme

### *Regressive*

Asafoetida
Chili peppers, hot
Fenugreek
Garlic, raw
Mace
Marjoram
Onion, raw

## CONDIMENTS

### *Minor*

Cilantro
Coconut milk
Coconut, roasted
Daikon, grated
Gomasio, mild
Horseradish
Lemon juice
Lime juice
Mayonnaise, noncommercial
Olives, black
Pickles, ginger or lime
Rock salt
Rose water
Sea salt
Tamari
Vinegars, brown rice or herbal
Wasabi
Yogurt, spiced

### *Regressive*

Ketchup
Mayonnaise, commercial
Mustard, commercial
Preservatives and additives, chemical
Salt, iodized
Vinegar, commercial

## SEAWEEDS

*Use mostly in fall (September to end of November).*
*Soak and rinse seaweeds thoroughly before use.*

### *Minor*

Agar-agar
Arame
Blue-green algae
Dulse
Hijiki
Kelp
Kombu
Riverweeds
Seaware
Wakame

## BREWS AND BEVERAGES

### *Major*

Apricot juice
Berry juice, sweet
Coconut milk
Cow's milk or drinks, sweet
Date and fig shakes
Fruit juices, sweet (cherry, grape, mango, peach, pomegranate, sweet orange, prune)
Lassi (sweet yogurt drink)

### *Minor*

Aloe vera juice or drinks
Apple juice
Chicory blends
Carob drinks
Carrot juice
Cow's milk or drinks, hot spiced
Grapefruit juice
Mildly salted or sour brews
Mixed vegetable juice
Papaya juice
Pear juice

### *Regressive*

Alcohol
Caffeinated drinks
Carbonated drinks
Chocolate drinks
Pungent beverages
Tomato juice

## TEAS

***Do not use chamomile if you are allergic to ragweed.***

### *Major*

Bancha (twig)
Birch
Cardamom
Chamomile
Elder flowers
Fennel
Hops
Lavender
Lemon balm
Lemon grass
Peppermint
Raspberry leaves
Rose flowers
Spearmint
Wild cherry bark

### *Minor*

Ajwan
Barley
Blackberry
Borage
Burdock
Chrysanthemum
Cinnamon
Cloves
Comfrey
Eucalyptus
Ginger
Hibiscus
Jasmine
Mexican bark tea
Passionflower
Red clover
Strawberry

# PITTA-KAPHA

## VEGETABLES

*Use fresh and seasonal vegetables.*

### *Major*

Artichokes
Arugula
Asparagus
Bell peppers
Broccoli
Broccoli rabe
Burdock root
Cabbage
Carrot tops
Cauliflower
Celery
Collards
Corn, fresh
Dandelion
Endive
Green beans
Jerusalem artichoke
Jicama
Kale
Karela
Lambsquarter
Landcress
Leeks, cooked
Lettuce
Lotus root
Mushrooms
Mustard greens
Okra
Onion, cooked
Parsley
Parsnips
Plantain
Potatoes, white
Pumpkin
Sprouts
Summer squash (yellow crookneck)
Turnip greens
Winter squash (acorn, buttercup, butternut, spaghetti)

### *Minor*

Bamboo shoots
Brussels sprouts
Carrots
Cassava
Chili peppers, mild
Cucumber
Daikon
Eggplant
Escarole
Kohlrabi
Pokeroot
Rutabaga
Spinach
Sweet potatoes
Watercress
Zucchini

### *Regressive*

Beets
Beet greens
Chili peppers, hot
Horseradish
Onion, raw
Radishes, raw
Taro root
Tomatoes

## FRUITS

*Use seasonal fruits.*

### *Major*

Apples
Apricots
Berries
Cherries
Coconut
Dried fruits
Mango
Pears
Pomegranate
Prunes
Quince
Raisins
Strawberries
Watermelon

### *Minor*

| | | |
|---|---|---|
| Avocado | Lemons | Peaches |
| Dates | Limes | Persimmon |
| Figs, fresh | Melons | Pineapple |
| Grapes | Oranges | Plums |
| Kiwi | Papaya | Tamarind |

### *Regressive*

| | | |
|---|---|---|
| Bananas | Rhubarb | Sour fruits, in excess |
| Cranberries | Soursop | Sweet fruits, in excess |
| Grapefruit | | |

## GRAINS

***Since most dry goods are available throughout the year, grains are categorized by season for the dual types.***

### *Winter/Spring (December to end of April)*

| *Major* | *Minor* | *Regressive* |
|---|---|---|
| Barley | Millet | Amaranth |
| Basmati rice, brown | Quinoa | Brown rice, medium- or short-grain |
| Oats, whole | Wild rice | Buckwheat |
| Wheat | | Corn |
| | | Rye |

### *Spring/Summer (May to end of August)*

| *Major* | *Minor* | *Regressive* |
|---|---|---|
| Barley | Brown rice, medium-grain or sweet | Amaranth |
| Basmati rice, brown or white | Millet | Buckwheat |
| Wheat | Wild rice | Quinoa |
| | | Rye |

### *Fall (September to end of November)*

| *Major* | *Minor* | *Regressive* |
|---|---|---|
| Barley | Brown rice, all grains | Amaranth |
| Basmati rice, brown or white | Millet | Buckwheat |
| Brown rice, sweet | Oats, whole | Corn |
| Wheat | Quinoa | Rye |
| | Wild rice | |

## PROCESSED GRAINS (ALL YEAR)

### *Minor*

Barley cereals
Barley flour
Bulgur
Couscous
Oats, rolled or steel-cut
Pasta, whole wheat
Rice cereals
Udon noodles
Wheat bran
Whole wheat flour

## LEGUMES, BEANS, PEAS, AND SOYBEAN DERIVATIVES

### *Major*

Aduki beans
Black beans
Black-eyed peas
Chickpeas
Lima
Muth beans
Urad dhal
White beans

### *Minor*

Kidney
Lentils, brown
Mung dhal, split or whole
Navy beans
Pinto beans
Soybeans
Tempeh
Tofu
Toor dhal

### *Regressive*

Lentils, brown or red

## NUTS AND SEEDS

### *Minor*

Coconut
Poppy seeds
Pumpkin seeds, roasted
Sesame seeds, roasted
Sunflower seeds, roasted

### *Regressive*

All nuts may be used occasionally in cooking

## DAIRY

### *Major*

Ghee

### *Minor*

Butter, unsalted
Cottage cheese
Cow's milk, certified raw
Goat's milk
Yogurt, mildly spiced

### *Regressive*

Buttermilk
Cheese
Dairy products, commercial or powdered
Ice cream, homemade
Sour cream

## OILS

### *Major*

| | | |
|---|---|---|
| Canola | Soy | Sunflower |

### *Minor*

| | | |
|---|---|---|
| Avocado | Corn | Safflower |
| Coconut | Olive | Walnut |

### *Regressive*

| | | |
|---|---|---|
| Almond | Mustard | Sesame, dark or light |
| Apricot | | |

## SWEETENERS

### *Major*

| | | |
|---|---|---|
| Amasake (rice milk) | Dried sweet fruits (apples, apricots, figs, mango, raisins) | Fruit juice concentrates |

### *Minor*

| | | |
|---|---|---|
| Barley malt | Dates | Sucanat |
| Brown rice syrup | Honey, raw and uncooked | Sugarcane juice |
| Brown sugar, unrefined | Maple syrup | |

### *Regressive*

| | | |
|---|---|---|
| Fructose | Sugar substitutes (saccharin, Sweet 'n Low, and NutraSweet) | White sugar |
| Honey, cooked | | |
| Molasses | | |

## HERBS, SPICES, AND FLAVORINGS

### *Major*

| | | |
|---|---|---|
| Black cumin | Fennel | Peppermint |
| Black pepper | Garam masala | Rose water |
| Coriander | Kudzu | Saffron |
| Cumin | Mint | Spearmint |
| Curry leaves | Orange peel | Turmeric |
| Dill leaves | Parsley | Wintergreen |

### Minor

Allspice
Anise
Basil
Bay leaf
Caraway
Cardamom
Chives
Cinnamon
Cloves
Coltsfoot
Curry powder
Dill seed
Garlic, cooked
Ginger, fresh or dried
Horseradish
Marjoram
Mustard seeds
Nutmeg
Oregano
Paprika
Pippali
Rosemary
Sage
Salsify
Star anise
Tamarind
Tarragon
Thyme
Vanilla

### Regressive

Asafoetida
Fenugreek
Garlic, raw
Mango powder
Onion, raw
Sorrel

## CONDIMENTS

### Major

Black pepper
Chutney, coconut
Cilantro
Coconut, fresh roasted
Coconut milk
Curry leaves
Daikon
Lemon juice
Mint leaves
Mustard
Rose water
Sprouts

### Minor

Chili pepper
Chutney, mango
Daikon, grated
Gomasio, mild
Horseradish
Mustard, noncommercial
Orange peel
Pickles, mild
Rock salt
Sea salt
Vinegar, brown rice or mild herbal
Wasabi
Yogurt, mildly spiced

### Regressive

Garlic, raw
Ketchup
Mayonnaise
Miso
Olives, black or green
Onion, raw
Pickles, strong
Preservatives and additives, chemical
Pungent or salty or sour items, in excess
Salt, iodized
Sesame seeds, black
Soy sauce
Tamari
Yogurt, plain

## SEAWEEDS

***Use seaweeds sparingly and mostly in the fall (September to end of November). Soak and rinse thoroughly before use.***

### *Minor*

Agar-agar
Arame
Blue-green algae
Dulse
Hijiki
Kelp
Kombu
Riverweeds
Seaware
Wakame

## BREWS AND BEVERAGES

### *Minor*

Amasake (rice milk)
Carob drinks
Carrot juice
Carrot-ginger juice
Chicory blends
Coconut milk
Cow's milk, spiced, in small amounts
Goat's milk, warm spiced
Lassi (sweet yogurt drink)
Mixed vegetable juice
Soy milk, warm spiced
Yogurt drink, mildly spiced

### *Regressive*

Alcohol
Caffeinated drinks
Carbonated drinks
Chocolate drinks
Fruit juices, sweetened
Ice cold or very hot drinks
Salted drinks, in excess

## TEAS

***Do not use chamomile if you are allergic to ragweed.***

### *Major*

Bancha (twig)
Barley
Birch
Blackberry
Borage
Burdock
Chamomile
Chicory
Chrysanthemum
Dandelion
Elder flowers
Fennel
Hibiscus
Hops
Jasmine
Lavender
Lemon balm
Lemon grass
Licorice
Nettle
Passionflower
Peppermint
Raspberry leaves
Red clover
Rose flower
Saffron
Spearmint
Strawberry
Violet
Wintergreen
Wild cherry bark
Yarrow

### *Minor*

Basil
Cardamom
Cinnamon
Cloves
Comfrey
Eucalyptus
Ginger, dried
Lotus
Orange peel
Osha
Sarsaparilla
Yerba maté

**PITTA-KAPHA**

*Regressive*

Ginger, fresh
Ginseng
Rosehips
Sassafras

# KAPHA

## VEGETABLES

*Major*

Arugula
Asparagus
Beets
Bell pepper
Bok choy
Broccoli
Brussels sprouts
Burdock root
Cabbage
Carrots
Carrot tops
Cauliflower
Celery
Chili peppers, hot
Collards
Corn, fresh
Daikon
Eggplant
Endive
Green beans
Jerusalem artichoke
Jicama
Kale
Karela
Landcress
Leeks
Lettuce
Mushrooms
Mustard greens
Okra
Onion
Parsley
Peas
Pokeroot
Spinach
Sprouts
Turnips
Turnip greens
Watercress

*Minor*

Artichoke
Cassava
Gourd squash
Parsnips
Plantain
Summer squash (yellow crookneck or zucchini)

*Regressive*

Beet greens
Cucumber
Pumpkin
Rutabaga
Sweet potatoes
Taro root
Tomatoes
Winter squash (buttercup, butternut, acorn, spaghetti)

## FRUITS

*Use seasonal fruits.*

*Major*

Apples
Apricots
Berries
Cherries
Dried fruits from major category
Figs, dried
Peaches
Pears
Persimmon
Pomegranate
Quince
Raisins

### *Minor*

Grapes
Kiwi
Lemons
Limes
Mango
Oranges
Strawberries
Tangerine
Tamarind

### *Regressive*

Avocado
Bananas
Coconut
Cranberries
Dates
Figs, fresh
Fruits, excessively sweet or sour or watery
Grapefruit
Melons
Papaya
Pineapple
Plums
Rhubarb
Soursop
Watermelon

## GRAINS (ALL YEAR)

### *Major*

Barley
Buckwheat
Corn
Millet
Rye

### *Minor*

Amaranth
Basmati rice, brown or white
Quinoa

### *Regressive*

Brown rice, all grains or sweet
Oats, whole cooked
Rice flour
Wheat
Whole wheat flour

## PROCESSED GRAINS (ALL YEAR)

### *Minor*

Barley cereals
Barley flour
Buckwheat flour
Corn grits
Cornmeal
Millet cereals
Millet flour
Oat bran
Pasta, rye
Rye cereals
Rye flakes
Rye flour
Soba noodles
Udon noodles

## LEGUMES, BEANS, PEAS, AND SOYBEAN DERIVATIVES

### *Major*

Aduki beans
Black beans
Chickpeas, black or yellow
Lentils, red
Lima beans
Muth beans
Navy beans
Pinto beans
Split peas, green or yellow

### *Minor*

Black-eyed peas
Mung dhal, split or whole
Tofu, cooked
Toor dhal
Urad dhal
White beans

### Regressive

Kidney beans
Lentils, brown
Soybeans
Tempeh

## NUTS AND SEEDS

### Minor

Coconut
Poppy seeds
Pumpkin seeds, roasted
Sesame seeds
Sunflower seeds, roasted

### Regressive

All nuts

## DAIRY

*Dairy products are to be used sparingly by K types.*

### Minor

Ghee
Goat's cheese, unsalted
Goat's milk
Yogurt drinks, spiced

### Regressive

Butter
Buttermilk
Cheese
Cow's milk, certified raw
Dairy products, commercial or powdered
Ice cream, homemade
Sour cream
Yogurt

## OILS

### Minor

Canola
Corn
Mustard
Safflower
Sunflower

### Regressive

Almond
Apricot
Avocado
Coconut
Olive
Sesame, dark or light
Soy
Walnut

## SWEETENERS

*Honey is the best sweetener for K types, but all sweets are to be used sparingly.*

### Major

Honey, raw and uncooked

### Minor

Amasake (rice milk)
Barley malt
Brown rice syrup
Dates
Dried fruits
Fruit juice concentrates
Maple syrup

### *Regressive*

Brown sugar, unrefined
Fructose
Honey, cooked
Molasses
Sucanat
Sugarcane juice
Sugar substitutes (saccharin, Sweet 'n Low, and NutraSweet)
White sugar

## HERBS, SPICES, AND FLAVORINGS

### *Major*

Ajwan
Allspice
Anise
Asafoetida
Basil
Bay leaf
Black pepper
Caraway
Cardamom
Cayenne
Cinnamon
Cloves
Coriander
Cumin
Curry leaves
Curry powder
Dill leaves or seeds
Eucalyptus
Ginger, dried
Garlic
Garam masala
Horseradish
Hot peppers
Marjoram
Mustard seeds
Neem leaves
Nutmeg
Onion
Orange peel
Oregano
Paprika
Parsley
Peppermint
Pippali
Rosemary
Saffron
Sage
Spearmint
Star anise
Tarragon
Thyme
Turmeric

### *Minor*

Fennel
Fenugreek
Ginger, fresh
Mace
Mint
Mugwort
Tamarind
Vanilla
Wintergreen

### *Regressive*

Mango powder

## CONDIMENTS

### *Minor*

Black pepper
Chili pepper
Cilantro
Daikon, grated
Endive
Garlic
Horseradish
Kudzu
Lettuce
Lime juice
Mint leaves
Mustard, noncommercial
Rose water
Rock salt
Sea salt
Sprouts
Vinegar, brown rice or herbal
Wasabi
Yogurt, spiced

### *Regressive*

Almond extract
Coconut milk
Cow's milk, certified raw
Gomasio
Miso
Olives, black or green
Salt, iodized
Tamari
Vinegar, commercial
Yogurt

## SEAWEEDS

***All seaweeds are highly salted, so use sparingly. Rinse and cook seaweeds thoroughly before eating.***

### *Minor*

Agar-agar
Arame
Dulse
Hijiki
Kelp
Kombu
Riverweeds
Seaware
Wakame

## BREWS AND BEVERAGES

***Fruit juices should be diluted with water for K types.***

### *Major*

Aloe vera juice or drinks
Amasake
Apple juice
Apricot juice
Berry juice
Carob drinks
Carrot juice
Cherry juice
Coconut milk
Cranberry juice
Mixed vegetable juice
Peach nectar
Pear juice
Pineapple juice
Pomegranate juice
Prune juice
Soy milk

### *Minor*

Alcohol
Almond drink
Almond milk
Caffeinated drinks
Grape juice
Mango juice
Vegetable broth, unsalted
Yogurt drink, spicy

### *Regressive*

***Drink fruit juice in small quantities. Excess fluids, very rich drinks, dairy drinks, alcohol (on a regular basis), and excess caffeine are all regressive for K types.***

Banana shake
Carbonated drinks
Chocolate drinks
Coconut milk
Cold drinks
Fig shake, with dates
Grapefruit juice
Lemonade
Orange juice
Papaya juice
Salted and sour drinks
Tomato juice

## TEAS

***Do not use chamomile if you are allergic to ragweed.***

### *Major*

Ajwan
Alfalfa
Bancha (twig)
Barley
Basil
Chamomile
Chicory blends
Chrysanthemum
Cinnamon
Cloves
Dandelion
Ginger, dried
Elder flowers
Eucalyptus
Hibiscus
Hops
Jasmine
Lavender
Lemon balm
Mormon tea
Nettle
Orange peel
Pennyroyal
Peppermint
Raspberry
Rose flower
Saffron
Sage
Sassafras
Spearmint
Violet

### *Minor*

Borage
Burdock
Fennel
Ginger, fresh
Ginseng
Hyssop
Lotus
Rosehip

### *Regressive*

Comfrey
Licorice
Marshmallow
Pungent teas

# KAPHA-VATA

## VEGETABLES

***Use fresh and seasonal vegetables.***

### *Major*

Arugula
Asparagus
Beets
Beet greens
Bok choy
Broccoli
Broccoli rabe
Brussels sprouts
Burdock root
Cabbage
Carrots
Cauliflower
Celery
Collards
Corn, fresh
Eggplant
Endive
Green beans
Jerusalem artichoke
Jicama
Kale
Karela
Kohlrabi
Landcress
Lettuce
Lotus root
Mustard greens
Okra
Onion, cooked
Parsnips
Pokeroot
Potatoes, white
Radishes, cooked
Rutabaga
Shiitake mushrooms
Spinach
Sprouts
Watercress

### *Minor*

| | | |
|---|---|---|
| Bamboo shoots | Papaya, green | Sweet potatoes |
| Bell peppers | Peas | Turnips |
| Cassava | Plantain | Turnip greens |
| Escarole | Pumpkin | Winter squash (acorn, buttercup, butternut, spaghetti) |
| Gourd squash | Snow peas | |
| Lambsquarter | Summer squash (zucchini) | |
| Mushrooms | | |

### *Regressive*

| | | |
|---|---|---|
| Swiss chard | Taro root | Tomatoes |

## FRUITS

### *Major*

| | | |
|---|---|---|
| Apples | Grapefruit | Pomegranate |
| Apricots | Mango | Quince |
| Berries | Peaches | Raisins |
| Cherries | Pears | Strawberries |
| Cranberries | Persimmon | Tangerine |

### *Minor*

| | | |
|---|---|---|
| Avocado | Kiwi | Papaya |
| Bananas | Lemons | Pineapple |
| Coconut | Limes | Plums |
| Dried fruits | Melons | Tamarind |
| Grapes | Oranges | |

### *Regressive*

| | | |
|---|---|---|
| Dates | Rhubarb | Sweet fruits, in excess |
| Dried fruits, in excess | Sour fruits, in excess | Watermelon |
| Figs | Soursop | |

## GRAINS

***Since most dry goods are available throughout the year, grains are categorized by season for the dual types.***

### *Winter/Spring (December to end of April)*

| *Major* | *Minor* | *Regressive* |
|---|---|---|
| Barley | Amaranth | Brown rice, medium- or short-grain or sweet |
| Buckwheat | Basmati rice, brown or white | Oats, whole cooked |
| Millet | Brown rice, long-grain | Wheat |
| Quinoa | Corn | |
| Rye | | |

### *Spring/Summer (May to end of August)*

| *Major* | *Minor* | *Regressive* |
|---|---|---|
| Amaranth | Basmati rice, brown or white | Brown rice, medium- or short-grain or sweet |
| Barley | Brown rice, long-grain | Oats, whole cooked |
| Buckwheat | Corn | Wheat |
| Millet | Rye | |
| Quinoa | Wild rice | |

### *Fall (September to end of November)*

| *Major* | *Minor* | *Regressive* |
|---|---|---|
| Amaranth | Brown rice, medium- or long-grain or sweet | Brown rice, short |
| Barley | Buckwheat | Oats, whole cooked |
| Basmati rice, brown or white | Corn | Wheat |
| Millet | | |
| Quinoa | | |
| Rye | | |

## PROCESSED GRAINS (ALL YEAR)

### *Minor*

Barley cereals
Barley flour
Corn grits
Cornmeal
Millet cereals
Millet flour
Pasta, whole wheat or rye
Rye flakes
Rye flour
Soba noodles
Udon noodles
Wheat bran
Whole wheat flour

## LEGUMES, BEANS, PEAS, AND SOYBEAN DERIVATIVES

### *Major*

Aduki beans
Black beans
Black-eyed peas
Chickpeas, black or yellow
Lentils, red
Lima beans
Muth beans
Navy beans
Pinto beans
Split peas, green or yellow
Toor dhal
Urad dhal
White beans

### *Minor*

Lentils, brown
Mung dhal, split or whole
Tofu

### *Regressive*

Kidney beans
Soybeans and soy derivatives, except tofu

## NUTS AND SEEDS

*Minor*

Coconut
Pumpkin seeds, roasted
Sesame seeds, roasted
Sunflower seeds, roasted

*Regressive*

All nuts

## DAIRY

*Major*

Goat's milk

*Minor*

Butter, unsalted
Cow's milk, certified raw
Ghee
Yogurt

*Regressive*

*Small amounts of cheeses and sour cream are permitted in fall (September to end of November).*

Butter, salted
Buttermilk
Cheeses, hard or soft
Cottage cheese
Dairy products, commercial or powdered
Ice cream, homemade
Sour cream

## OILS

*Major*

Canola
Corn
Sunflower

*Minor*

Almond
Apricot
Avocado
Mustard
Olive
Safflower
Sesame, dark or light
Walnut

*Regressive*

Animal oils or lard
Coconut
Soy
Vegetable, mixed

## SWEETENERS

*Major*

Dried fruits (apricots, berries, cherries, dates, mangoes, figs, peaches, raisins)
Fruit juice concentrate
Honey, raw and uncooked

### *Minor*

Amasake (rice milk)
Barley malt
Brown rice syrup
Maple syrup

### *Regressive*

Brown sugar, unrefined
Fructose
Molasses
Sucanat
Sugarcane juice
Sugar substitutes (saccharin, Sweet 'n Low, and NutraSweet)
White sugar

## HERBS, SPICES, AND FLAVORINGS

### *Major*

Allspice
Anise
Asafoetida
Basil
Bay leaf
Black cumin
Black pepper
Caraway
Cardamom
Cinnamon
Cloves
Coriander seeds
Cumin
Curry powder
Dill leaves
Eucalyptus
Fenugreek
Garam masala
Garlic, cooked
Ginger, dried or fresh
Mace
Marjoram
Mint
Mustard seeds
Neem leaves
Nutmeg
Onion, dried
Orange peel
Oregano
Paprika
Parsley
Peppermint
Rosemary
Saffron
Sage
Savory
Spearmint
Star anise
Tarragon
Thyme
Turmeric

### *Minor*

Ajwan
Almond extract
Cayenne
Dill seed
Fennel
Garlic, raw
Horseradish
Kudzu
Mango powder
Mugwort
Orange extract
Tamarind
Vanilla

## CONDIMENTS

### *Major*

Black pepper
Chili pepper, hot or mild
Cilantro
Coconut or coconut milk
Daikon, grated
Garlic
Horseradish
Lemon juice
Mint leaves
Mustard, noncommercial
Onion, raw
Orange peel
Pickles, ginger
Rose water
Sprouts
Tamari
Yogurt, spiced

*Minor*

| | | |
|---|---|---|
| Chutney, coconut or sweet mango | Pickles, cucumber or lime or mango | Vinegar, brown rice or herbal or umeboshi |
| Gomasio, mild | Rock salt | Wasabi |
| Mayonnaise, noncommercial | Sea salt | |
| Olives, black | | |

*Regressive*

| | | |
|---|---|---|
| Mayonnaise, commercial | Preservatives and additives, chemical | Salt, iodized |
| Miso | | Vinegar, commercial |
| Mustard, commercial | | |

## SEAWEEDS

***Use sparingly in the fall (September to end of November). Soak and rinse seaweeds thoroughly before use.***

*Minor*

| | | |
|---|---|---|
| Agar-agar | Hijiki | Riverweeds |
| Arame | Kelp | Seaware |
| Dulse | Kombu | Wakame |

## BREWS AND BEVERAGES

***Juices should be diluted with water for K-V types.***

*Major*

| | | |
|---|---|---|
| Aloe vera juice or drinks | Carrot-ginger juice | Mixed vegetable juice |
| Apple juice | Cherry juice | Peach juice |
| Apricot juice | Chicory drinks | Pear juice |
| Berry juice | Goat's milk, warm spiced | Pomegranate juice |
| Carob drinks | Mango juice, unsweetened | Soy milk, warm spiced |
| Carrot juice | | |

*Minor*

| | | |
|---|---|---|
| Almond drink or milk | Coffee | Orange juice |
| Apricot juice | Grape juice | Pineapple juice |
| Banana drink | Mildly salted or sour brews | Pungent brews |

*Regressive*

| | | |
|---|---|---|
| Alcohol | Chocolate drinks | Fruit juices, sweetened |
| Caffeinated teas | Cold drinks | Tomato juice |
| Carbonated drinks | | |

## TEAS

*Do not use chamomile if you are allergic to ragweed.*

*Major*

Ajwan
Alfalfa
Bancha, twig)
Barley
Basil
Chamomile
Chicory
Chrysanthemum
Cinnamon
Clove
Dandelion
Elder flowers
Eucalyptus
Ginger, dried or fresh
Hibiscus
Hops
Hyssop
Jasmine
Lavender
Lemon balm
Lemon grass
Mexican bark tea
Nettle
Orange peel
Osha
Pennyroyal
Peppermint
Raspberry
Red clover
Rose flower
Saffron
Sage
Spearmint
Violet

*Minor*

Comfrey
Ginseng
Licorice
Sarsaparilla

# KAPHA-PITTA

## VEGETABLES

*Use fresh and seasonal vegetables.*

*Major*

Arugula
Asparagus
Beet greens
Bell peppers
Broccoli
Broccoli rabe
Brussels sprouts
Burdock root
Cabbage
Carrots
Carrot tops
Cauliflower
Celery
Collards
Corn, fresh
Daikon
Dandelion
Eggplant
Endive
Green beans
Jerusalem artichoke
Jicama
Karela
Kohlrabi
Landcress
Leeks
Lettuce
Mushrooms
Mustard greens
Okra
Onion, cooked
Parsley
Pokeroot
Potatoes, white
Spinach
Sprouts
Summer squash
(yellow crookneck)
Turnips
Turnip greens
Watercress
Winter squash (spaghetti)

*Minor*

| | | |
|---|---|---|
| Artichokes | Onion, raw | Sweet potatoes |
| Chili peppers, hot | Plantains | Winter squash (acorn, buttercup, butternut) |
| Cucumber | Pumpkin | |
| Horseradish | Rutabaga | Summer squash (zucchini) |

*Regressive*

| | | |
|---|---|---|
| Beets | Radishes | Tomatoes |

## FRUITS

*Use seasonal fruits.*

*Major*

| | | |
|---|---|---|
| Apples | Mango | Pomegranate |
| Apricots | Peaches | Prunes |
| Berries | Pears | Quince |
| Cherries | Persimmon | Raisins |
| Figs, dried | | |

*Minor*

| | | |
|---|---|---|
| Avocado | Kiwi | Pineapple |
| Cranberries | Lemons | Plums |
| Dates | Limes | Strawberries |
| Figs, fresh | Melons | Tamarind |
| Grapes | Oranges | |

*Regressive*

| | | |
|---|---|---|
| Bananas | Papaya | Soursop |
| Grapefruit | Rhubarb | Sweet fruits, in excess |
| Grapes, green | Sour fruits, in excess | Watermelon |

## GRAINS

*Since most dry goods are available throughout the year, grains are categorized by season for the dual types.*

*Winter/Spring (December to end of April)*

| *Major* | *Minor* | *Regressive* |
|---|---|---|
| Barley | Amaranth | Basmati rice, white |
| Basmati rice, brown | Buckwheat | Brown rice, medium- or short-grain |
| Quinoa | Corn | Oats, whole |
| Wild rice | Millet | Wheat |
| | Rye | |

*Spring/Summer (May to end of August)*

| ***Major*** | ***Minor*** | ***Regressive*** |
|---|---|---|
| Barley | Amaranth | Brown rice, medium- or short-grain or sweet |
| Basmati rice, white | Basmati rice, brown | Oats, whole |
| Corn | Buckwheat | |
| Millet | Rye | |
| Quinoa | Wheat | |
| Wild rice | | |

*Fall (September to end of November)*

| ***Major*** | ***Minor*** | ***Regressive*** |
|---|---|---|
| Barley | Amaranth | Brown rice, medium- or short-grain |
| Basmati rice, brown or white | Brown rice, long-grain or sweet | |
| Corn | Buckwheat | |
| Rye | Oats, whole | |
| Millet | Wheat | |
| Quinoa | | |
| Wild rice | | |

## PROCESSED GRAINS, (ALL YEAR)

*Use processed grains sparingly.*

***Minor***

Barley cereals
Barley flour
Cornmeal
Millet cereals
Oat bran
Pasta, whole wheat
Soba noodles
Udon noodles

## LEGUMES, BEANS, PEAS, AND SOYBEAN DERIVATIVES

***Major***

Aduki beans
Black beans
Black-eyed peas
Chickpeas
Lentils, red
Lima
Muth beans
Navy
Pinto
Split peas, yellow or green
Urad dhal
White beans

***Minor***

Mung dhal, split or whole
Tofu, cooked
Toor dhal

***Regressive***

Kidney
Lentils, brown
Soybeans and soy by-products, except cooked tofu

## NUTS AND SEEDS

*Minor*

Coconut
Poppy seeds
Pumpkin seeds, roasted
Sunflower seeds, roasted

*Regressive*

All nuts
Sesame seeds, roasted

## DAIRY

*Major*

Ghee
Goat's milk

*Minor*

Cottage cheese
Yogurt, mildly spiced

*Regressive*

Buttermilk
Cheeses, hard or soft
Cow's milk, certified raw
Dairy products, commercial or powdered
Ice cream, homemade
Sour cream

## OILS

*Major*

Canola
Sunflower

*Minor*

Almond
Corn
Mustard
Safflower
Soy

*Regressive*

Apricot
Avocado
Coconut
Olive
Sesame
Walnut

## SWEETENERS

***Sweeteners are to be used sparingly by K types.***

*Major*

Dried sweet fruits (apples, apricots, figs, mangoes, and raisins)
Fruit juice concentrates
Honey, raw and uncooked

### *Minor*

Amasake (rice milk)
Barley malt
Brown rice syrup
Maple syrup

### *Regressive*

Brown sugar, unrefined
Dates
Fructose
Honey, cooked
Molasses
Sucanat
Sugarcane juice
Sugar substitutes (saccharin, Sweet 'n Low, and NutraSweet)
White sugar

## HERBS, SPICES, AND FLAVORINGS

### *Major*

Allspice
Anise
Bay leaf
Black cumin
Black pepper
Caraway
Cardamom
Cinnamon
Cloves
Coriander
Curry leaves
Curry powder
Cumin
Dill leaves or seed
Garam masala
Garlic, cooked
Horseradish
Mace
Marjoram
Mint
Mustard seeds
Nutmeg
Orange peel
Oregano
Paprika
Parsley
Peppermint
Pippali
Rosemary
Saffron
Sage
Spearmint
Star anise
Tarragon
Thyme
Turmeric
Vanilla
Wintergreen

### *Minor*

Ajwan
Asafoetida
Fennel
Fenugreek
Garlic, raw
Ginger, dried
Kudzu
Savory
Tamarind

### *Regressive*

Mango powder

## CONDIMENTS

### *Major*

Black pepper
Cilantro, fresh
Daikon, fresh
Mint leaves
Orange peel
Rose water
Sprouts

### *Minor*

Chili peppers
Chutney, coconut or mango
Coconut, fresh or roasted
Coconut milk
Gomasio, mild
Lemon juice
Mustard, noncommercial
Pickles, mild
Rock salt
Sea salt
Vinegar, brown rice or mild herbal
Wasabi
Yogurt, mildly spiced

### *Regressive*

Black sesame seeds
Garlic, raw
Ketchup
Mayonnaise
Miso
Olives, black or green
Onions, raw
Pickles, strong
Salt, iodized
Salty condiments, in excess
Sour condiments, in excess
Soy sauce
Tamari
Yogurt, plain

## SEAWEEDS

***Use seaweeds sparingly and mostly in the fall (September to end of November). Rinse and soak thoroughly before use.***

### *Minor*

Agar-agar
Arame
Dulse
Hijiki
Kelp
Kombu
Riverweeds
Seaware
Wakame

## BREWS AND BEVERAGES

***All fruit juices should be diluted with water or milk for K-P types.***

### *Major*

Aloe vera juice/drinks
Apple juice
Apricot juice
Banana drinks
Berry juice
Carob drinks
Carrot juice
Carrot-ginger juice
Cherry juice
Chicory drinks
Cranberry juice
Goat's milk, spiced
Grape juice
Lemonade
Mixed vegetable juice
Orange juice
Papaya juice
Peach nectar
Pear juice
Pineapple juice
Pomegranate juice
Prune juice
Vegetable broth
Yogurt drinks, mildly spiced

### *Minor*

Almond drink or milk
Amasake (rice milk)
Caffeinated drinks
Coconut milk
Lassi (sweet yogurt drink)
Mango juice
Soy milk, warm spiced

### *Regressive*

Alcohol
Carbonated drinks
Chocolate drinks
Fruit juice, sweetened
Iced and very hot drinks
Salted drinks
Tomato juice

## TEAS

***Do not use chamomile if you are allergic to ragweed.***

### *Major*

Ajwan
Alfalfa
Bancha (twig)
Barley
Basil
Blackberry
Borage
Burdock
Cardamom
Catnip
Chamomile
Chicory
Chrysanthemum
Cinnamon
Cloves
Cornsilk
Dandelion
Elder flowers
Eucalyptus
Ginger, dried
Hibiscus
Hops
Hyssop
Jasmine
Lavender
Lemon balm
Lemon grass
Mexican bark
Mormon tea
Nettle
Orange peel
Osha
Passionflower
Pennyroyal
Peppermint
Raspberry
Red clover
Rose flower
Saffron
Sage
Spearmint
Strawberry
Violet
Wild cherry bark
Wintergreen

### *Minor*

Fennel
Ginger, fresh
Ginseng
Lotus
Sarsaparilla
Sassafras
Yarrow
Yerba maté

### *Regressive*

Comfrey
Marshmallow
Licorice
Rosehips

# TRIDOSHA CHART

***This chart lists some of the foods common to all constitutional types. While these foods may be used when cooking for large groups, this chart should not be used by any one body type exclusively. It lacks variety and thus does not have the healing potential that can be derived from the chart appropriate to your particular type.***

## VEGETABLES

*Use fresh and seasonal vegetables.*

| | | |
|---|---|---|
| Artichoke | Jerusalem artichoke | Spinach |
| Asparagus | Jicama | Sprouts |
| Bok choy | Kale | Summer squash |
| Broccoli | Landcress | (yellow crookneck |
| Broccoli rabe | Mustard greens | or zucchini) |
| Carrots | Onion, cooked | Sweet potatoes |
| Collards | Okra | Watercress |
| Corn, fresh | Parsley | Winter squash |
| Daikon | Parsnips | (buttercup, butternut, |
| Green beans | Potatoes, white | spaghetti) |

## FRUITS

*Use seasonal fruits.*
*All fruits should be tree-ripened and fresh.*

| | | |
|---|---|---|
| Apricots | Lemons | Pomegranate |
| Berries | Limes | Raisins |
| Cherries | Mango | Strawberries, sweet |
| Grapes, dark | Peaches | Tamarind |

## GRAINS

*Since most dry goods are available throughout the year, grains are categorized by season.*

*Winter/Spring (December to end of April)*

| | | |
|---|---|---|
| Barley | Millet | Quinoa |
| Basmati rice, brown | | |

*Spring/Summer (May to end August)*

| | | |
|---|---|---|
| Barley | Basmati rice, white | Wheat |
| Basmati rice, brown | | |

*Fall (September to end November)*

Basmati rice, brown
Brown rice, short-grain
Oats, whole cooked
Wheat
Wild rice

## PROCESSED GRAINS (ALL YEAR)

*Minor*

Barley cereal
Barley flour
Bulgur
Corn grits
Cornmeal
Couscous
Millet cereal
Mochi (pounded sweet rice)
Oat bran
Oats, rolled or steel-cut
Pasta, spinach or whole wheat
Rice flour
Rye flakes
Rye flour
Soba noodles
Udon noodles
Wheat bran
Whole wheat flour

## LEGUMES, BEANS, PEAS, AND SOYBEAN DERIVATIVES

Aduki beans
Mung dhal, whole
Tofu
Urad dhal

## NUTS AND SEEDS

Nuts may be used sparingly
Pumpkin seeds
Sunflower seeds

## SWEETENERS

Amasake (rice milk)
Barley malt syrup
Fruit juice concentrate
Honey, raw and uncooked
Maple syrup

## HERBS, SPICES, AND FLAVORINGS

Black pepper
Cardamon
Cinnamon
Coconut
Coriander
Cilantro
Cumin
Dill leaves or seeds
Fennel
Garlic, cooked
Ghee
Ginger, cooked
Ginger, fresh
Lemon
Mint leaves
Mustard
Nutmeg
Orange peel
Parsley
Rose water
Saffron
Sea salt
Tamarind
Tarragon
Turmeric
Vanilla
Wintergreen

## DAIRY

*Use organic dairy products.*

| | | |
|---|---|---|
| Butter, unsalted | Ghee | Yogurt, spiced |
| Cottage cheese | | |

## OILS

| | |
|---|---|
| Canola | Sunflower |

## BEVERAGES

| | | |
|---|---|---|
| Aloe vera juice | Berry juices, sweet | Mango juice |
| Apple juice | Carob drinks | Peach nectar |
| Apricot juice | Carrot-vegetable juice | Soy milk, spiced |
| Amasake (rice milk) | Grape juice | Yogurt drinks, spiced |

## TEAS

*Do not use chamomile if you are allergic to ragweed.*

| | | |
|---|---|---|
| Bancha (twig tea) | Barley (grain tea) | Raspberry |
| Barley | Hops | Rice (grain tea) |
| Chamomile | Jasmine | Rose flower |
| Chicory | Lemon balm | Saffron |
| Chrysanthemum | Lemon grass | Sarsaparilla |
| Cinnamon | Lotus | Spearmint |
| Cloves | Mexican bark | Violet |
| Elder flower | Orange peel | Wintergreen |
| Fennel | Peppermint | |

CHAPTER 7

# EATING WITH THE CYCLES OF NATURE— SEASONAL MENUS

According to Ayurveda, there are six seasons—every two months is considered a season. The Vata seasons are early fall (the rainy season), mid-July to mid-September; and autumn, mid-September to mid-November. Mid-November through mid-March, early through late winter, mark the two seasons of Kapha. Spring and summer, spanning mid-March through mid-July, are considered the two Pitta seasons.

Because each dosha is increased in its own season, these particular times of year are crucial for each body type: Vata is increased in the rainy season and autumn; Kapha is increased in both the early and late parts of winter; and Pitta is increased in the spring and summer.

The period of time when the seasons are changing is also very critical for all the types. According to Charaka: "All diseases begin at the junctions of the seasons," and so all types are cautioned to be especially aware during the seasonal transitions. The fortnights surrounding mid-September and mid-November are the most crucial periods during the Vata seasons. Vata types are advised to cultivate infinite patience and to initiate gentle, grounding sadhanas and use Vata-nurturing foods during these periods. The fortnights surrounding mid-January and mid-March are the most critical days for Kapha types, who are cautioned to be stoic and firm with their sadhanas and food choices during these periods. The fortnights surrounding mid-May and mid-July are the most vunerable days during the Pitta seasons. Pitta types are asked to be especially patient and observant of their sadhanas and food choices during these periods.

The doshas are at their zenith during a certain time of day and time of life. Two to six in the early morning and afternoon is Vata's peak time. Six to ten in the morning and evening is Kapha's heightened time. Ten to two in the day and evening is when Pitta is most intense.

The childhood years from birth to fourteen are considered the Kapha years. Twenty-seven to forty-two are considered the Pitta years, and fifty-six to seventy-seven are the prime Vata years. Fourteen to twenty-seven are the Pitta-Kapha years; forty-two to fifty-six the Vata-Pitta years; seventy-seven to life's end, the Vata-Kapha years.

The prevalent times of each dosha generally reflect the time when that dosha needs to be nurtured and nourished to balance its heightened state. During its prevalent time, a Vata type would seek light, warm, and moist temperatures, as well as substantial Vata-nurturing foods. The sadhanas most appropriate to balance Vata are gentle and consistent activities, which include listening to mellow and harmonious sounds.

The Pitta type would seek tranquil and cool temperatures. Wholesome, fragrant, and calming foods reduce the intensity of Pitta. The most appropriate sadhanas are restful, meditative, and gentle activities, which include observing forms that are visually wholesome and beautiful.

Kapha types need to stir and rise in great motion and activity. The temperature needs to be warm, dry, and crisp. Kapha should repast on small portions of stimulating and warming foods. The best sadhanas for Kapha are in the kitchen, cleaning house, parting with many years of collectibles, as well as hiking, biking, and so on.

## SEASON, CONDITION, AGE, AND TIME WHEN EACH DOSHA IS MOST PREVALENT

### VATA

Rainy season, mid-July through mid-September (early fall)

mid-September through mid-November (fall)

Dewy season (late winter)

56–77 years of age

2:00–6:00 A.M. and P.M.

### KAPHA

mid-November through mid-March (winter)

Cold and humid season

Moonlight

Birth–14 years of age

6:00–10:00 A.M. and P.M.

### PITTA

mid-March through mid-July (summer)

Excess heat

Sunlight

27–42 years of age

10:00 A.M.–2:00 P.M.; 10:00 P.M.–2:00 A.M.

### PITTA-KAPHA and KAPHA-PITTA

14–27 years of age
Change from spring to summer

### VATA-PITTA and PITTA-VATA

42–56 years of age
Change from summer to fall

### VATA-KAPHA and KAPHA-VATA

77 years to life's end
Change from fall to winter
Seasonal extremes

## AVERAGE DAILY FOOD PROPORTIONS FOR ALL TYPES

| | | |
|---|---|---|
| Grains | 1 cup (cooked) | 18% |
| Beans | 1/2 cup (cooked) | 9% |
| Vegetables | 3 cups | 40% |
| Fruits | 2 cups | 25% |
| Desserts | 1/2 cup | 8% |
| | | 100% |

## SEASONAL USE OF GRAINS FOR ALL TYPES

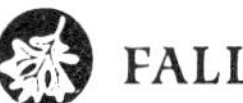

### FALL

| | | |
|---|---|---|
| Amaranth | Bulgur | Medium-grain brown rice |
| Barley (hulled and pearl) | Cracked oats | Millet |
| Basmati rice (brown and white) | Grain flours | Quinoa |

### WINTER

| | | |
|---|---|---|
| Amaranth | Hulled barley | Wheat berries |
| Basmati rice | Quinoa | Whole oats |
| Buckwheat | Rye | |
| Grain flours | Short-grain brown rice | |

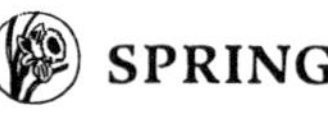

### SPRING

| | | |
|---|---|---|
| Barley (hulled and pearl) | Cracked oats | Grain flours |
| Basmati rice (brown and white) | Cracked rye | Long-grain brown rice |
| Bulgur | Cracked wheat | Millet |

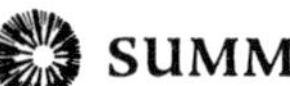

### SUMMER

| | | |
|---|---|---|
| Basmati rice (brown and white) | Grain flours | Noodles and pastas |
| Couscous | Long-grain brown rice | Pearl barley |
| Cracked wheat | Millet | |

## AYURVEDIC IDEAL

In making the transition to the Ayurvedic diet, you may begin by eating the quantity of food that feels satisfying to you, without overeating. Many of us have grown accustomed to consuming two to three times more food than we need. Within the realm of Ayurveda, certain principles are normally recognized and honored when it comes to eating. According to the Ayurvedic master Vagbhata, after a meal the stomach should be filled as follows: 1/3 solid food, 1/3 liquid, and 1/3 empty. Over the following six months, you may gradually reduce your intake of liquids and solids by about 25 percent to reflect this ideal. Water may be taken occasionally during the meal; taking a small amount of warm water before each meal is actually an Ayurvedic prescription.

Ultimately, the desired number of meals per day is two—one taken between 8 and 10 A.M. and the other between 6 and 8 P.M. (Those engaged in hard, physical labor may take three large meals a day.)

## TRANSITIONAL MEALS

When making a transition to a healthy and balanced diet, people often feel deprived of their unhealthy habits and foods. For this reason we need to move forward gingerly and gently into this new phase of life. Understanding that our old attachments and habits, even though resolved, can intrude on new beginnings makes it easier to cope with them. Because of the vulnerable nature of the mind and body during transitional phases, the quantity and frequency of meals recommended in the menus that follow exceed the Ayurvedic ideal. It is important to cosset the mind by providing frequent small meals that are visually stimulating. The five meals provided on each of the following menus are actually two snacks and three small meals. When we allow plentiful and enriching foods, the mind and senses are more readily compelled to let go of old expectations. Essentially we are flooding the organism with love in the form of vital food energies, in the same way we would nurture a battered child until the old wounds heal.

## TASTES AND TEXTURES OF A MEAL

In the Vedic culture, the six tastes were combined and used in every meal. Depending on body type, the tastes in one meal may vary from sweet to pungent. For example, a Pitta breakfast might typically include the sweet taste (a sweet porridge of grains or tapioca, or sweet vegetables or fruits, such as melon or carrots) and even a touch of bitter (as found in karela or endives). A Vata breakfast might typically include the sweet taste (rich, creamy grains) with an occasional spicy touch of an idli and sambar. A typical Kapha breakfast might be light and dry with a pungent taste, such as a rye crisp or roasted grains with a mint masala condiment.

When eating a meal, foods that are hard in character should be eaten at the beginning, soft foods during the middle, and liquid toward the end. Some ancient Ayurvedic schools maintain that the sequence of tastes in a meal should progress in the order of sweet, salty, sour, pungent, bitter, and astringent. More recent Ayurvedic thinking, however, supports a sequence similar to that followed in the West: Begin with salty and sour, progress to pungent followed by bitter and astringent, and end with sweet. In the preparation of these menus, I have followed the more current viewpoint.

In the Festivities category of the following menus, the six tastes are demonstrated in an exotic and dynamic way, reflecting the enormous variety of life, joy, and love that you may experience in your foods. The six tastes in Ayurveda serve to garner the spirit of allowance, kindness, joy, and plenty within the bodily organism, so that we may learn about our true nature.

As you practice this dynamic science of well-being, you will gradually notice principles of balance manifesting within yourself and in your home. Eventually, as you maintain a consistent routine, you will develop ease and grace with your food preparation.

Remember that these guidelines are only tools to support and augment your own commitment to excellent health and spirit. Once the essence of Vedic teaching is grasped, you will blossom with rapidity into your own splendor.

Be aware. Do not become attached to your learning tools—use them for a while, and thereafter refer to them from time to time. The heart of this teaching is that you make it your own. Ayurvedic cooking is not Indian cooking. It is a universal principle of absolute wellness, and thus may be translated into all cultures.

Allow the balance achieved in the act of cooking to become a reflection of the greater achievement of balance in self, universe, and God. I encourage you to share the wisdom you have learned. May Isvara grant abundant grace to you, your family, and your friends.

*Note: Menu items that are capitalized refer to recipes that can be found in this book (see the index for page references). Many of the other items can be found in natural food stores. When a specific type of fruit lassi is specified, substitute a fruit appropriate to your body type. Remember to add honey to tea only after it has cooled.*

*Some recipes appropriate for your body type may contain small amounts of an ingredient that is not recommended by the food charts. Small amounts of these foods will not hinder the overall dosha-benefiting aspects of that dish.*

## MENUS FOR VATA TYPES

### VATA, VATA-PITTA, VATA-KAPHA

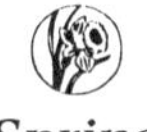

#### *Spring*

**BREAKFAST (7–8)**

Cream of Wheat Porridge with raisins

**LUNCH (12–1)**

Carrot and Broccoli Soup with moist wheat bread
fresh fruits (grapes, mango, melon) with yogurt

**TEA (4–4:30)**

1 cup lemon balm tea
ginger cookies

**DINNER (6–7)**

Seitan, Daikon, and Carrot Stew
brown basmati rice
Daikon Pickle (Mula Achar)
Almond and Hazelnut Cream Pie
1 glass spring water

**EVENING BREW (7–7:30)**

1 cup Warm Saffron Milk

## MENUS FOR VATA TYPES (continued)

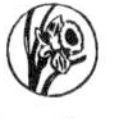

### *Spring*

**BREAKFAST (7–8)**

Soft Rice with Gomasio

1/2 melon with touch of lime juice

1 cup Spice Tea

**LUNCH (12–1)**

Masala Dosa or Rice Idli

with Green Ginger and Coconut Chutney

yogurt and fruits

**TEA (4–4:30)**

1 cup chamomile tea

Marzipan Date Cake

**DINNER (6–7)**

Sesame and Onion Sauce

Tofu and Broccoli

Cinnamon Spiced Wheat

1 glass spring water

**EVENING BREW (7–7:30)**

Warm Almond and Nutmeg Brew

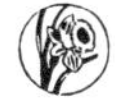

### *Spring*

**BREAKFAST (7–8)**

Hot Milk Tea (Chai)

puffed rice cereal with almond milk

orange slices

**LUNCH (12–1)**

Plain Dhal and Chapati

Pressed Red Radish Salad

1 glass spring water

**TEA (4–4:30)**

peach nectar diluted with sparkling spring water

**DINNER (6–7)**

Spiced Yogurt Drink

Tamarind Rice

Dried Masala Okra

**EVENING BREW (7–7:30)**

1 cup rose flower tea

Amasake and Cardamom Pie (or pudding)

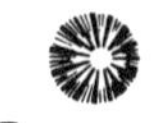

### *Summer*

**BREAKFAST (7–8)**

mixed fruits (bananas, nectarines, oranges), or

whole wheat bread soaked in almond milk with honey, or

puffed rice or wheat cereal with hot milk and dates

**LUNCH (12–1)**

whole wheat noodles with Pesto for V Types

Sautéed Asparagus with sprinkle of mirin

**TEA (4–4:30)**

1 cup peppermint tea

Fruit Cobbler

**DINNER (6–7)**

Almond and Carrot Rice Salad

Carrot and Oat Sauce

Vegetable Stir-Fry with Vata vegetables

**EVENING BREW (7–7:30)**

Warm Spiced Soy Milk

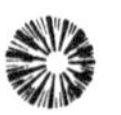

### *Summer*

**BREAKFAST (7–8)**

puffed wheat cereal with warm milk

1 cup twig tea with unrefined brown sugar

1/2 grapefruit

**LUNCH (12–1)**

White Basmati Kichadi

Lime Pickle (Nimbu Achar)

1 glass spring water

**TEA (4–4:30)**

1 cup fennel and peppermint tea

Blueberry Pudding Cake

## MENUS FOR VATA TYPES (continued)

**DINNER (6–7)**

Barley and Pea Salad with Orange and Fennel Dressing
Oil Roti with Ghee
1 glass spring water

**EVENING BREW (7–7:30)**

Warm Almond and Peach Nectar
1 mango

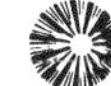

### *Summer*

**BREAKFAST (7–8)**

whole wheat toast soaked in amasake
with sprinkle of orange zest
1 cup lemon balm tea

**LUNCH (12–1)**

udon noodles with mild tamari sauce
Mustard Greens and Asparagus with Hollandaise Sauce
1 glass spring water

**TEA (4–4:30)**

wild ginger and spearmint tea with milk
fresh fruits

**DINNER (6–7)**

Creamed Squash with Chapati
Watercress and Sesame Seeds
1 almond cookie
1 glass spring water

**EVENING BREW (7–7:30)**

almond tea

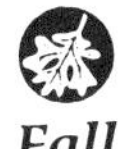

### *Fall*

**BREAKFAST (7–8)**

Whole Mung Dhal with Chapati
bancha tea with lime

**LUNCH (12–1)**

Leek and Potato Soup
sprouted whole wheat bread
1 cup ginseng tea

**TEA (4–4:30)**

peppermint tea
Peppermint and Walnut Mousse

**DINNER (6–7)**

Linguini with Beet Sauce
1 glass spring water
seasonal fruits (fresh or cooked)

**EVENING BREW (7–7:30)**

Warm Sandalwood Milk Brew

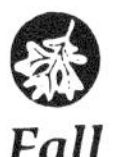

### *Fall*

**BREAKFAST (7–8)**

Wheat Berries and Cloves and Gomasio
1 cup peppermint tea with milk

**LUNCH (12–1)**

Collard Nori Roll
1 cup Japanese green tea

**TEA (4–4:30)**

1 cup chamomile tea
Clay Pot Baked Pears, or roasted sunflower and pumpkin seeds with tamari

**DINNER (6–7)**

Carrot and Broccoli Soup
whole oat bread
Stripped Tarragon Seitan

**EVENING BREW (7–7:30)**

1 cup raspberry tea

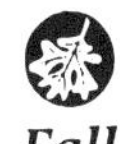

### *Fall*

**BREAKFAST (7–8)**

fresh whole wheat bread with Ghee and jam of choice
1 cup Hot Milk Tea (Chai)

**LUNCH (12–1)**

Rice Idli with Imli (Tamarind) Chutney
Zucchini and Cucumber with Oil & Vinegar Dressing
1 glass spring water

## MENUS FOR VATA TYPES (continued)

**TEA (4–4:30)**

1 cup rosehips tea

choice of pistachio, hazelnuts, or walnuts

**DINNER (6–7)**

Karikai (Carrots and Plantain)

brown basmati rice

fresh Mango Chutney

fresh mango with yogurt

**EVENING BREW (7–7:30)**

Warm Saffron Milk

### *Winter*

**BREAKFAST (7–8)**

Cream of Wheat Porridge

1 cup hot Morning Booster

**LUNCH (12–1)**

Tofu Lasagna

mustard greens sautéed in sesame oil

**TEA (4–4:30)**

avocado sandwich with soybread toast (no crust)and Ghee

1 cup warm Spice Tea

**DINNER (6–7)**

Sweet Rice and Aduki Beans with Mango Chutney

Glazed Carrots

**EVENING BREW (7–7:30)**

1 cup eucalyptus and mint tea

Date Bread Pudding

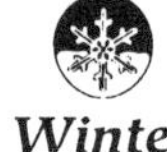

### *Winter*

**BREAKFAST (7–8)**

Soft Rice with Gomasio

Spicy Home Fries (sweet potatoes) or

Sloppy Joe (scrambled tofu)

1 glass Energy Shake

**LUNCH (12–1)**

Creamed Squash with Steamed Artichokes

Cumin Quinoa

**TEA (4–4:30)**

1 cup chicory tea with dash of cinnamon

blueberry muffin

**DINNER (6–7)**

Spinach and Tofu Curry (use seitan instead of tofu)

Caraway Rice

Split Pea Dhal

Lime Pickle (Nimbu Achar)

**EVENING BREW (7–7:30)**

1 cup ginger tea

Raspberry Tart

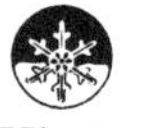

### *Winter*

**BREAKFAST (7–8)**

Squash and Seaweed Soup

Soft Rice

1 cup hot bancha tea

**LUNCH (12–1)**

Leek, Potato, and Barley Soup with Chapati

cooked fruits

**TEA (4–4:30)**

1 cup Hot Milk Tea (Chai)

salted cashews

**DINNER (6–7)**

Aduki and Shallot Dhal

Sesame Rice

Cilantro and Parsley Chutney

Sweet and Sour Landcress (may substitute watercress)

**EVENING BREW (7–7:30)**

1 cup Almond and Peach Nectar

Almond and Hazelnut Cream Pie

## MENUS FOR VATA TYPES (continued)

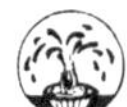

### *Festivities (brunches, celebrations, holidays)*

**BREAKFAST (7–8)**

*Select from among the following:*

Masala Dosa with Green Ginger and Coconut Chutney or Mango Chutney

whole wheat pancakes with maple syrup and fresh blueberries or sweetened jelly and fresh fruits

Rice Idli with Spinach Sambar or Orange Rasam

Eggless French Toast with fresh buttermilk

Squash and Seaweed Soup with sprouted wheat berry bread

Carrot, Celery, and Ginger Juice

Morning Booster

amasake

hot milk, tea, or coffee

---

**LUNCH (12–1)**

*Select from among the following:*

Nori Rolls

Plantain Kuttu

Sautéed Asparagus served with yogurt

Arame and Carrot Tempura

Squash and Potato Soufflé served with sour cream

Vata teas or fresh coffee with milk

amasake

Warm Soy Chai

blueberry muffins

Raspberry Tart

Mocha Mousse

fresh fruits with cottage cheese or whipped cream

tea sandwiches (avocado or jam) with Ghee or unsalted butter

**DINNER (6–7)**

*Select from among the following:*

Chickpea and Seitan Stew or Stuffed Seitan

Carrot and Broccoli Soup

Vegetable Dumpling Soup

Mustard Greens and Asparagus with Hollandaise Sauce

Spinach and Tofu Curry

Karikai (Squash Curry) with white basmati or wild rice

Tofu Lasagna

Linguini with Pesto for V Types

Shepherd's Pie

---

**DESSERTS**

*Select from among the following:*

Universal Trifle

Date Bread Pudding

Fruit Cake or Fruit Cobbler

---

**EVENING BREW (7–7:30)**

*Select from among the following:*

Warm Almond and Nutmeg Brew

Warm Saffron Milk

Sago Payasam (tapioca)

# MENUS FOR PITTA TYPES

## PITTA, PITTA-VATA, PITTA-KAPHA

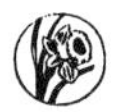

### *Spring*

**BREAKFAST (7–8)**

Sago Payasam (tapioca)
1 cup mint tea

**LUNCH (12–1)**

Steamed Artichokes with Couscous and Carrots
sweet fresh fruits, in season
1 glass spring water

**TEA (3–4)**

1 glass apple juice diluted with spring water
yogurt with maple syrup

**DINNER (6–7)**

Barley and Mung Kichadi with Mint Chutney
steamed leafy greens
radicchio leaves
Raspberry Tart

**EVENING BREW (8–8:30)**

1 cup comfrey tea brewed in milk and water

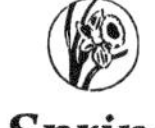

### *Spring*

**BREAKFAST (7–8)**

granola or wheat bran cereal in Warm Spiced Soy Milk
1 cup chrysanthemum tea

**LUNCH (12–1)**

Sautéed Asparagus
Glazed Carrots with Saffron Basmati Rice
Mango and Melon Custard
1 glass spring water

**TEA (3–4)**

1 cup peppermint tea
ricotta chesse and fruit dessert

**DINNER (6–7)**

Barley and Pea Salad with Orange Fennel Dressing
Clay Pot Baked Pears

**EVENING BREW (8–8:30)**

1 cup Warm Saffron Milk

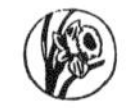

### *Spring*

**BREAKFAST (7–8)**

wheat flakes cereal with milk
1 cup orange peel tea

**LUNCH (12–1)**

Arugula Salad with Orange Fennel Dressing
(omit the orange)
Carrot and Raisin Stuffed Tofu
1 glass spring water

**TEA (3–4)**

1 cup fennel tea
melon or papaya with whipped cream

**DINNER (6–7)**

Soybean and Red Cabbage Dhal
Saffron Basmati Rice
broccoli, cauliflower, and Brussels sprouts with pepper, sautéed in Ghee

**EVENING BREW (8–8:30)**

1 cup coriander tea

### *Summer*

**BREAKFAST (7–8)**

puffed oats cereal with Warm Saffron Milk
1/2 cup aloe vera drink

**LUNCH (12–1)**

Carrot and Cucumber Aspic
sprouted wheat berry bread
1 glass spring water

## MENUS FOR PITTA TYPES (continued)

**TEA (3–4)**

1 glass sweetened lemonade

Pineapple Kanten with almond cookies

**DINNER (6–7)**

Aduki and Shallot Dhal with Chapati

Dried Masala Okra

sautéed mushrooms and green peppers in soy oil

1 glass spring water

date balls rolled in shredded coconut

**EVENING BREW (8–8:30)**

1 cup mint tea

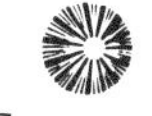

### *Summer*

**BREAKFAST (7–8)**

melon with lime juice

shredded wheat in Soy and Orange Peel Brew

1 apple

**LUNCH (12–1)**

chickpea humus with an avocado

fresh Belgian endive

whole wheat toast

1 glass spring water

**TEA (3–4)**

1 cup cool orange peel tea

grapes and tangerine

maple syrup cookies

**DINNER (6–7)**

baked potatoes with Ghee and coriander

Ratatouille

Amasake and Cardamom Pie

**EVENING BREW (7–7:30)**

1 cup dandelion tea

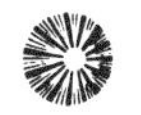

### *Summer*

**BREAKFAST (7–8)**

Coconut Oatmeal Porridge

1 cup peppermint tea

**LUNCH (12–1)**

Sautéed Broccoli Pasta

Bibb lettuce with wheat crisps

1 glass spring water

**TEA (3–4)**

1 cup fennel and coriander tea

blueberry muffin

**DINNER (6–7)**

Tofu Stuffed Squash

Broccoli Rabe with Lemon

Bulgur and Peas

sliced fresh fennel bulb

homemade ice cream

**EVENING BREW (8–8:30)**

1 cup lemongrass tea

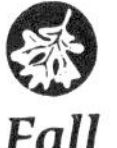

### *Fall*

**BREAKFAST (7–8)**

Cream of Wheat Porridge

1 cup chamomile tea

**LUNCH (12–1)**

Couscous and Carrots

Steamed Broccoli, Cauliflower, and Carrots with Carrot and Oat Sauce

pear juice diluted with mineral water

**TEA (3–4)**

1 cup peppermint tea

fruits in season, or

roasted sunflower seeds with turmeric

**DINNER (6–7)**

Tofu Tempura

boiled buttercup squash with daikon radish

radicchio and cucumber salad

**EVENING BREW (8–8:30)**

1 cup fennel tea

## MENUS FOR PITTA TYPES (continued)

### *Fall*

**BREAKFAST (7–8)**

Wheat berries and Cloves with Dry Coconut Chutney
1 cup Morning Booster

**LUNCH (12–1)**

Bulgur and Peas
cauliflower and endive salad with Orange Fennel Dressing
1 cup barley tea

**TEA (3–4)**

1 cup Cardamom, Coriander, and Fennel Tea
sweet berries with cream

**DINNER (6–7)**

Stuffed Mushrooms with Brown Gravy
white basmati and wild rice (equal amounts)
Peppermint and Walnut Mousse
1 glass spring water

**EVENING BREW (8–8:30)**

1 cup lavender tea, brewed in milk

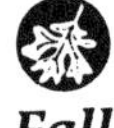

### *Fall*

**BREAKFAST (7–8)**

cooked rolled oats and figs
with milk and unrefined brown sugar
1 glass pear juice

**LUNCH (12–1)**

Split Pea Dhal
Dosa (wheat and chickpea) or Chapati
3 radicchio leaves
1 cup comfrey tea

**TEA (3–4)**

Pear Lassi
rice cakes

**DINNER (6–7)**

Chickpea and Seitan Stew
couscous
steamed broccoli rabe and collard greens

**EVENING BREW (8–8:30)**

1 glass apple cider mixed with fresh apple pulp

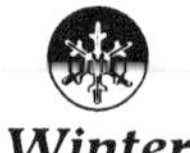

### *Winter*

**BREAKFAST (7–8)**

Sago Payasam (tapioca)
1/2 melon
1 glass vegetable juice

**LUNCH (12–1)**

whole wheat pasta with Sunflower Seed Sauce
Watercress and Sesame Seeds
(substitute sunflower for sesame seeds)

**TEA (3–4)**

1 cup spearmint tea
Fruit Cobbler

**DINNER (6–7)**

Lima Bean Soup
Aviyal (spicy vegetables)
Cumin Basmati Rice
Clay Pot Baked Apples

**EVENING BREW (8–8:30)**

Warm Barley Brew

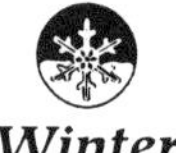

### *Winter*

**BREAKFAST (7–8)**

Cream of Wheat Porridge
1 glass warm spring water

**LUNCH (12–1)**

Fennel Roasted Eggplant
pita bread or Oil Roti
Black Bean Chili
1 glass apple juice diluted with water

**TEA (3–4)**

1 cup peppermint tea
dried fruits with roasted pumpkin seeds

## MENUS FOR PITTA TYPES (continued)

**DINNER (6–7)**

Brown Rice Kichadi
Stripped Tarragon Seitan
steamed mustard greens
Cherry Strudel

**EVENING BREW (8–8:30)**

Warm Sandalwood Milk Brew

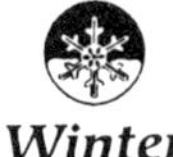

### *Winter*

**BREAKFAST (7–8)**

Soft Rice and Mint Chutney
1 cup Energy Shake

**LUNCH (12–1)**

Karhi (Yogurt Soup) with Chapati
fresh plums
1 glass spring water

**TEA (3–4)**

1 cup lavender tea
vanilla cookies

**DINNER (6–7)**

Karikai (Squash Curry)
Barley and Mung Kichadi
Plain Dhal
Amasake Payasam

**EVENING BREW (8–8:30)**

1 cup rose flower tea, steeped in milk

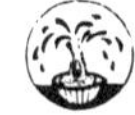

### *Festivities (brunches, celebrations, holidays)*

**BREAKFAST (7–8)**

*Select from among the following:*
whole wheat blueberry pancakes with maple syrup
Wheat and Split Pea Dosa with Mango Chutney
Sloppy Joe (scrambled tofu)
whole wheat toast and Spicy Home Fries
Eggless French Toast
Pear Lassi or Warm Spiced Soy Milk

**LUNCH (12–1)**

*Select from among the following:*
Ricotta and Tofu Quiche
steamed leafy greens or Vegetable Tempura
with Mild Tamari Sauce
Nori Rolls with a Carrot and Cucumber Aspic
Stuffed Mushrooms (with Wheat Bread Crumbs)
Peppered Barley Idli with Orange Rasam
mineral water or Pitta teas

**TEA (3–4)**

*Select from among the following:*
Pitta teas, Pear Lassi, Amasake Payasam,
hot Morning Booster, or fresh juices
fruits, Saffron and Apple Pie, Cherry Strudel
tea sandwiches (cucumber, watercress, buttercup
squash and avocado, or jams) with
Ghee or unsalted butter

**DINNER (6–7)**

*Select from among the following:*
whole wheat pasta dishes with Sunflower Seed Sauce
Tofu Tempura or Chickpeas and Seitan Stew
kichadi and Karikai (Squash Curry)
Coconut Rice
Lime and Raisin Rice
Shepherd's Pie
Mustard Greens and Asparagus with Hollandaise Sauce
Steamed Artichokes with Cilantro and Coconut Sauce

**DESSERTS**

*Select from among the following:*
Hazelnut Carob Mousse
Rosewater Pudding
Fruit Cake
Universal Trifle

**EVENING BREWS (8–8:30)**

*Select from among the following:*
Warm Saffron Milk
Cardamom, Coriander, and Fennel Tea
Warm Sandalwood Milk Brew

# MENUS FOR KAPHA TYPES

## KAPHA, KAPHA-VATA, KAPHA-PITTA

*Note: Kapha types should substitute certified raw goat's milk for cow's milk.*

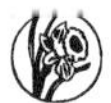

### *Spring*

**BREAKFAST (8–9)**

fresh strawberries
puffed millet cereal in warm apple juice with dash of cinnamon
1 cup Warm Spiced Soy Milk

**LUNCH (1–2)**

steamed vegetables (Brussels sprouts, leafy greens, carrots, daikon) with Basil Dressing
Millet and Corn
½ glass spring water

**TEA (4–4:30)**

1 glass Carrot, Celery, and Ginger Juice
rice cakes

**DINNER (6–7)**

Barley and Mung Kichadi with Green Ginger and Coconut Chutney
sautéed leafy greens
1 cup raspberry tea

**EVENING BREW (7:30–8)**

1 cup warm goat's milk with cardamom

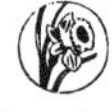

### *Spring*

**BREAKFAST (8–9)**

granola with raisins
1 cup hot Morning Booster

**LUNCH (1–2)**

Arugula Salad or endive salad
Sautéed Asparagus with Hollandaise Sauce
Millet Croquettes
1 glass spring water

**TEA (4–4:30)**

1 cup barley and cardamom tea
dried fruits

**DINNER (6–7)**

Stuffed Mushrooms (with Rye Bread Crumbs)
wild rice
Sautéed Red Cabbage
Clay Pot Baked Apples

**EVENING BREW (7–7:30)**

1 cup warm apple cider with fresh mint leaves

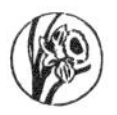

### *Spring*

**BREAKFAST (8–9)**

Roasted Breakfast Grain with sprinkle of Pudina (Mint) Masala
½ glass Carrot, Celery, and Ginger Juice

**LUNCH (1–2)**

Peppered Corn on the Cob
Clear Ginger and Corn Soup with 3 radicchio leaves
Quinoa and Carrots
½ glass spring water

**TEA (4–4:30)**

1 glass pear juice with pinch of dried ginger, or fruits in season

**DINNER (6–7)**

Split Pea Dhal
Peppered Barley Idli
Broccoli Rabe with Lemon or sautéed mustard greens

**EVENING BREW (7–7:30)**

1 cup cardamom and coriander tea

## MENUS FOR KAPHA TYPES (continued)

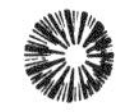

### *Summer*

**BREAKFAST (8–9)**

puffed millet cereal with warm goat's milk and dash of cardamom

½ glass spring water with pinch of ginger

**LUNCH (1–2)**

Buckwheat and Pea Salad (substitute snow peas for peas)

1 cup chamomile tea

1 apple

**TEA (4–4:30)**

1 glass mango and lime juice

rice cakes

**DINNER (6–7)**

udon noodles with Pesto for K Types garnished with fresh radicchio leaves or fennel bulb

Raspberry Gel Pie

**EVENING BREW (7–7:30)**

1 cup chrysanthemum and fennel tea brewed in soy milk with touch of honey

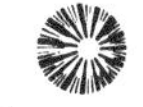

### *Summer*

**BREAKFAST (8–9)**

apricots and peaches

1 cup blackberry tea

**LUNCH (1–2)**

steamed leafy greens

Lemon Broccoli Tofu

Millet and Snow Pea Salad

1 glass spring water

**TEA (4–4:30)**

1 cup cooled rose flower tea

roasted pumpkin seeds

**DINNER (6–7)**

Corn Balls and Red Peppers

lightly sautéed zucchini

**DESSERT**

Pineapple Kanten

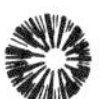

### *Summer*

**BREAKFAST (8–9)**

corn flakes and pears in warm soy milk

1 glass orange juice

**LUNCH (1–2)**

Barley, Onion, and Carrot Salad with Orange Fennel Dressing

fresh endives

1 glass spring water

**TEA (4–4:30)**

1 cup lemon balm tea

Popcorn Crunch Crustless Pie

**DINNER (6–7)**

Lima Bean and Cauliflower Soup

steamed watercress

Chapati

**DESSERT**

fresh strawberries

**EVENING BREW (7–7:30)**

1 cup warm goat's milk

### *Fall*

**BREAKFAST (8–9)**

Sloppy Joe (scrambled tofu) with rye crisp

1 cup dandelion tea

**LUNCH (1–2)**

Millet Nori Roll

steamed mixed vegetables (string beans, carrots, mustard greens)

½ glass apple and cranberry juice

**TEA (4–4:30)**

1 cup Warm Soy Chai

Popcorn Crunch Crustless Pie or fresh peaches

## MENUS FOR KAPHA TYPES (continued)

**DINNER (6–7)**

Aduki and Shallot Dhal
Millet and Corn
Arugula Salad or sliced red radishes with Basil Dressing

**DESSERT**

1/2 cup raspberry gel

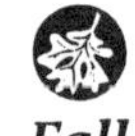

### *Fall*

**BREAKFAST (8–9)**

puffed barley or puffed rice cereal
goat's milk spiced with dash of cinnamon and diluted with water
1/2 glass prune juice diluted with water

**LUNCH (1–2)**

Millet and Quinoa Salad with Carrot and Oats Sauce
1 cup blackberry tea

**TEA (4–4:30)**

1 cup alfalfa and clove tea

**DINNER (6–7)**

Mung and Buckwheat Soup
Baked Spiced Tofu
steamed broccoli with Cumin Dressing

**DESSERT**

Peppermint and Walnut Mousse

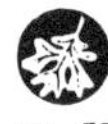

### *Fall*

**BREAKFAST (8–9)**

oat bran muffin
1 cup elder flower tea

**LUNCH (1–2)**

Leek and Chickpea Soup
Escarole and Garlic
2 leaves of lettuce
Quinoa and Carrots (substitute amaranth for quinoa)
1/2 glass spring water

**TEA (4–4:30)**

1 cup chrysanthemum tea steeped in water (3 parts) and amasake (1 part)

**DINNER (6–7)**

soba noodles with Burdock and Mushroom Sauce

**EVENING BREW (7–7:30)**

1 cup eucalyptus tea with a few saffron strands

### *Winter*

**BREAKFAST (8–9)**

Soft Rice with Mint Chutney
1 cup hot apple cider

**LUNCH (1–2)**

Ramp and Tofu Stew
Mola Hora
Pressed Red Radish Salad
1/2 glass spring water

**TEA (4–4:30)**

1 cup Amasake Payasam

**DINNER (6–7)**

Cassava Masala
Cumin Millet
steamed Brussels sprouts

**DESSERT**

1 oatmeal cookie

**EVENING BREW (7–7:30)**

1 cup Warm Spice Tea

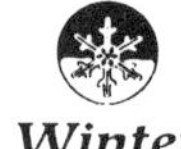

### *Winter*

**BREAKFAST (8–9)**

Split Pea Dhal with a Chapati
1 cup Hot Milk Tea (Chai)

## MENUS FOR KAPHA TYPES (continued)

**LUNCH (1–2)**

steamed winter squash (buttercup, butternut, spaghetti, etc.)
Spicy Roasted Eggplant
Cumin and Basmati Rice

**TEA (4–4:30)**

1 cup Spice Tea

**DINNER (6–7)**

Leek and Potato Soup with rye croutons
Vegetable Stir-Fry with mild Tamari and Ginger Sauce

**EVENING BREW (7–7:30)**

1 cup blackberry tea

### *Winter*

**BREAKFAST (8–9)**

Soft Millet and Carrots
Rasam Masala
1 cup Spice Tea

**LUNCH (1–2)**

Lima Bean Soup
wheat crisp
sautéed collard greens and watercress
1 cup dandelion tea

**TEA (4–4:30)**

1 cup peppermint tea
cooked fruits of choice

**DINNER (6–7)**

Mixed Vegetable Sambar
Barley and Whole Mung Beans
Dried Masala Okra

**EVENING BREW (7–7:30)**

1 cup barley tea

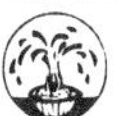

### *Festivities*
### *(brunches, celebrations, holidays)*

**BREAKFAST (8–9)**

*Select from among the following:*
Rye and Urad Dhal Dosa with Mango Chutney or Dry Coconut Chutney
Sloppy Joe with whole wheat toast
buckwheat pancakes with fresh blueberries and unsweetened jam
fresh juice and fruit, or vegetable juice
Pear Lassi

**LUNCH (1–2)**

*Select from among the following:*
vegetable sandwiches (cucumber, radicchio, or lettuce) on warm grain bread or in Chapati
sautéed onion sandwich with eggless mayonnaise or peppered oil and Ghee on warm grain bread or in Chapati
Vegetable Dumpling Soup or Clear Noodle Soup
Millet and Corn Soup
pressed salad or Cauliflower and Potato Soufflé
Ricotta and Tofu Quiche

**TEA (4–4:30)**

*Select from among the following:*
Warm Soy Chai
hot Morning Booster
Kapha teas
Energy Shake
apple lassi
fresh juices (with or without mineral water)
tea sandwiches (cucumber, fresh watercress, steamed leafy greens, sautéed onions with peppered oil, or unsweetened jams and sunflower seed butter)
cookies sweetened with fruit juices
Collard Nori Rolls

## MENUS FOR KAPHA TYPES (continued)

**DINNER (6–7)**

*Select from among the following:*

Toor Dhal and Eggplant Kuttu with Chapati

Tofu Lasagna with Carrot and Oat Sauce

Squash and Potato Soufflé

Vegetable Stir-Fries

Arame and Carrot Tempura

Shepherd's Pie with brown or white basmati rice or wild rice

Natto Stuffed Tofu

Seitan, Daikon, and Carrot Stew

Kichadi

Buckwheat and Pea Salad with Garlic and Ginger Sauce

steamed asparagus or artichoke

**DESSERTS**

*Select from among the following:*

Saffron and Apple Pie

Clay Pot Baked Apples (or pears)

Popcorn Crunch Crustless Pie

Vanilla Flan

Raspberry Tart

Pineapple Kanten

**EVENING BREW (7–7:30)**

*Select among the following:*

Warm Barley Brew

Warm Spiced Tea

Warm Goat's Milk with Cardamom

CHAPTER 8

# FOOD SADHANAS

During my vigilant post-cancer years, I spent a great deal of time working with food—in the kitchen, at the farmers' market, in the health food stores, and in my garden. I discovered the simple act of wholesome cooking to be crucial in the invocation of cognitive memory. This is the only sadhana that takes us through a complete cycle, from the earth and back to earth.

It all begins with a good seed—a seed that remembers its essential DNA, its memory of all time; a seed that has not been tampered with or genetically manipulated; a seed from which a healthy and happy plant will sprout. The healthy plant is prepared into food, and the waste and roughage return to earth after the food body is nourished. In time the food body itself exhausts its ration of breath, completes its living cycle, and naturally returns to earth.

When we learn to grow, prepare, and cook our own foods, to sustain excellent memory, and thus to have the glow of health, we are able to know the living harmony. Our individual potential, as a single bead relating to the cosmic mala, is fulfilled.

The art of cooking gives us endless practice to refine the food body. This sadhana does not exclude the millions of other wholesome activities; rather it is the hub around which everything falls into balance. When this sadhana is culled, all irrelevant activities, attitudes, and invalid memories dissolve. Foods are a means of re-learning nature.

These principles of living are not implacable doctrines. They are meant to remind us of a time in the past when humans melded with the earth, and a time in the future when we will once more know the ineffable bliss of this melding. While I hold the ancient traditions about food in high esteem, I have not blindly relied on their teachings. All the sadhanas recommended in this book have been processed through the sonority of my own experience. Today many controversies exist surrounding the land and its foods. Some truths have been plied and altered to serve selfish ends. Only our own hearts and our own practice can tell us which of these tenets still ring true. When the self becomes strongly linked to the essential memory of this planet, it becomes our true guide. By attending to our

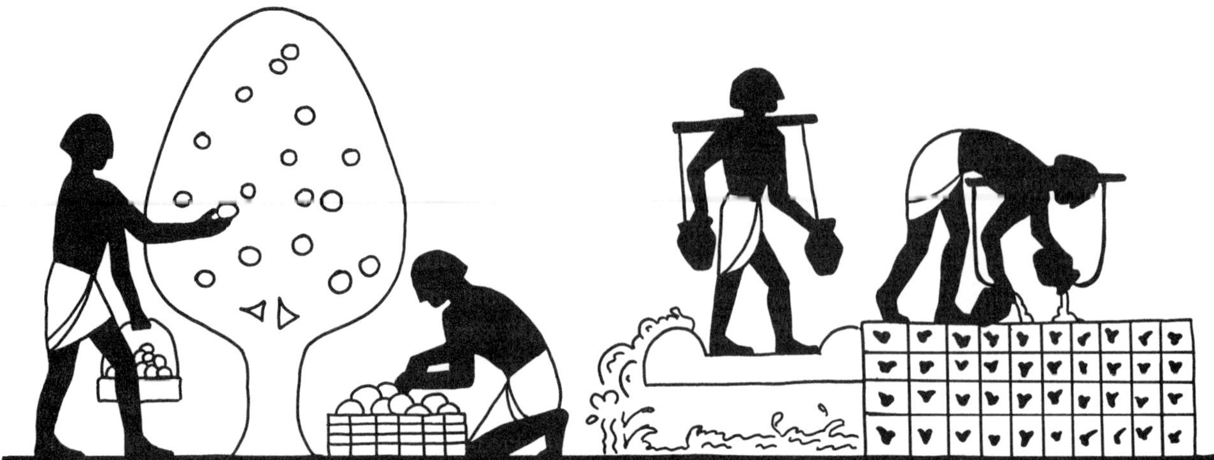

**Egyptian Garden Scene—The community at work planting the seed, watering the sprouts, and celebrating the fruits. From tomb painting, 2,000 B.C.**

life and our practice, by allowing wholesome living to permeate our being, by allowing it to sit in our hara, we will discover the truth in everything.

## THE FOOD BODY

*From the earth came herbs, from herbs came food, and from food came the seed which gave life to the humans.*
*Taittirya Upanishad (11.1)*

Our food, our body, and nature are one entity. The flesh of our body is the same as the flesh of a winter squash; the bodily fluids are the same as the coconut milk. The network of fibers in our body is the same as the loofah of the gourd squash. The heart of an artichoke is the same as our heart. The kidney bean is the same as our kidneys. The leaves of a tree are the same as our lungs, and its bark the same as our skin. When the trees are cut, they bleed. When they are uprooted, they die.

But we perceive ourselves as different from trees and plants, from the animals and birds, from the single-celled organisms. We see them as outside of ourselves. Similarly, we perceive foods as products separate from ourselves. In truth, our very perception exists within the same light of consciousness as do food, animals, and all principles of the cosmos. The same light of consciousness that makes us visible makes the foods we eat visible.

Nature is so fine and its pattern so intricate that if we were to use our foods intelligently, it would be like intimately knowing the symphony of nature's vast spectrum of light, color, sounds, scents, and salves. The essential threads of our cognitive memory would be plied and we would begin to remember, to balance Life within our lives, like the confluence of a river and streams.

It is normal to overdo in the first few years of learning a new discipline. With time our comfort factor adjusts and we become at ease with our new lifestyle. Until this happens, we need to be alert and consistent so as not to regress. Food is our sustenance and as such deserves great reverence. Over the years, however, I have often seen people distort this principle and become obsessively addicted to particular diets. Addictive behavior, even in the context of well-intentioned dietary and lifestyle changes, invariably turns to fanaticism. I have seen grown men and women actually focus their entire existence on dissecting the positive and/or negative qualities of certain foods. While it is valuable to know what is clean and healthy for our bodies and minds and what is not, we must remember that eating is not our ultimate aim as human beings. In becoming obsessed with food, we become obsessed with the body. This obsession is destructive.

## SADHANAS FOR THE HEART

### *Grace in Receiving Sustenance*

To be gracious does not mean one has to be religious or trained in social etiquette. Essentially it means to pay reverence to the creator of the wise earth, to the farmers, and to the cooks who bring us our daily bread. Reverence dissolves dissent and coaxes the acids of peaceful digestion. Graciousness is shown in many ways. Preparing meals, assisting with clean-up after meals, attending the needs of the mother or cook—these are all attitudes of divine goodwill that foster graciousness. Traditionally, a small portion of each cooked food is offered to the fire with a prayer to the Lord, the giver of all food. This ritual is observed before the food is tasted or served. The first offering is given to the universe as a token of perpetual gratitude for our provisions. Since most of us do not have an open fireplace in which to perform this offering, a small fire lit in an earthen pot may be kept in the kitchen for this purpose, or a simple prayer will suffice. Pine kindling should be used for the burning of the sacred tender.

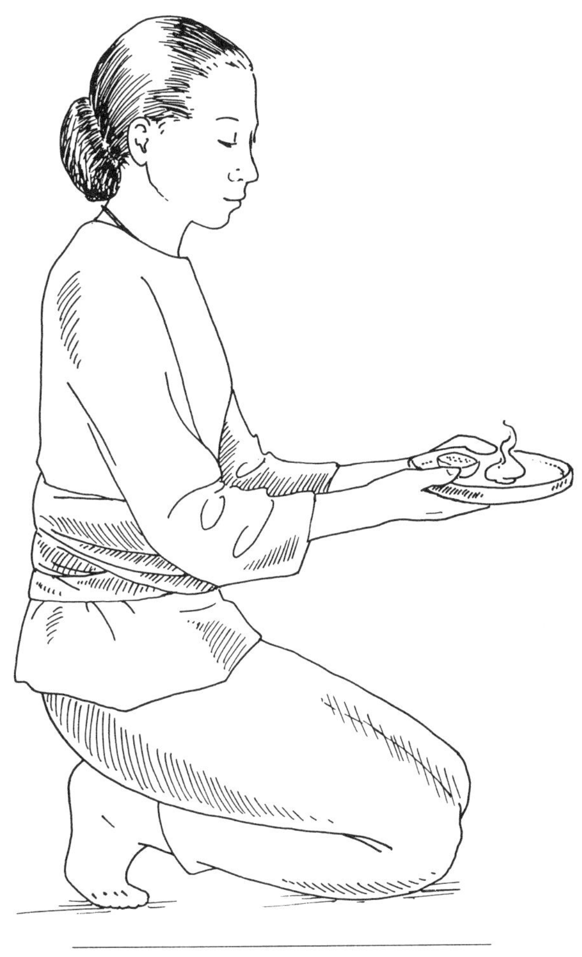

**Offering Food to the Fire—
Sadhana of Gratitude**

Any form of prayer may accompany the offering. The following is a Sanskrit prayer to Brahman, the Absolute one, or pure Consciousness, from the Bhagavad Gita.

*Brahmarpanam Brahma Havih*
*Brahmagnau Brahmana Hutam*
*Brahmaiva Tena Gantavyam*
*Brahmakarma Sanadhina*

Brahman is the Offering
Brahman is the Oblation
Poured out by Brahman into the fire of Brahman
Brahman is to be attained by the one
who contemplates the action of Brahman.

### *Harmony in Eating*

Sweet foods turn sour in our digestive tracts when the emotions present during the meal are negative. Never eat while you are upset. It is an insult to the food, to the giver of foods, and to your body.

While silence is the best sadhana to maintain during meals, gentle, wholesome conversation is also acceptable. It is important to maintain a mealtime schedule that is consistent: meals should be eaten at the same time each day. Although there is a beneficial eating time for each body type, it is often difficult to coordinate these times within a family situation. People concerned with weight gain should never sleep directly after a meal. A few other Ayurvedic precepts follow.

- Allow a few hours between meals and bedtime.
- Take a gentle walk after meals to soothe digestion.
- Never eat and run.
- Never stand up, lie down, or watch television while eating.
- Fill the stomach—which holds about two-and-a-half handfuls of food—one third full of food and one third full of liquid. The remaining third should remain empty, to allow space and energy for proper digestion.

Many ancient peoples sat directly on an earthen floor, or on the skin of an animal that died naturally. Sitting in the half-lotus position and leaning forward to eat from a utensil placed on the ground provides a natural and involuntary limit to our intake of food. The pressure caused by moving forward restricts the quantity of food to be eaten.

While rules are allowed to be broken from time to time, we do need to be vigilant of our behavior. By gradually observing these precepts, we can over time promote and facilitate an excellent state of mind.

## Savoring Food

Taste is primal to the eating process. When the juices of the mind and appetite whet the tongue, we are ready to receive the blissful memories each food gives. The first step of digestion is chewing. The digestive water of the tongue aids in the breakdown of food. As we take the time to ruminate, we remember. Memories of the entire universe are held in the savoring of our food. Chewing food to a pulp facilitates digestion and lightens the load on our organs of assimilation. By being considerate toward the agni of digestion, we are rewarded with a calmer mind. We cannot remember the truth of being if we are agitated.

Chewing is a delicate sadhana. When we do not chew properly, we deprive the body of its nutrients and shut down the channels of memory. Conversely, when eating becomes a tedious and jaw-breaking chore, we defeat the process of assimilation. We must practice quietude and relaxation while we eat. We must nurture a wholesome attitude and chew with awareness.

Recently, I was present at a national health conference attended by many holistic practitioners. During lunch I was seated with a well-known "chewing" master. Before the wave of conversation began at our table, the master quickly began to play a recording of subliminal music. This was supposed to assist the mind in its contemplation of the chewing process. Next to him was a stopwatch, with which he kept time of each mouthful being chewed.

Given the circumstance, everyone graciously acquiesced and chewed in self-conscious tedium. Seeing that in this unnatural and tense situation a perfectly good meal was being wasted, I quietly excused myself and joined a group of students who were enjoying their meal. However slight the chewing and however loud the chatter, the students were clearly receiving the grace and joy of their food.

## Love, Kindness, and Sharing of Foods

Love and kindness are the two most important ingredients in any meal. Without these, the ojas, the energy of food after it is digested, is vastly diminished. Whatever circumstances we find ourselves in at cooking time, we must never project our negative emotions onto the foods. While we may be angry, sad, disappointed, stressed, or fatigued, if we are conscious of our state the essence of our love can shine through. There is a certain gentleness, which can be learned, that needs to prevail through all manners of crisis when we are holding food. It must be picked up, washed, prepared, and cooked with a firm care. Should negative emotions prevail, leave the kitchen. Go outside or to another room, scream, kick up a storm, pound on the walls—allow the emotions to dissolve and then return with a softness and delicacy to the kitchen.

The sharing of food goes back in time to when every household fed the mendicants. In India, a small portion of food is always placed on the altar before each meal is eaten as an offering to the deity. Today we continue this sharing of food with our friends and family. It is vital to remember that the toil of the wage-earning family member makes this sharing possible. Thus, this person's name should be included in the grace, with thanks.

The sharing of food has always produced powerful emotional bonding. When we are able to control all stages of food preparation, the wholesome results help bond us with our universal kin. As we adhere to the dharma of harmonious behavior within our home and during our meals, we forge a healthy tie with each family member and with our friends. When we neglect this natural human urge, we seek to fulfill this need in other ways. As a result, we develop attachments to foods, to substances, and to material things.

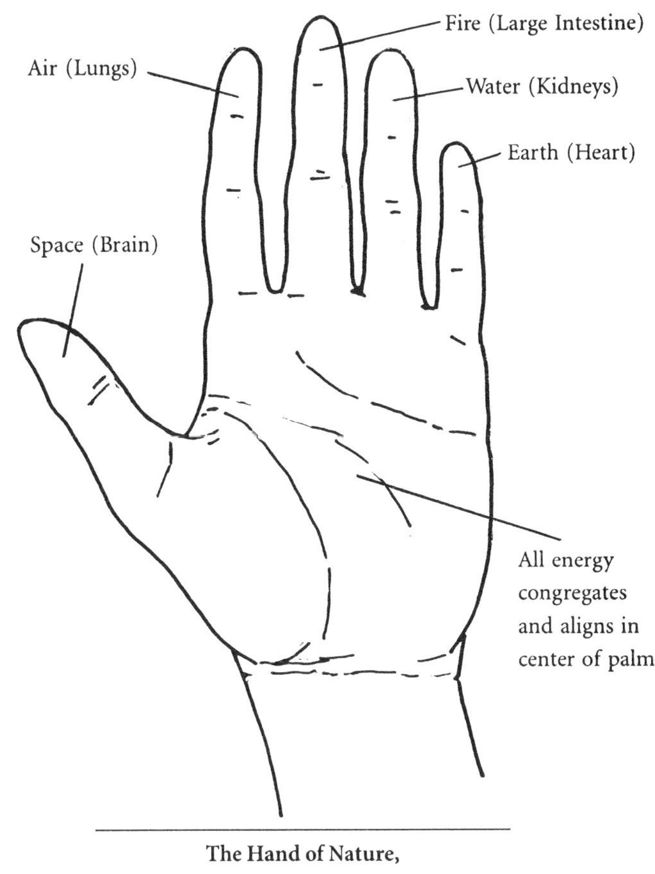


**The Hand of Nature, our continuous dance with the five elements**

## THE LIMBS OF GRACE—SADHANAS OF THE HAND AND FOOT

Eating food with our hands is as old as time itself. The mere touching of food with the fingertips stimulates the five elements. Each finger is an extension of one of the five elements. Each serves to aid in the transformation of food before it passes on to internal digestion. One broad and numinous stroke extends from the beginning of the food preparation to its final invitation into our bodies.

The sadhana of feeding ourselves from hand to mouth enhances our vital memory. It begins from the day of our birth. According to Ayurveda, a newborn should be given a mild emetic made from rock salt and medicinal ghee. This is administered by placing the emetic in the right hand of the newborn and assisting the hand to the child's mouth. This procedure even precedes breast-feeding.

In the Vedas, the hands and feet are referred to as the "organs of action." By using our organs of action, we engage in the moment-to-moment remembering of the five elements of our nature. Our hands are vital extensions that enable us to touch, and be in touch with, creation. Ayurveda exhorts us to use our body as the ruler and measuring cup for all our needs. We are born with all the tools needed to exercise our gifts for sadhanas, including those needed to feel and measure foods as we prepare them.

In keeping with this principle, you need to become comfortable using your hands and eyes for all measuring. In Sanskrit, the term *anjali* refers to the volume that can be held by your two hands cupped together. Two anjalis of grain or vegetables from your own hands is designed by Nature to fill your own stomach. When you are cooking for others use two anjalis for each adult, and one anjali for each child. Likewise gauge your spices or accents with your own pinch. Like your handful, it is tailored to provide a suitable amount for your own personal body needs. *Angula* refers to the distance between the joints of each finger. This unit of measure is cosmically designed to gauge spices and herbs, such as cinnamon sticks and ginger.

| | |
|---|---|
| Amount in your cupped hands | = your equivalent of 1 cup |
| Size of your pinch | = your equivalent of $^1/_{16}$ teaspoon |
| Liquid in your palm | = your equivalent of 1 tablespoon |
| Length of your finger joint (1 angula) | = your equivalent of $^3/_4$ inch |

Sadhana means your participation with everything. Use only those tools that are absolutely necessary. As soon as possible, give up using measuring cups, spoons, and useless kitchen paraphernalia. These adjuncts are distracting and interrupt your direct energetic exchange with the food.

It may be difficult at first to take this conscious step, to trust the accuracy of your own physical-spiritual apparatus. With time, you will become comfortable enough to return to the original and most natural system of measurement. Unfortunately today's publishers, in deference to their readers, will not accept a cookbook manuscript unless it has precise measurements. For this reason, I have, with reluctance, included them in this book. I urge you to translate all the tedious measurements in this and other cookbooks and use your own personalized measures, based on your limbs, hands, and fingers.

Your hands should partake fully in all food preparation. Knead your energy into the dough, massage your hands with the grains, pat the chapatis and roll the rice balls between your palms. Allow the universal energy to mix with and transmute your own energy. Puree sauces and mash potatoes with your hands. Tear leafy greens gently with your fingertips. When the hands must have a medium, use the grinding stone or mortar and pestle for grinding, the *suribachi* for the positive energy provided by clockwise motion. This is sadhana. The closer to nature each utensil or apparatus, the more connected the prepared food will be to the energy of the cosmos.

The motion of a hand grinder compels cognitive remembering. This motion transports us to the realm of timelessness, to the sadhana of meditation. We were given these hands and feet so that we may bond gently with the earth. We are meant to use both our hands and feet in providing for our own sustenance. This is the most important of all sadhanas. From planting the seed to nourishing the dhatus and releasing bodily waste, reinvested into the soil to continue its complex cycles of fertilization, we are tending to only one sadhana. When we squat close to the land to sow and dig into her soil, we begin to know God by the smell of the black earth deep within. When we leave the garden, we are transformed by this soil and water. For as long as we maintain this sadhana, we are forever changed. All God's creatures will light upon us without flinching.

Before juicing machines were invented, pulped fruits were juiced in big vats by the feet of villagers in the same way that grapes were stomped on to make wine. In ancient times, farmers used their feet to pack the soil, and bakers used their feet to knead large amounts of dough for the community. In those days, people died from old age or the plague, not from the degenerative diseases, such as cancer or heart disease, or from AIDS and mental disorders, as now.

A hand filled with sadhana is a hand that will heal others. It is charged with the prana of the five elements, which when used harmoniously is in constant touch and exchange with nature. This exercise gives poignant vitality to our subtle energies, held within the core of the universe's memory until we are ready to use them. The hands and feet are at either extreme of the physical body. Together they span the boundaries of our relationship with the universe: Our hands touch the wind, space, and fire; our feet tread water and earth. Both are in continuous communion with the five elements. Our feet carry us from place to place. Our hands embrace, offer, and receive. Every fiber of memory strives toward motion, as a young life begins to walk and touch the objects of the world. We are propelled only by collective memory. We need to remember, to reconnect as a collective whole.

As we learn to receive the earth's energy directly through our physical form, by means of our organs of action, we will be more able to harness our extraordinary potential for wholeness of memory and feel unison with our earth and universe. My maternal grandfather was a farmer who had migrated from South India to British Guiana. The British were recruiting natives to plant the rice paddies and work the banana plantations. He spent his time amid the vast fields and under the shade of broad banana leaves that rustled beneath the fiery tropical skies of the Corentyne Coast. He seldom went home. Long years of sadhana on his farm in India had seasoned every sinew of his lithe and tiny frame. He was formed from the wind and the earth. I remember him as a farmer—his gleam and his chiseled features, and especially his magic touch. He cured many by his touch and was known to fix a sprain or a broken ankle or arm by firmly holding and manipulating it. In later years, as I grew up, I observed my mother performing the same magic. My excellent retention of academic material in school was due to the head massages she gave me with her eloquent hands while I studied for exams. This magic is still with me today, helping me understand the energy and depth of our love and faith made tangible through sadhana.

Each one of us has ancestors who possessed, in varying degrees, these simple and serene skills. Our forefathers were much closer to the living earth than we are. They truly epitomized nature. They did not forget. We must not blame the creator for what is lacking in our lives; we were provided with a pure and unbiased creation. It is we who have chosen to forget the primacy of nature.

Sadhanas bring us full circle to regain the spirit of fraternity and community of our ancestors. Even within urban areas, we must find a way to become a community. We need to encourage cooperative efforts, such as finding a small plot of earth to work and sowing the seeds of our vegetables and herbs. We must make of the word *rural* a state of mind. It is a beautiful sight to watch the elderly perform their morning t'ai chi amid the early quiet of Manhattan's Chinatown. Heaps of garbage are piled high on concrete streets but have no bearing on our ability to commune with nature. Great beauty exists everywhere, and wherever we find ourselves for a period of time must be our home. To perform sadhana, we must first learn to sit comfortably in ourselves. When we are truly with ourselves, we see ourselves not as solitary but as a collective entity. When we are truly with ourselves, we are collectively with nature and her species.

The universe's only purpose is to enable us to embrace our magnificent true nature. All of creation vibrates with magnetism. We are in a continuous state of exaltation. To know this love is to become this love. We are not fish, bird, animal, human, microbe, and molecule. We are energy in a gross and subtle state at once. When we learn to tame and garner our forces, we become love. Love is not an emotion, it is our ultimate state of being. When I sit in myself and direct my love to you, you will receive it, and whatever ill feeling you may have had will dissipate. All sadhanas refine us to this end. When you prepare a wholesome meal for yourself and your family, it is love. When a seed bulges through the earth and sprouts into virgin green, it is love. Every natural movement in nature is sadhana, love. The creation, in its impeccable wisdom, bequeathed us its heart, which throbs through the fingers and toes of our organs of action. We are constantly engaged in mental and biological interactions with nature. In maturing, we give in to accepting with our hearts. The human species is approaching its time of first maturity. Let us open our hearts with joy and bask in the vibrations of the universe.

## SADHANAS FOR YOUR KITCHEN

The direction in which our homes, kitchens, temples, and schools are laid out is vital for the culling of positive energies from the earth. To ensure harmonious living, ancients' dwellings were positioned compatibly with the energy field of the earth. The Vedas contain extensive information about the energy field of the universe, and how it affects all living organisms. When we observe the migration of birds and animals, we can see that these life-forms have an instinctual sense of the energy field of the planet. The native American tribes refer to the female buffalo as the Wife of the South Wind, representing all that causes growth on the earth.

The term *sadhana* implies that which is close to the earth. In India, the ancient ones lived on the earth itself. They made their beds on heavy floor coverings and slept with their heads pointing East or South. Their shrines for prayer and meditation faced South:

within them, the teachers faced South and students faced North.

As I was growing up, I often watched my mother daub the cooking fireplace with cow dung brought in from the fields. This manure was also used to rub down the floors and walls of the huts of elderly relatives. Manure from a healthy cow—rich in antiseptic properties—absorbs negative energies and produces negative ions in the atmosphere. Once daubed in this way, the huts were naturally buffered against radiation and toxicity. They maintained their cool temperature through the long, hot days. Rubbing down the mud and brick fireplace was a daily sadhana. A prayer would be offered, and frequently a floral pattern made of freshly ground flour would decorate the newly cleaned fireplace.

Our cooking fireplace faced West. After the cocks sounded their sharp announcement that the day had begun, my mother would make the early repast—freshly baked roti, fresh chana dhal, and cream of wheat or tapioca with fresh, hot milk were among the morning panoply. But the constant fare was the serenity and beauty of my mother's face in that early morning light as she cooked at the wood-burning fireplace.

Years later, I was taught by my father how to cook in the Vedic tradition. He had come to visit me in my Greenwich Village apartment. I discovered, in my little urban kitchen, that I had a good talent for cooking. Perhaps I had imbibed this skill from my mother during those early years. Father was a solid Pitta-Kapha man. He taught me how to grind the bread grains very fine, and how to knead, roll, and bake the dough into rotis, chapatis, and dosas. He shared with me some ancient secrets of baking—one of them was about my grandmother's bread. She would first make a fire on the earth; then she would place fresh dough in a small dugout in the earth and cover the hole with the coals from the kindling wood of her fire. An hour or so later, she had bread that was baked in the earth.

As I became less involved with my design career, father and I began to spend timeless weeks shopping in the Chinese open markets and natural foods stores, and preparing wholesome Vedic meals. In the early mornings and evenings, he would unfold the knowledge contained in the Vedas. I would hurry home from work early to find him either cooking or poring over his cherished books and hand-wirtten notes in the pink light of Manhattan's dusk. He often appeared translucent, as if I could reach through him. The transmission of the lineage had begun. He had thrown me the ball and I had caught it, unbeknownst to me at the time.

One day, upon coming home, I found father scrubbing soot off his hands and face—he looked like a chimney sweep. It turns out that while cooking the kichadi, he had misplaced the pressure cooker nozzle and spent several hours looking for it in the basement incinerator. I reassured him that nozzles were easy things to replace and that he was not. The kichadi that evening was superb. Spoonful after spoonful, I reveled in my father's qualities—the beauty of that statesman, that erudite pundit who was so loved by the thousands of people whose lives he had touched. And here he was teaching me how to cook and scurrying about in an incinerator looking for a nozzle! My very next spoonful was surprisingly heavy. The nozzle had somehow found its way into the kichadi.

A few months later father died. In retrospect, I see that he had come to help me onto my path. Through his teachings I was able to transform my life completely. Today I still feel his numinous energy, and I am grateful. Much of my love for the ancient kitchen and cooking methods was instilled by his love.

### *The Ancient Kitchen*

1. Earth or a clear wood floor
2. A wood-burning cooking stove built directly on the earth, facing West
3. Iron holders for storage of such things as baskets and utensils, facing South
4. Racks for food staples and spices, facing North
5. A nearby stream or well to get water for washing the utensils, facing South

The floor was the work table. This encouraged the optimum posture of squatting, sitting in the thunderbolt pose (Vajrasana), or the lotus or half-lotus.

### *Utensils of Ancient Times*

1. A stone mortar and pestle for spices (about 6" in diameter)
2. A stone mortar and pestle for seeds and nuts (about 10" in diameter)
3. A large mortar and pestle (of stone or wood) for grains and beans (about 4 feet in diameter)
4. A flat and slightly concave grinding stone with a smaller hand-held stone
5. Several straw baskets, cloth bags, and airtight wooden or stone barrels for storing food staples
6. A sifting basket for separating hulls, stems, and stones from grains
7. Sieves, tea strainers, and food steamers, all made from bamboo

## *Pots and Pans*

The stomach linings of animals were used in ancient times as containers for heating and cooking foods. Later, tightly woven grass baskets containing hot rocks were used for cooking foods. Pots made of earthenware came afterward, followed by cast-iron, copper, and bronze cookware. Today, our utensils are made primarily of stainless steel, enamel, glass, and that poisonous material which was welcomed by many during the war years but which unfortunately we continue to use—aluminum.

## *Ancient Eating Utensils*

In ancient times, the status of a person determined what utensils he or she used during a meal. The wealthy used mainly those made of gold, while the poor and the sages ate from earthenware, leaves, or wooden bowls, which are said to enhance simplicity. Wooden plates aid in the secretion of phlegm. Food served on gold platters is more nurturing to all doshas. The element gold also helps reduce disorders of the eyes. Silver plates, bowls, and pans cool the bodily fire, regulate the digestive fire, promote hepatic function, and generally soothe aggravated Pitta conditions. A service on zinc plates improves the appetite and sharpens the intellect. Brass utensils promote heat and wind in the body. Brass is also a vital metal for curing phlegmatic disorders and alleviating Kapha disorders. Copper is recommended mainly for drinking vessels; it awakens the tissues and assists the apana prana to evacuate boldily waste. Glass, especially crystal, and stainless steel help heal jaundice and chlorosis, and serve also to purify and cool the system. Fresh lotus leaves, which are still used today in many parts of India as plates, serve as an antidote to poison. Stone and clay receptacles, used mostly by the poor, are said to induce poverty. The best containers to drink from are those made of copper, earthenware, and glass. The best containers to drink from, based on body type, are gold and zinc for Vata; silver, crystal, and glass for Pitta; brass, copper, and wood for Kapha. All three types may use gold or lotus leaves, and on occasion earthenware or wooden plates and bowls. We may continue to use these various types of eating and drinking utensils to enhance the desired qualities in our lives.

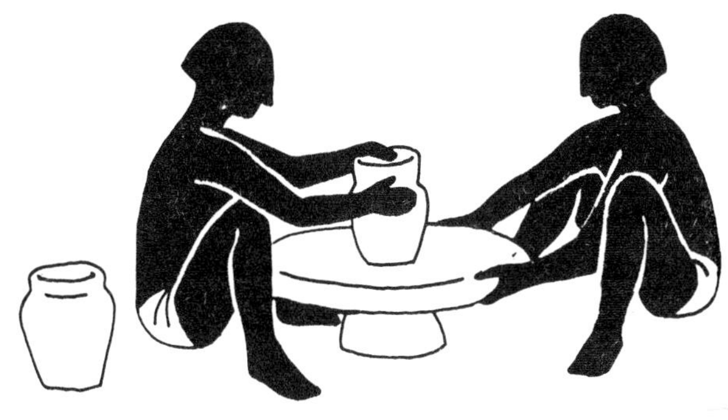

**Two Men at Potter's Wheel**

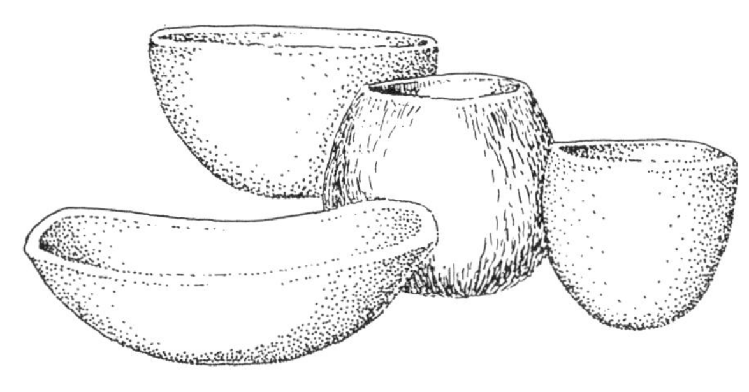

**The Shapes of Ancient Pottery**

## *Modern Utensils*

The pressure cooker and enamelware pot are definite improvements over the stomach lining of an animal. However, our modern stand-up work tables and stoves have deprived us of an essential sadhana—working in various crouching positions. These provided excellent stimulation of the vital organs and tissues as well as a means of receiving the earth's energies through the womb and/or hara.

Similarly, a gas and electric stove deprives us of the direct exchange with the fire of transformation that we would experience with a wood-burning stove. Of the two, a gas burning stove is far better than an electric stove since the direct flame still provides some benefit. Electrical applicances generate noise pollution and are drying to the internal and external organism. When electricity passes through food it damages the tanmatra, or energy quanta of the food, which aggravates all three doshas, and Vata in particular. Microwave cooking is hazardous to one's health. It transmutes and distorts the energy structure of a food, depleting food of its ojas-producing potential and of its memory. Electric blenders, food processors, dough-kneading machines, and so on have definitely removed the most important aspect of food sadhanas from our lives: the handling of fresh grains, beans, vegetables, and spices, and their transformation through processing by our own hands and feet. Dissonant machinery cannot refuel and refine the exchange of energy between the human body and nature.

Hand grinders certainly generate results more quickly than the hard-to-find giant mortar and pestle. Hand grinders are valid kitchen tools because our hands are still engaged to a certain degree. Even the occasional use of a blender or an electric coffee mill is acceptable. While I'm not proposing that we revert back to 500 B.C., we do need to make conscious choices, ones that allow for the maximum amount of human exchange with nature. The sadhanas reaped from preparing foods with hand tools are irreplaceable. These are the peaceful weapons that were given to humans so that we could live in harmonic vigor with nature. Walk gingerly through the maze of cooking inventions. Consider what portion of your vital and cognitive memory you are willing to sacrifice to the insipid conveniences of modern life. The principle of sadhana is so simple that it becomes impalpable. We need to retrieve our innocence. We need to learn through remembering. We need to trust that the journey of time holds the essence of all knowing. We need to embrace our ineffable nature. We need to find our stillness amid the pother and welter of daily life. We need to ponder these things.

## *Making the Transition*

The suggestions listed below will prove helpful at the beginning of your food transition.

1. Simplify your kitchen. Get rid of all utensils that are not being used.
2. Discard all old spices, frozen food, and canned food.
3. Keep your cooking space neat and uncluttered.
4. Gradually eliminate most electrical appliances, as you increase your inventory of hand-operated utensils.
5. Familiarize yourself with your new foods. Begin with the most familiar and appealing items. Secure the basics: spices, oils, grains, and beans. If possible, buy vegetables daily and be alert to their quality. Use as many fresh, organically grown vegetables and herbs as you can.
6. Be conscious of maintaining variety in your menu. Take pride in the pleasing and artistic presentations of your food. Visually pleasing foods stimulate the appetite and can be a successful way to impress your family with a new way of life. Always discuss the food changes with your family and provide them with information on the wholesome benefits and the personal and universal need for these changes. Conscious awareness needs to be taught gently. Your changes will succeed only when they are well presented and backed by reason and thoughtfulness. When a feeling of deprivation is invoked, all else fails. Remember that the only thing you are being deprived of is harmful

and regressive foods. Your attitude as the chef will make the difference between "Yuk!" and "Wow!"

7. Be alert to your energies. At stressful times, take a few minutes to silence your mind by sitting in a comfortable place and taking a few deep breaths. In the beginning, take the support of soothing music, soft lights, and "saging" the air (burning dried sage). These are all tools for inviting stress and misery to leave your kitchen. Never cook when you are dominated by anger or grief. Emotions permeate the energies of the foods you are handling.
8. Consult the Food Charts (pages 74-130) daily on meal preparation, food, taste, and color combinations. Use these as guidelines to help you knowledgeably orchestrate meals.
9. Use the Seasonal Menus (pages 135-148). These are organized according to body type and are specifically designed to help you in making your food transition.
10. Clean your kitchen thoroughly after each meal. This functions as a beautiful invitation to return to it. Enlist the help of your family, and establish routine cleaning duties for every member who shares in the meals.

The Puranas are replete with stories that elucidate our forgetfulness of the self. There is an ancient story of a guru who was crossing a river with his disciples. The ten of them set out together on a journey to the forest. After they crossed a turbulent river, the guru stopped and took count of his students. He counted only nine and began to grieve. Very often when we cross a bridge in our life, we assume new ideals but inadvertently leave behind our most relevant self. For example, when we eat healthy, organic food but have no part at all in its gathering and preparation—this is like leaving the self behind. There are many degrees possible in a transition. With time and practice, our crossings do become complete. Sadhanas are the means of remembering the presence of the self.

The transitional phase is especially disconcerting when we are coming from a fast, modern, meat-based diet. Like any fine-crafted art, the skillful blending of the six tastes, the prime colors, and the subtle combinations of foods needs to be learned. Your attitude in approaching this transition is most important. The change needs to be recognized as a necessity. Unfortunately, many of us who make a major dietary change come to it only after a severe illness. While this may be the most compelling reason to change our lifestyle, we need not wait until our health collapses to embrace a wholesome way to personal and universal wellness.

Approach dietary transitions one step at a time. If you are changing from a modern, meat-based diet, begin by personalizing the food charts: Find the foods within each category best suited to your body type and mark those that you prefer. Start reducing all fats, meats, and salts. Substitute fresh vegetables and herbs for canned, frozen, and dried ones; white meats and fish for red meats; vegetable oils for animal fats and commercial butters; rock or sea salt for iodized salt; whole grains for commercial breads and flour products; and fruits for sugar and dairy-laden desserts. Maintain cooking styles that are familiar to you, but adjust the quality and quantity of such things as fats, salts, and sugars. Make an effort to attend seminars on the Ayurvedic principles of health and cooking. If you are in the moderate to advanced stages of a disease, consult with an Ayurvedic physician.

Those who are making a less radical transition, as from macrobiotic or lacto-vegetarian and vegetarian regimens, will discover that the adjustments you make will be subtle, but powerful. Ayurveda reinforces all authentic information found in alternative health regimens. However, its highly personalized guidelines significantly increase each individual's chances for wellness.

### *Ablutions for the Cook*

1. Wash your hands, feet, and face. Comb your hair and tie it back.
2. Keep your nails clipped and unpolished.
3. Wear clean and uncluttered clothing.
4. Remove all jewelry.
5. Do not taste the food during its preparation and cooking.

6. Do not enter the kitchen, cook, or prepare foods during your menstrual period.
7. Do not handle foods for three hours after sexual intercourse.
8. Observe a few minutes of silence before entering the kitchen.
9. Listen to wholesome sounds while cooking, or cook in silence.

### *Scheduling Your Sadhanas*

Reserve two hours every weekend for your cooking sadhanas. The first weekend you may begin with picking through your grains and beans (see page 167), and washing and hand grinding the amounts that you will need for a fortnight. The following weekend you might spend the two hours drying fresh herbs, stone grinding spices, and mixing masalas for a fortnight's use. During the last few weekends of summer, you may want to set aside an additional hour for such things as preparing fall and winter pickles, or learning how to preserve your own fruits and vegetables.

After a few months, you'll be able to build a routine with your sadhanas and begin to deeply enjoy your practice. The results will be tremendously pleasurable, both in the preparation and taste of your foods, as well as in your personal health and appearance.

## SADHANAS OF GRAIN

The backbone of every culture since the beginning of time, grains knit humankind together as a species. They are also the most holy of foods. They are birthed in water, as the embryo of cosmic life. There are a thousand times more seeds of grain in the world than any other kind of seed. The wholesome husbandry and preservation of such grains as rice, wheat, barley, and millet is an excellent beginning to harnessing the energy of the planet. Each type of grain serves a specific purpose. The tiny, translucent grain of quinoa gave the Incas strength to scale the mountains and keep warm as they labored; the hard, beady millet enabled the desert nomads in Africa to fortify themselves and bend with the harsh winds; the light, golden wheat provided the fat and strength to the European farmers to sow virgin lands and leave a legacy of green fields; the American maize allowed the indigenous people to keep the soil and water alive through reverence and sowing of the land. In all cultures throughout all time, human dignity was maintained through the grain.

From the perspective of sadhana, the grain is the seed of memory. It was brought to life by Gaja, the eternal elephant, who carries the memory of plants and herbs. This memory has been kept alive in the ahamkara of all elephants on the planet. In order for humans to sustain the memories of grains, vegetables, fruits, or herbs, the elephant must remain a thriving species. While the form of these plants may exist after the elephant becomes extinct, the spirit of cosmic memory, which each seed holds from the beginning of time and which is transmuted in the vital energy system of humans and other living creatures, will die. And, in time, so will the human species.

We must begin to perceive all plants, and the sadhana of planting, as reaching as far as the galaxies and stars. This process is not only about topsoil, composting, companion planting, sowing, maintaining, and then reaping the bounty of nature for wholesome survival. Hold a seed in your hand and know that it unfolds from within itself the entire creation, that this seed is the linkage to all memory of this plant from the beginning of time. The magical quality of healing that resides in a grain or an herb comes from the very memory of its seed, whose potency has been collected for more than twenty billion years of original existence. Food is memory, and the grains hold the nectar of this memory.

### *Rice: The Holy Grain*

It is said in the Vedas that the entire universe is held within each grain. Rice has been the primary food for most ancient cultures. It is the most widely consumed grain in the world—more than thirty thousand varieties of rice are currently cultivated. Ninety percent of the rice in the world is grown in India, China, and Japan.

The components of a grain of rice—the husk, bran/germ, and endosperm—symbolize the cosmic gunas

of sattva, rajas, and tamas, respectively the harmony or protection, dynamism, and inertia of the living universe. The grain endures the seven stages of life, from seed to sprout, to seedling, to young plant, to mature plant, to flowering plant, to fruitful plant.

In the Asian countries, a spiritual aura surrounds the planting, harvesting, and preparing of rice. In India, it is cooked in hundreds of ways and used as an offering to the gods during religious ceremonies. Rice is the first food an Indian bride offers to her husband at her nuptials; it is the first solid food an Indian mother offers her newborn. In India, the grains of rice are regarded as two brothers, close but not stuck together. In China, the word for rice is synonymous with food. A typical Chinese salutation upon greeting someone is "Have you had your rice today?" In Japan, cooked rice is the same word for meal. Japanese children are encouraged to eat every grain of rice by calling each grain a little Buddha. In Thailand, the dinner bell is expressed by the resounding words, "Eat rice!"

During the Vedic period in India, the inedible husk was removed and the remaining whole grain—with bran and germ intact—was eaten. This was called brown or unpolished rice. There was no oiling, bleaching, parboiling, pearling, or powdering. Later, during the time of the Moguls, rice had to be polished or white before it was considered edible. Even though India is still not bleaching, pearling, or powdering its rice, there is excessive use of white and parboiled rice. Today only the very poor villagers avail themselves of brown rice. Generally, its quality is excellent, since it has been husked and winnowed by the energies of the hand and heart.

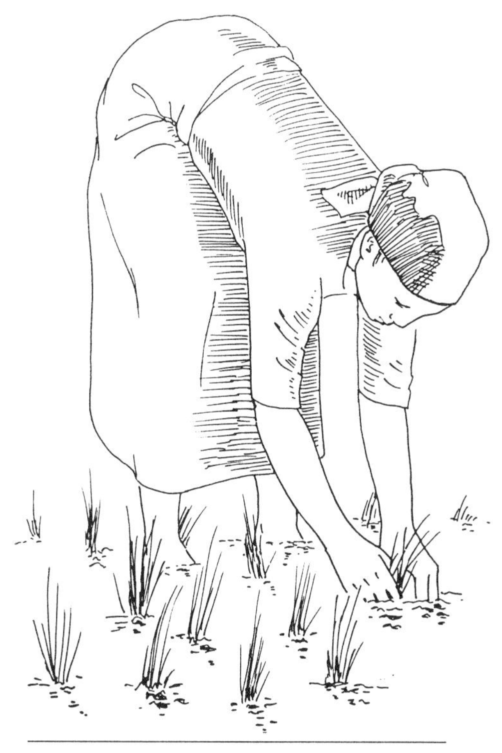

**Planting Rice—
Sadhana to Invite Humility**

***Rice Bran.*** The bran is the nutrient-rich outer layer of a rice kernel. When this bran remains on the kernel, the rice is brown; when it is removed by milling, the rice is white. Bran has a sweet, nutty flavor and is an excellent source of rice-oil, minerals, and fiber. Until recently, most of the rice sold in the United States was white, with the separated bran used exclusively as an animal feed supplement. Rice bran needs to be used shortly after its removal from the grain, since its oil content causes it to turn rancid quickly.

***Parboiled Rice.*** Research reveals that rice was being parboiled in northern India more than two thousand years ago. In parboiling, the rice is steamed and dried before milling, forcing some of the nutrients from the bran layer to penetrate the endosperm. Parboiling a grain makes it easier to digest, although many nutrients are sacrificied in the process.

***Instant or Precooked Rice.*** This rice is milled and polished to remove the bran layers and germ and is then completely cooked and dried. While this rice takes very little time to prepare, it has little or no nutritive value.

***White Rice.*** White rice has the life-supporting bran and germ removed and is milled and polished. Commercial white rice is often coated with glucose and vegetable oil to make it more appealing. Generally the iron, B vitamins, niacin, and thiamin are reintroduced into it, after its innate nutrients have been stripped, thus the term *fortified white rice.* This product offers little or no contribution to health.

***Flaked Rice.*** Although dried, steamed, and flattened, rice flakes are a gentle breakfast cereal good for all body types.

Each type of rice bears a subtle difference in color, shape, aroma, and taste. There are infinite varieties in India—pearl, ivory, pink, red, brown, taupe; long, short, oval, fat, thin, and wispy. The following is a variety of the most commonly known rices, ranging from the staple rice to the most exotic.

### Basmati Rice

An aromatic, nutty flavored rice, basmati has been cultivated for centuries in North India and Pakistan. Some villages in northern India conduct a harvest ritual of hulling and winnowing the grain by hand, with all villagers sharing in this sadhana. Basmati is renowned for its long, slender shape, which lengthens instead of swelling when cooked. The word *basmati* translates literally as the "queen of fragrance." This sattvic grain remains unrivalled among the aromatic rices, due to its exquisite scent, which has been likened to the jasmine flower and the exotic walnut.

Due to an Indian preference for rice that cooks somewhat dry and that separates well, basmati is usually aged up to two years before being used. Traditionally, this rice is used on ceremonial occassions and in the preparation of rice pilafs.

Basmati is available in both white and brown. White basmati is easy to digest, cooling to the digestive fires, and is held in high regard Ayurvedically as a cleansing and healing food for all body types. Brown basmati, like other brown rice, retains both the bran and the germ of the rice kernel, giving it greater healing properties than most other types of rice.

### Black Japonica

This medium-grain rice, which has a black bran, is grown in small quantity by the Lundberg farms in California. It is used in many gourmet rice blends because of its flavor. Black japonica is sweet and slightly pungent in taste. Good for Vata types; may be used occasionally by Kapha and Pitta types.

### Brown Rice

Brown rice comes in long-, medium-, and short-grain. This rice has only the hull removed; both the bran layer and germ layer are left intact, clinging to the kernels. Brown rice has a cream color and a chewy texture, due to its high gluten content. It is superbly rich in minerals and vitamins and has three times the fiber of white rice. Generally, the medium and short grains have more amylopectin (a waxy starch), which gives them a chewier and stickier character than long-grain rice; they also take longer to cook. The long-grain brown rice is fluffier and lighter when cooked. All types of brown rice must be well-cooked and chewed properly to facilitate proper digestion. Brown rice is best for Vata types. On rare occasions, Pitta and Kapha types may indulge.

### Calmati

Basmati has recently been cross-seeded with an American long-grain variety in northern California to produce this popular brown basmati.

### Italian Rices

Arborio, vialone nano, carnaroli, and padano, the most popular rices in Italy, are grown in the regions of Piedmont and Lombardy. Most Italian and Spanish rice is medium-grain and high in starch, which makes the grains stick together. When cooked these varieties become soft, translucent, and yet retain a firm central core; they also yield a top layer of rice cream. Arborio is often used to prepare the well known Italian rice dish called risotti. Italian rice may be substituted occasionally in any recipe calling for short- or medium-grain rice. These are good for Vata types, may be used occasionally by Pitta types, and seldom by Kapha types.

### Jasmine Rice

Native to Thailand, this rice resembles the basmati grain. It has a rich fragrance and is silken to the touch. This grain goes through a water-milling process, which leaves it smooth and long. Unlike basmati, this rice is not aged and usually expands into a moist and medium-grain shape when cooked. Jasmine rice is now grown successfully in the United States. Its cooling energy during digestion makes it useful for cleansing by those of all types on a healing diet. As part of a regular diet, like most rice, jasmine is suited to the Vata types.

### Sushi Rice

This short-grain white rice, used in Japan for making sushi, can be found in most Oriental food stores and some natural food stores. When cooked it is softer and stickier than most other types of rice because of its high starch content. Best for Vata types, sushi rice may be used occasionally by Pitta and Kapha types.

### Sweet Brown Rice

This sticky cream-colored short-grain rice is used in East Asian cuisines for making desserts. Its taste is naturally sweeter than short-grain brown rice. Native to both India and Japan, it can be found in some Oriental or natural food stores. Best for Vata types, sweet brown rice may be used occasionally by Pitta and Kapha types.

### Texmati Rice

A hybrid of Indian basmati rice and American long-grain white rice, texmati is also called American basmati. Its aroma and popcorn-like flavor favor the basmati, but its cooking texture is softer and stickier, partly because the rice is not aged before use. The rice is named after the state in which it grows, Texas, and its resemblance to the basmati rice. Available in both white and brown, texmati is a good substitute for basmati rice. White texmati may also be used for cleansing or healing diets by all three doshas. As a regular part of the diet, texmati is best for Vata types and may be used occasionally by Pitta and Kapha types.

### Valencia Rice

A medium-grain rice native to Spain, this rice is soft and flavorful. It is similar to the Italian rices in that it retains a firm central core after being cooked. Valencia is used in the traditional Spanish rice dish known as paella. This rice is good for Vata types and may be used occasionally by Pitta and Kapha types.

### Wehani Rice

This long-grain rice with a rust-colored bran layer partially splits when the rice is cooked, exposing an earth-red kernel. Considered an aromatic rice, like Jasmine and basmati, wehani is named after the Lundberg brothers—Wendell, Eldon, Harlan, Homer—and their father, Albert, from the Lundberg family farms in California.

### Wild Rice

This rich and long dark brown rice is actually not a rice at all, but the seed of a grass, native to Minnesota, where it grows profusely in rivers, lowlands, and lakes. It was harvested by Native Americans as early as the 1600s. In Minnesota, it is still harvested by the traditional "canoe and flail" method: one person stands and poles the canoe while the other maneuvers two sticks—a long one to bend the stalks into the canoe, and a short one to thrash out the seeds.

Today, much of the wild rice harvest occurs in California where the crop is seeded by airplanes and harvested by machine. Wild rice has an earthy and pungent flavor and was used with game and wild meat by the native people. Wild rice is best for Vata and Kapha types.

## *Other Holy Grains*

### Wheat

Like rice, wheat is an ancient grain whose use can be traced to the beginning of time. Wheat flour has been a staple of Indian cuisine for over five thousand years. In India, wheat is used in as many ways as there are dialects. The ancient flatbread known as chapati is still the primary grain served with meals in North India. Chapati is made from a low gluten, soft-textured, cream-colored wheat flour known as *atta.* In this flour, the whole kernel, bran, germ, and endosperm are all milled to a fine powder, which offers no resistance to being rolled into a dough. An even finer strain of flour known as *pisi lahore* is sometimes used to yield a soft, silken chapati. Semolina, known as *sooji* in India, is a granular meal made from the endosperm of the durum wheat. Its glutinous character makes it a perfect ingredient for a South Indian dish called uppama. Sooji is available in three textures—fine, medium, and coarse; it is used in sweets, such as halva, and in breakfast porridge.

Many varieties of yeasted and unyeasted whole wheat breads and wholesome wheat berry soups are made by the Nords and the cultures of Europe and the Middle East. More glutinous than rice, it is infinitely versatile. Wheat berries are wheat kernels with the inedible hulls removed. One of the most ancient wheat recipes in existence is mentioned in the Vedas. In it, the whole kernels of wheat are placed in an earthen pot with water and cooked over a slow fire for many hours. It yielded the most exquisite wheat cream, which, no doubt, was the staple breakfast food of many ancient cultures.

The people of the Middle East turned wheat into bulgur by boiling the whole wheat grain and leaving it to parch in the sun. The sun-dried grains are then crushed with a mortar and pestle. A finer grind of bulgur is used in the traditional dish known as tabouli. A coarse grind of bulgur is used in another popular dish called *kibbi.*

Although it is cooling in energy (best for Pitta types), wheat is a rich, vital, and sweet grain which supports Vata as well as Pitta.

### Cracked Wheat

This split whole kernel of wheat is slightly different from bulgur. The cracked wheat is not precooked or parched in the sun before it is broken. However, both bulgur and cracked wheat may be used interchangeably. Farina is a finely ground wheat kernel that generally is used for breakfast porridge.

### Couscous

This grain is made from semolina, the endosperm of durum wheat. To make couscous, semolina flour is mixed with salted water, then tossed and rubbed into tiny pellets. The pellets are then steamed on a cotton sheet over simmering water until they swell. This step can also be accomplished by steaming the pellets twice over a hot, bubbling pot of stew.

Couscous is native to the diets of Moroccans, Algerians, Tunisians, and Egyptians. In North Africa, the term *couscous* describes a variety of dishes.

### Oats

Of the common grains, oats are among the highest in nutritional value. Samuel Johnson, with much prejudice, defined oats in the English dictionary more than two centuries ago as "a grain which is generally given to horses, but in Scotland supports the people."

Oats are one of the few grains to have been used whole as a breakfast food throughout most of Europe and the United States. In nineteenth-century Scotland, universities observed "Oatmeal Monday"—a day when the parents of poor students gave their children a sack of oatmeal to insure their health through the brutal Scottish winters.

This wonderfully sustaining food is available in many forms today. The whole grain is threshed to remove the inedible husks. The remaining grain, with the bran and germ left intact, is referred to as groats. These groats, or whole kernels, may be further reduced by being split with a sharp steel blade to make steel-cut oats, also called Scottish or Irish oatmeal.

To make old fashioned rolled oats, the groats are slightly softened by steaming and then flattened with steel rollers; this makes for a faster cooking cereal. As a result of intensive processing, dehydrated instant oats, unlike old-fashioned rolled oats, have little nutritive value.

Although heating in energy (best for Vata types) the rich, sweet taste of oats supports Pitta as well as Vata.

### Barley

Known as *jawar,* barley has been cultivated in India since the Vedic period. Once the husk is removed, the remaining grain—referred to as hulled barley—is nutritionally intact. It consists of a layer of germ and protein known as aleurone. In the West, the hulled barley is known as pot or scotch barley. When the aleurone layer is stripped, the ivory colored pearl barley remains. In India, the silken, freshly ground barley flour, which has a low-gluten content, is often mixed with atta, or chapati flour. Barley flour performs like white flour, except it is much more nutrititious and wholesome.

Barley is truly a universal grain that has played a role in most cultures. Until the late 1500s in Europe, loaves of barley bread were more common than loaves of whole wheat. In England, nannies fed barley water to their wards to strengthen their constitution. English women still credit their flawless complexions to the use of barley water. The Japanese make a famous tea from roasted barley called *mugicha,* and Scandinavian cooks make barley into breakfast porridge and dessert puddings. The Chinese stuff cooked ducks with barley and lotus seeds.The Scots use it as a "bottom" for their world-famous whisky, and for nutrition in their thick (and equally famous) barley and leek stew.

Until recently in the United States, more than eighty percent of the barley crop has been used as feed for pigs and cows, with a small amount used for brewing alcoholic beverages.

Barley is best for Pitta types and also supports Kapha types. Although cooling in energy, Kapha does well with this grain due to its dryness.

## Millet

Known as *bajra* in North India and *ragi* in South India, millet is widely harvested from several cereal grasses. The two most popular kinds are finger millet and pearl millet, the kind found most often in natural food stores. Millet is the third most used grain in India, after rice and wheat. It grows well in sandy and poor soil, and in hot, harsh climates, thriving where wheat may be too frail. Freshly ground millet flour is often mixed with other flours into flat breads or mixed with vegetables.

This delicious buff-yellow grain is the most underestimated on earth. It possesses more protein than either oats, rice, or corn and at the same time is a perfect grain for losing weight. In northern India and China, millet is used predominately by the poor, who make delightful thin pancakes, porridge, and pilafs with this regal golden bead. In Africa and Ethiopia, freshly ground millet flour is made into a spongy crepe that forms the basis of a meal. In the United States, millet is used mostly to feed the birds. However, with the recent increase in awareness of the whole foods market, millet is gaining popularity among humans.

Millet is best for Kapha types. If it is cooked softly, it may be used occasionally by Vata types. This grain is heating in energy.

## Rye

Among the grains produced by grasses or cereal grains, rye—along with millet and barley—is sorely underestimated. Rye grows better in cold, wet climates where wheat fares badly. Its rich pungency is best demonstrated in German pumpernickel bread. The Russians and Scandinavians seldom repast without freshly baked slices of dark rye bread. Scandinavian rye crisp bread, or *knache*, a favorite among health food advocates, is baked from unsifted whole rye flour. The English and early New Englanders enjoyed hot whole rye porridge for breakfast, as well as rye pancakes, muffins, biscuits, and popovers. This was before the use of whole grains went out of fashion, due to the unfortunate invention of instant, lifeless, breakfast foods. Rye is also available in its cracked form, which is similar to cracked wheat or steel-cut oats. Through a drying, steaming, and flattening process the rye berries are made into rye flakes, which make a gentle and nutritive breakfast dish. Rye is a deliciously pungent food suited to Kapha types.

## Buckwheat

This edible fruit seed has been used as a cereal grain for centuries in Asia and Europe. A beautiful field of white or pink buckwheat in full bloom is still a common sight in the Himalayas, Russia, China, and Nepal. Related to rhubarb, garden sorrel, and the dock family, buckwheat is known as *kutu* or *phaphra* in India. Much like a wheat berry, buckwheat has a hard outer shell which when removed yields a seed called a groat. In India this is traditionally ground fine and used in a pakora or tempura-style batter, used as a dough for poori (a thin fried chapati), and used for making sweets, such as halva.

When the groats are roasted, they are called *kasha*. In Russian and Jewish cuisines, kasha holds a place of reverence. Kasha varnishkas, or varnitchkas (a combination of kasha and noodles), as well as the blini (a paper thin crepe served hot) have left an indelible mark on universal cuisine. In Japan, soba, a rich tasting noodle made from buckwheat flour, is another great addition to the buckwheat panoply.

Perhaps buckwheat is the only "grain" that held a place of true esteem in Early American cuisine. Mark Twain reportedly became homesick for buckwheat cakes while visiting Europe in the 1870s. Freshly made buckwheat cakes served with pure maple syrup was among the finest of America's first foods.

The groats, whole or crushed, roasted or unroasted, are available through most health food stores. Buckwheat groats are best suited to Kapha types because of their somewhat pungent nature. However, when the groats are mixed with wheat and a natural sweetener, both Pitta and Vata types may indulge occasionally.

## Corn

Native to India and the American continents, corn is a special grain. In India the freshly ground flour is known as *makkai atta*. Low in gluten, it is mixed with whole wheat flour to lend a different texture to flatbreads. Like millet and barley, corn is used mainly by the peasants in rural India. In ancient times, aboriginal tribes depicted the corn goddess as a symbol of fertility for both food and humans. There is no sight holier than a field of rice or a golden field of corn.

Native Americans lived on corn as their main grain. When the English settlers arrived in Virginia in 1607, they found Native Americans eating foods they had never seen before. One of these foods was *rockahominie*, the native word for dried white field corn. The settlers were instructed to soak the dried corn in a wood ash solution to loosen the husk, and then to cook in water until tender. The settlers shortened the name to hominy. Finely ground, this dried corn is called hominy grits.

The Italians began harvesting corn in the mid-seventeenth century. The peasants of rural Italy discovered that the coarsely ground cornmeal made tasty polenta, a porridge made from a variety of grains since Roman times. Corn is planted abundantly in the north of Italy, where corn polenta often replaces the humble bread of the mountain people.

Corn is excellent for Kapha types, and if it is cooked porridge style or fresh as corn on the cob, slathered with organic butter or ghee, an occasional repast of this food will also benefit Vata types.

## Triticale

The newest of grains, triticale is a crossbreed of wheat and rye. Its name is derived from *triticum* and *secale*, the Latin words for wheat and rye, respectively. Since it contains the characteristics of both, triticale may be used in place of either wheat or rye. Although Ayurvedic thinking does not support crossbreeding in general, much less that of different species, the triticale marriage has produced an unusual and pleasant grain.

Triticale can be an occasional food for all types. It is most specifically suitable for Kapha in the summer and fall, for Pitta in the fall and winter, and for Vata in the winter and spring.

## Quinoa

Called the Mother Grain by the Incas, quinoa was first harvested more than three thousand years ago in South America. After the Spanish conquest, the Incas began to harvest European grains and ceased to use their native quinoa for more than four centuries. Quinoa is a distant relative to the beet, spinach, and Swiss chard family. In fact, the leaves of the quinoa plant are cooked and used like spinach.

Like buckwheat, quinoa is technically the fruit of a plant from the Chenopodiaceae family. While quinoa comes in an array of colors—pink, orange, and red—the variety available in the United States is a buff color. The resurgence of this stoic grain affords us many vital nutritients. Quinoa, similar in composition to milk, is the only grain that contains the eight essential amino acids (proteins) in perfect proportion. Some of these eight amino acids, such as lysine, methionine, and cystine, are scarce in most plant sources. Quinoa is sweet, astringent, and pungent, with a heating energy. An excellent grain for Vata and Kapha types, it may also be used occasionally in the fall and winter by Pitta types.

## Amaranth

Amaranth was discovered in the crevices of fallen caves of Mexico. It is believed that this grain was harvested by the indigenous people of Mexico more than six thousand years ago. A relative of the tumbleweed plant, it has similar properties to quinoa but is smaller in size. Amaranth has the highest lysine (an amino acid) content of all grains. Sweet and astringent, with a heating energy, amaranth is excellent for

Vata and Kapha types and may be used occasionally by Pitta types.

## Sorting, Cleaning, and Washing Grains

### Sorting and Cleaning

1. Spread out a clean piece of natural burlap or canvas on a clean kitchen or dining room floor. If these cloths are not available, you may use a shallow, flat basket instead.
2. Place the unwashed grain—at the most a fortnight's worth—in the center of the cloth and squat or sit in a comfortable position.
3. Separate out a few handfuls and sift through to find debris—such as stones, husks, and stems. Place the debris in a container until you can return it to the soil in your yard. While you may invite your family or friends to join you in this activity, be alert, and maintain quiet. Do not allow the children to play with the grain, or fight and become excited. You may also choose this as your still time and perform this sadhana alone.
4. Brush and fold the cleaning cloth and store in a clean place until your next use. Place the sorted grain in a glass jar with a tight-fitting lid and store in a cool, moisture-free location.

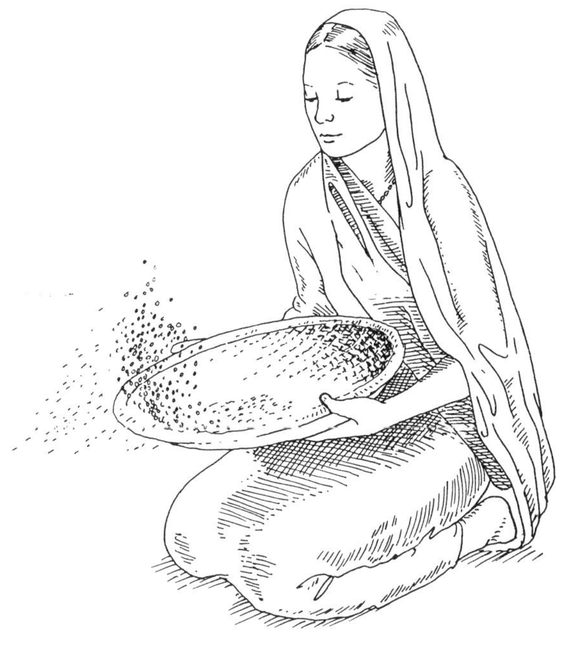

**Woman in Diamond Position Sifting Rice in Straw Basket—Sadhana to Invite Resolve**

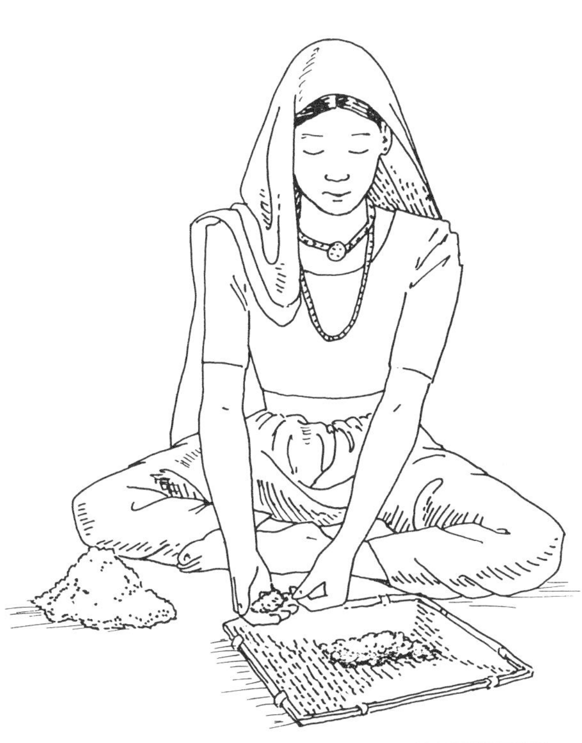

**Woman in Lotus Position Cleaning Grain—Sadhana to Invite Resolve**

### Washing

1. Grains should be washed during meal preparation time and not beforehand. Fill a large bowl with cold water and the amount of rice you need. Massage your hands with the grains and remove any remaining bran or husks that float to the surface.
2. Drain and rinse several times until the water runs clear; follow instructions for soaking or cooking.

## Soaking and Cooking Grains

*Short and medium-grain brown rice, rye and wheat berries, hulled barley, and whole oats:* These grains will benefit from soaking for 3 hours. If you need mildly

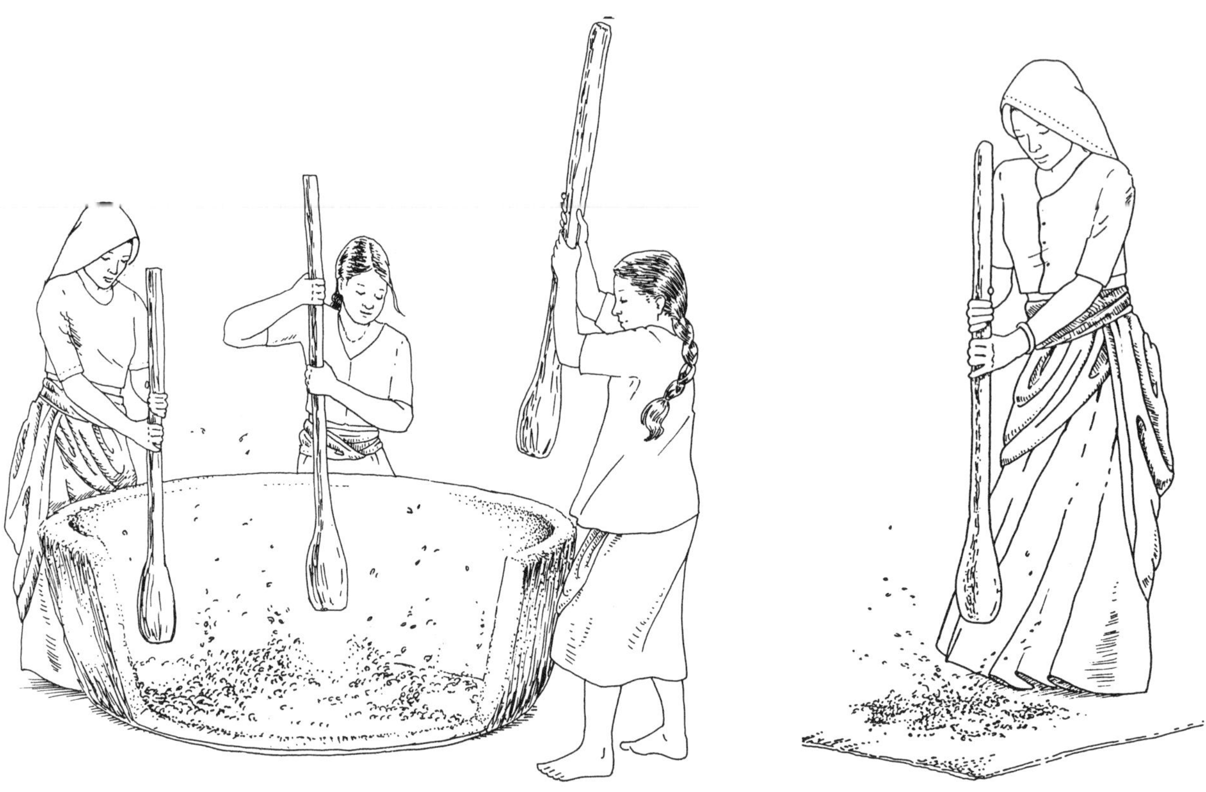

**Rhythmic Pounding:**
**Hulling Grain in Stone Mortar—**
**Sadhana to Invite Harmony of Body, Mind, and Heart**

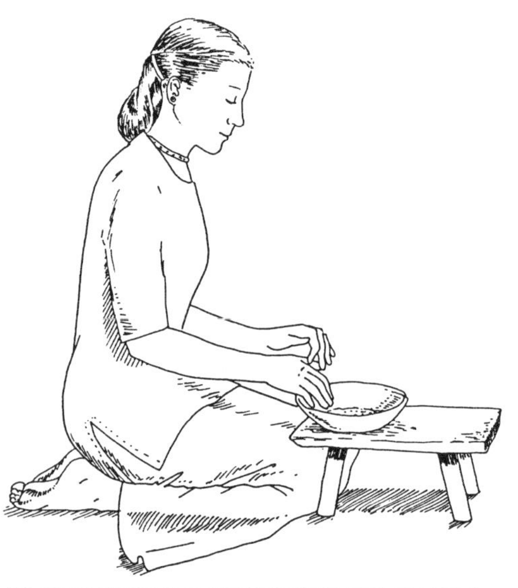

**Woman in Diamond Position**
**Massaging Hand with Grain—**
**Sadhana to Invite Exhilaration**

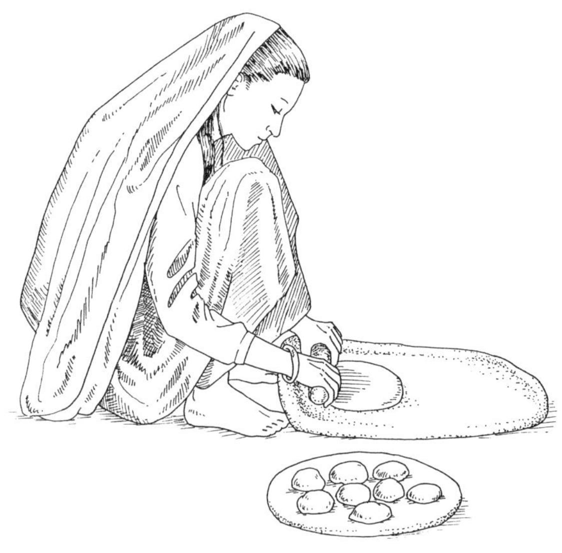

**Woman in Squatting Position**
**Rolling Chapati Dough—**
**Sadhana to Invite Earth's Energy to the Womb**

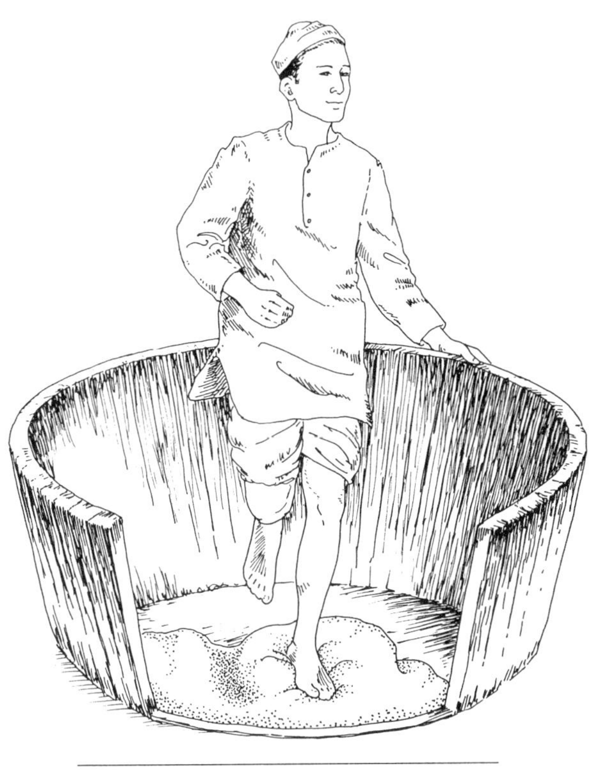

**Kneading Dough with Feet—
Sadhana to Invite Potency**

fermented rice to make Indian pancakes (dosa) or idli (see pages 205 and 206), soak the rice overnight. *Whole wheat and whole oats* may be soaked overnight.

Grains may be cooked in a pressure cooker, or in any of the following types of pots: cast-iron, stainless steel (heavy), clay, or enamelware. Whatever pot you use must have a tight-fitting lid. Among the grains, wheat berries, whole oats, and short- and medium-grain brown rice are best cooked in a pressure cooker (or a heavy cast-iron pot) because of their density. The chart below lists the recommended grains for pressure cooking. Millet, hominy grits, pearl barley, long-grain brown rice, Italian rices, sushi rice, and bulgur may also be pressure cooked for both a firm and porridge-like consistency. Adjust water and cooking time to yield the desired result.

## PRESSURE COOKING CHART (TO 1 CUP GRAIN)

| GRAIN | CUPS WATER | TIME (MINUTES) | CUPS YIELD |
|---|---|---|---|
| Barley, pot | 3 | 40–45 | 3 |
| Barley, grits | 2 1/2 | 20–23 | 3 |
| Corn, dried whole | 4 1/2 | 75–80 | 3 |
| Cracked wheat | 2 1/2 | 25–30 | 2 1/2 |
| Oats, whole groats | 3 | 45 | 3 |
| Oats, steel-cut | 3 1/2 | 30–35 | 3 |
| Rice, short & medium brown | 2 1/4 | 25–30 | 3 |
| Rice, sweet | 2 1/4 | 25–30 | 3 |
| Rye berries | 3 | 45 | 3 |
| Rye, cracked | 3 1/2 | 30–35 | 2 1/2 |
| Triticale, whole berries | 3 | 40–45 | 2 1/2 |
| Wheat berries | 3 | 40–45 | 2 1/2 |

To cook, follow the instructions that accompany your pressure cooker.

## CONVENTIONAL COOKING CHART (TO 1 CUP GRAIN)

| GRAIN | CUPS WATER | TIME (MINUTES) | CUPS YIELD |
|---|---|---|---|
| Amaranth | 2 | 15 | 2½ |
| Barley, pot | 3½ | 50–55 | 3 |
| Barley, pearl | 2½ | 30–35 | 3 |
| Barley, grits | 3 | 30–35 | 3 |
| Buckwheat groats | 2 | 20–25 | 2½ |
| Buckwheat, kasha | 1¾ | 15 | 2½ |
| Corn, whole dried | 5 | 125 | 3 |
| Cornmeal polenta | 4 | 25 | 3 |
| Cornmeal, hominy grits | 4 | 25 | 3 |
| Millet | 3 | 25–30 | 3½ |
| Oats, whole | 3½ | 40–60 | 3 |
| Oats, steel-cut | 4 | 40–45 | 3 |
| Oats, rolled | 1½ | 10 | 2 |
| Quinoa | 2 | 15–20 | 3½ |
| Rice, long-grain brown | 2½ | 35 | 3 |
| Rice, short-grain brown | 2½ | 35–40 | 3 |
| Rice, medium-grain brown | 2½ | 35–40 | 3 |
| Rice, brown basmati | 2½ | 30–35 | 3 |
| Rice, white basmati | 2 | 15–20 | 2½ |
| Rice, wild rice | 2½ | 30–35 | 3 |
| Rice, sweet rice | 2½ | 35–40 | 3 |
| Rice, jasmine | 2 | 15–20 | 2½ |
| Rice, Italian rices | 2¼ | 20–25 | 3 |
| Rice, sushi | 2¼ | 20–25 | 3 |
| Rice, flaked | 1¼ | 5–8 | 2 |
| Rye berries | 3½ | 50–60 | 3 |
| Rye, cracked | 3 | 40–45 | 3 |
| Rye, rolled or flaked | 2 | 15–20 | 2 |
| Triticale, berries | 3½ | 50–55 | 2½ |
| Triticale, flaked | 2 | 15–20 | 2 |
| Wheat berries | 3½ | 50–55 | 2½ |
| Wheat, bulgar | 2 | 30 | 2½ |
| Wheat, cracked | 3 | 35–40 | 2½ |
| Wheat, couscous | 2 | 15 | 3 |
| Wheat, rolled/flaked | 2 | 15–20 | 2 |

To cook: Bring water and grain to a boil and add a pinch of salt. Cover and lower heat to medium low. Allow to simmer gently for the time indicated and serve.

## SADHANAS OF DHAL

The term *dhal* refers to beans, lentils, and dried peas. (It can also refer to a finished dish made with beans.) Dhals have been a vital food to all cultures since the beginning of time. They sustain energy and strength, owing to their high protein content, and yet give a light and cooling feeling to the body, unlike protein obtained from animals.

From the Vedic period, the king of dhal—the mung bean—has been used in a combination with rice called kichadi. This is the single most popular dish in the panoply of Ayurvedic healing and cleansing diets. Long known for their healing capacity, dhals have been used in medicinal plasters and poultices. They are also made in pastes combined with herbal medicines and used in the *svedana* (sweating) and *snehana* (oil massage) therapies, which are part of the panchakarma system of Ayurveda.

Traditionally in India dhal was served with rice and chapati at least once a day. This is still true today. In every culture where grain is found, the legume is sure to soon follow. Spanish rice is served with red beans; sweet rice in Japan is served with aduki beans; soybeans are serve with jasmine rice in Thailand and China; arborio rice is served with cooked dried peas in Italy; white rice is served with black-eyed peas in the United States. The union of these two foods has provided humankind's best sustenance.

Ayurvedically, dhals are the single most important food when it comes to combining the sweet and astringent tastes. While vital to maintaining the health of all body types, dhals are especially nurturing for Pitta and Kapha. The astringent taste helps to dissolve stomach acids and to temper the digestive fires, functions vital to the balancing of the Pitta dosha. The sweet taste of dhals lend a sattvic (calming and harmonious) energy to the mind and moderate the aggressive nature of Pitta.

Because of their astringent action within the body, beans do not contribute to Kapha's weight gain. Rather, the rasa derived from the assimilation of beans in the process of digestion aids in the breakdown of excessive fat and ama gathered in the bodily tissues. The combination of the sweet and astringent tastes provides a rush of stimulation essential to the Kapha type.

Vata types are cautioned to use the smaller beans, such as mung and aduki, and occasionally urad dhal and red lentils. Not only are these types of beans more sweet than astringent in nature, their protein content is more easily assimilated by the Vata types. Vata-nurturing spices, such as cardamom, ginger, black pepper, asafoetida, and cumin, added to a bean dish can counteract the astringency in the beans and alleviate their gas-producing potential.

### Aduki Bean

This bean is also known as adzuki or *feijao.* If mung is the king of beans, this is the queen. A small, reddish-brown bean, aduki is native to Japan and China. In Japan, the aduki is coarsely ground and used as a facial scrub. It leaves the skin glowing and silky. Rich in nutrients, it is considered, like mung, to be a tridoshic bean.

### Chana Dhal

A variety of the small chickpea, which is husked and split. This pale yellow dhal is among the most popular in Indian cuisine. It is roasted or fried for vegetable dishes, ground for chutneys, or fermented and ground with rice for making dosas (Indian pancakes). Best for Pitta and Kapha types, chana may be used occasionally by Vata types.

### Chowla

See Lobya.

### Kabli Chana

Chickpeas or garbanzo beans. Best for Pitta and Kapha types, these beans may be used occasionally by Vata types.

### Kala Chana

A smaller, older variety of the chickpea; it is dark brown. This bean, like the Japanese aduki and Indian mung, is ancient and thus much more potent energetically than other beans. Best for Pitta and Kapha types, these beans may be used occasionally by Vata types.

### Lobya

Black-eyed peas or cow peas. The split dhal is called chowla. Not recommended for Vata types. Best for Pitta and Kapha types.

### Masoor Dhal

This small legume closely resembles the red lentil. Generally it is used hulled and split in North Indian cooking. A relative of toor dhal, when split it is pinkish in color. Best for Pitta and Kapha types, these beans may be used occasionally by Vata types.

### Matar Dhal

The common split peas which are yellow or green.

### Mung Dhal

This dhal has been used since Vedic times. Also known as *masha* and *green gram,* they are available as whole mung (*sabat*), split form without the skin (*mung*), and split form with the skin (*chilke*). Mung is a tridoshic bean.

### Muth

Dew bean. These beans are used fresh, as a vegetable, or dried. They are greenish-brown in color. Muth may be used in any recipe that calls for lentils. Best for Pitta and Kapha types, these beans may be used occasionally by Vata types.

### Navy Beans

These large white beans are exceptionally good in stews and soup. Best for Pitta and Kapha types.

### Rajma Dhal

Kidney beans. These are mostly used in North Indian dhals. They may be used in all chili dishes. Best for Pitta and Kapha types.

### Soybean

Native to India, China, and Japan, the soybean is a medium-sized bean, either white or black in color. Both varieties are high in nutrients and have a cooling energy. The soybean has many derivatives: tofu, soy milk, soy granules. Soy milk is excellent for infants who are born lactose intolerant.

While both Kapha and Pitta types may use this bean, it is tailor-made for the Pitta type because of its cooling energy and high nutritive value. Vata types may indulge in soybean and soybean derivatives occasionally.

### Toovar Dhal

Also known as *toor* or *arhar* dhal, this golden dhal is popular in South Indian cooking. Best for Pitta and Kapha types, these beans may be used occasionally by Vata types.

### Urad Dhal

Urad is an ancient dhal also known as black gram. It is available in whole form (sabat), which is black; in split form without the skin (urad), which is white; or in split form with skin (chilke). Urad is a tridoshic bean.

## *Cleaning, Washing, and Soaking Dhals*

All dhals need to be sorted through to have stems, stones, and debris removed, then washed until the water runs clear. Follow instructions on page 167 for cleaning grains and washing grains.

Soaking times vary greatly for dhals, depending on what type of dish is being prepared and whether a pressure cooker is being used or not. While split peas and dhals do not need soaking, it is helpful to soak whole dhals to reduce their gas-producing qualities. Small legumes are soaked for 2 to 5 hours, medium ones for 5 to 8 hours, and large and hard legumes, overnight. If you do soak them, decrease the cooking time listed below by about 20 percent and use approximately 10 percent less water.

Like grains, dhals may be cooked in a pressure cooker, or in any of the following types of pots: enamel-coated cast iron, stainless steel (heavy), or clay. Whatever pot you use, it must have a tight-fitting lid. Since beans tend to boil over more easily than grains, use a taller pot to cook them in if possible. Whole dhals—such as whole mung, soy, or chickpeas—are best cooked in a pressure cooker or cast-iron pot because of their density. Split dhals, such as split peas, mung, or urad, may be cooked

## PRESSURE COOKING CHART (FOR 1 CUP DHAL)

| DHAL | CUPS WATER | TIME (MINUTES) | CUPS YIELD |
|---|---|---|---|
| Small whole beans (mung, aduki, urad, muth) | 2 | 25–30 | 3 |
| Medium whole beans (Navy, soy, lima, black-eyed peas) | 2½ | 40–45 | 3 |
| Large, hard beans (rajma, chickpea, kala chana) | 3½ | 65–75 | 3 |

## CONVENTIONAL COOKING CHART (FOR 1 CUP DHAL)

| DHAL | CUPS WATER | TIME (MINUTES) | CUPS YIELD |
|---|---|---|---|
| Small whole beans (mung, aduki, urad, muth) | 2½ | 35–40 | 3 |
| Small split beans | 2 | 20–25 | 2½ |
| Medium whole beans (navy, soy, lima, black-eyed peas, turtle) | 3 | 55–65 | 3 |
| Medium split beans (chana, split peas) | 2½ | 25–30 | 2½ |
| Large, hard beans (rajma, chickpea, kala chana) | 4½ | 120 | 3 |

without pressure. Adjust the water amount and cooking time to yield the desired result.

### *Sprouting*

The seed or grain is considered holy by the ancient peoples of all cultures. Each grain carries the potency of being the source of thousands of seedlings. When sprouted, it loses the ability to flourish into its full nature and produce many more seeds. For this reason, it is considered inauspicious to sprout grains.

In Vedic times, sprouting was not done—this practice has only gained popularity in recent times. However, since there is a such need in today's world for high potency minerals, a minimal amount of sprouting is acceptable. In attempting to honor the ancient value of grains, I recommend sprouting only legumes, such as mung or aduki. (For instructions on how to sprout, see page 195.)

## SADHANAS OF SPICES

In ancient times, the energies between human beings, food, and the earth were continually being revitalized on an endless wheel of exchange. The ancients recognized the sadhanas of sowing, reaping, and preparing foods to be highly conducive to inviting memory of the earth. Early humans cleansed their energies and

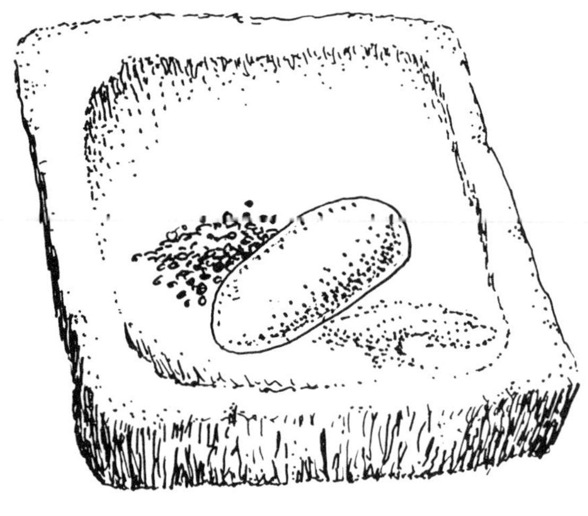

**Spice Grinding Stone with Small Rubbing Stone**

solidified their inherent bonding with nature through these practices.

The myriad of spices found throughout the world creates great and endless opportunities for stirring cognitive memory. The ancient grinding stone enabled humans to meld the spices and to work them in a back and forth motion with both hands. Stone grinding on stone stirs the memory and smell of the earth. The scent of each spice triggers a specific cognitive state of awareness with nature. With the invention of hand grinding tools, although the fragrance remained, the essential connection of the hand on a stone from the earth was lost. The grinding stone and the mortar and pestle are still the two best ways for us to grind our spices.

The motion of grinding soothes the space/air dosha of Vata. Each spice seed has a unique sound as it cracks. The life of the earth/water dosha—Kapha—comes alive with the rich aroma of each spice released during the grinding process. The sublime colors along with the calming motion of the hands working together bring an aliveness to the fire dosha of Pitta. Altogether, with these sadhanas of grinding and smelling spices, we garner the forces of all three doshas into quietude and communion with nature.(See Vedic Herbs, Spices, and Accents, pages 295–310, for spice recipes.)

## OILS*

True to the Sanskrit term *sneha,* which means "fat" as well as "lavish love," oil provides the essential lubricating love to the dhatus. Some people, such as Kapha types, are born with plentiful love in terms of natual bodily oils, and they need less lubrication from foods. Others, such as the Vata types, have the least amount of bodily love and need a profusion of warmth and lubrication from nature as well as from foods. Pitta types are endowed with intense, hot bodily oils from birth and need less lubrication and more coolant to balance their natures.

All foods contain natural oils to varying degrees. In addition to their warming and lubricating attributes, oils fortify, build tissues, soothe bodily membranes, and to some extent activate the digestive fire.

Oils should never be used excessively by any of the body types, although Vata types are allowed ample amounts for their cooking, bathing, and massaging needs. According to the density, taste, and energy of the different kinds of oil, each body type is allowed a good and variable selection from which to choose.

In order to accomodate all body types, sunflower oil—and occasionally sesame and corn—are the primary oils used throughout the recipes in this book. However, it is recommended that you use a variety of cooking oils that are suitable to your personal constitution.

Do not use oils that have been hydrogenated, commercially processed, refined, treated with coloring agents, or mixed with other types of oil. Quality oils can be purchased at health food, gourmet, and Indian and Oriental food stores.

Store all of your oils in a cool, dark place. Use them one month after opening, as oils turn rancid easily.

* Certain oils, such as walnut, sesame, almond, olive, and coconut, may appear in the regressive category of the food charts for some of the body types. In the above discussion, concessions are made for sparing use. While this cannot be easily generalized in the context of the charts, because of their healing qualities these oils can be used to advantage from time to time.

### Almond Oil

A delicate, sweet oil pressed from almond nuts. Rich and warming in character, it is used in many Ayurvedic health formulas and massage therapies for Vata types. It should be used as an accent rather than a daily cooking oil. Best for Vata types; Kapha types may use sparingly.

### Avocado Oil

A rich, thick oil pressed from the pulp of the avocado fruit. It is warming in character and, like olive oil, lends itself as a base to salad dressings and herbal pasta sauces. Best for Vata types; Pitta types may use sparingly.

### Canola Oil

A recently popular oil pressed from rape seeds. It is light and soothing in character, closely resembling sunflower oil. Recommended for regular use by all body types.

### Coconut Oil

An oil extracted from coconut flesh and used extensively in South Indian cuisine (where it is known as *noriya ka tel*). While it is the most cooling of all oils, it is also very high in fat. Pitta and Vatta types may use occasionally.

### Corn Oil

A golden-colored oil pressed from the germ of the maize grain. Of all the oils, it has the longest history of use. It is light and drying in nature and has a high smoking point, making it good for deep-frying. Best for Kapha types as a routine oil; Vatta and Pitta types may use sparingly.

### Mustard Oil

An oil pressed from either the amber-colored or the black (purplish-brown) variety of mustard seeds. It is used extensively in East and North Indian cuisines (where it is known as *sarson ka tel*), and has been valued since ancient times in Ayurvedic snehana (oil massage) therapies. Highly pungent in taste and heating in nature, it is a traditional ingredient in chutneys and pickles. Best for Kapha types, as an accent rather than a daily cooking oil; Vata types may also use as an occasional cooking oil by first heating to near-smoking point to decrease pungency.

### Olive Oil

A rich, thick, and mildly pungent oil pressed from ripe olives. Introduced by Mediterranean, Spanish, and Italian cuisines, it has gained tremendous popularity throughout the world. Olive oil is available in a wide range of colors, densities, and qualities. The greenish virgin or extra-virgin varieties may be used, unheated, by both Vata and Kapha types in salad dressings, herbal pasta sauces, and chutneys. The blond-colored varieties may be used occasionally for cooking by Vata types and sparingly (because of its richness) by Kapha types.

### Safflower Oil

A light and mild-flavored oil pressed from the seeds of the safflower plant, or the flowering saffron thistle. Because of its high smoking point, it is good for deep-frying. May be used occasionally by all body types.

### Sesame Oil

A rich, thick, and warm oil pressed from sesame seeds. It has been used since ancient times in both China and India (where it is known as tila oil or gingelly oil). It is available in a light amber color, pressed from the buff-colored seeds, or a deep brown when pressed from the black seeds. When pressed from roasted seeds, it is a deep tan color. Sesame oil is used extensively in Ayurvedic medicine and is considered the main cooking oil for Vata types. May also be used sparingly by Kapha and Pitta types.

### Sunflower Oil

A golden oil pressed from the seeds of the sunflower

plant. It is hailed as the best all-round oil for all body types, and especially for the Pitta types because of its gentle, cooling nature and mildly sweet taste.

### Walnut Oil

A deep amber-colored oil pressed from walnuts. It is delicate, nutty, and aromatic and may be used sparingly by all types to accent salads, dresings, greens, and desserts. Like almond oil, it is best for Vata types.

## THE SADHANA OF MILK

*And it will come to pass in that day . . . the hills shall flow with milk.*

*Joel 3:18*

*The cows yield butter and milk inexhaustible for thee set on the highest summit.*

*Rig Veda, IX 2.7*

I grew up in an idyllic village not far from the sea. In the still afternoons, women gathered on their kitchen verandas and sifted through grains and dhals, or picked nits off the hair of their children. The young ones gamboled under the relentless sun as the cool breezes wafted over the surface of the murky marsh waters. The occasional half-clad farmer with his sickle and hoe dotted the dirt roads on his way home. The lithe, ebony milkman, whose feet were always in flight, would arrive before tea and fill the milk buckets that were waiting for him on the landing below. The milk was delivered, buff-colored and foaming, within the hour of the milking. It was never preboiled. Milk was a vital and living food for as long as the ancestry could remember. The cows were gentle and happy. They grazed in the green pastures of fertile and rich land. They roamed by instinct, with their own rhythm. No one questioned why they should seek shelter from the blazing sun, or why they sat and gazed with those stupendous lotus eyes. It was the norm to find them sleeping in the middle of the roads. Bicycles and other vehicles careened around them until they were covered with dust. No child felt threatened by the presence of the cows. They were part of the dynamism of our life. A field without grazing cows would have been inconceivable in those evanescent afternoons.

We lived with a large extended family. Among father's many trades was his priesthood. His father, who was from a prestigious lineage of Brahmins, was one of the many transported by the British from North India to British Guiana. Most of the villages along the Corentyne Coast became little replicas of our motherland. The values of sadhanas, still intact in India during the time of my grandparents' migration, were maintained with stoic observation. They were the heart of the tradition. Millions of hearts were broken in that relatively short period of exodus. These ancient customs were the only salve for the bleeding journeymen.

Every day the milk was boiled three times and the cream was removed to make fresh yogurt, buttermilk, and butter. Ghee, the elixir of Vedic foods and an important carrier of herbs and medicines in Ayurvedic remedies, was made by a process of heating the fresh sweet butter. On special occasions, the milk would be ordered twice daily for preparation of ceremonial foods for the various *pujas,* the ceremonies of worship. Occasionally, fresh goat's milk would be ordered for a young child or for a special health condition. Even the most rare tiger's milk was used from time to time for a serious health problem. The tenets of the Vedas were practiced effortlessly by the village elders. These sadhanas were handed down and perpetuated until the country was swallowed in a miasma of political wars following her independence from Britain.

Years later, during my stay at an ashram in Pennsylvania, I was taking my daily walk past a cow pasture. I saw for the first time what I had for so long felt in my heart: the abiding grief of these cows. I have walked through the valleys and shadows of death twice in my life and never have I witnessed such gargantuan grief. How can we in the West hope to rationalize or address the present state of unwholesomeness of milk as a food? The primary issue we must confront is the holocaust of these animals.

In the last two decades, many humane voices have risen in an attempt to eliminate the brutalities to which cows are subjected in the dairy and beef industries. These crimes against life and freedom are pervasive and tenacious. They deeply afflict the natural innocence of lives and lands not only in the United States, but also in the poor countries that have been contracted to farm meat and milk for U.S. consumption. The world continues to be influenced by actions performed in this unique country, actions that deny the excellence and freedom of spirit embodied in her national symbol, the bald eagle.

## *The Sacred Cow*

In the Vedic tradition each animal is considered to be sacred, for it holds the complex memory of life on earth. This memory is safely stored by all species that do not expend breath unnecessarily. Because of the willful and breath-consuming nature of humans, we are the most porous containers of remembrances. The animals are a living reflection of our memory banks. They were created to provide reminders of our full potentiality. More than mere symbols of memory, they are the embodiment of memory. Through the reverent ken of the ancients, the customs of paying tribute to the animals began and were perpetuated through timeless eons.

The shamanic cultures also observed animals by chase, capture, and sacrifice, and identified themselves by the name essences of the animals. They recognized the manifest spirit of the animals to be the direct reflection of universal memory. They learned to know the earth through their humble relationship with the animals. They celebrated cleverness through the spider, gentle cunning through the fox, the terrors of the dark nature through the bear, and the numinous beauty of the earth through the totality of the bison. The movements and appearances of animals clarified their deepest quest for spiritual unity to the earth. Each animal possessed its own rhythm of grace, movement, and self-nourishing instincts. These are the qualities that the human has yet to learn of its innate nature.

In Sanskrit, every name portends the cosmic meaning of the bearer's relationship to the earth. The cow is called *go*. *Go* is also the name for the earth and the holy scriptures. Lord Krishna was called Gopala, the one who protects the cow. "Protecting the cow" is a common, and ancient, expression used to infer the protection of the scriptures, the nurturing of the land, and the celebration of the cow, who is the manifest keeper of the memory of the earth's spiritual dharmas.

The cow and the elephant have been the most celebrated and adorned animals in India. The cow is the keeper of the scriptural memory, and the elephant is the holder of the first memory of plants and herbs on the planet. If either became extinct, we would not be able to maintain the memory necessary for the survival of the earth. We can be certain, however, that while we keep these sacred lives in their present miasma of pain and grief, it does not bode well for us. The degree of each animal's suffering is paralleled by the agony of the earth and by human pain.

The insidious suffering of the cows is directly reflected in the diseases of our food body. It is no coincidence that every symptom the cow suffers in her captivity is mirrored in the present condition of the human species.

In the agribusiness of dairy and beef farming, the cattle wallow in freezing mud and excrement during the ice-cold rains, they are rarely provided with shade or shelter, and they are held in the permanence of darkness and death without mobility, sunlight, or space, just to inhibit energy output and increase fat for the butcher. They are pumped with more than two thousand different chemicals, antibiotics, and hormones, in addition to stimulants and poisons such as arsenic. The diet of a milk cow consists of highly concentrated, roughage-less, mold-filled feed with chemical condiments of these antibiotics, pesticides, nitrate fertilizers, and herbicides.

The system victimizes animals, farmers, the world community, the land, and, in the last analysis, the perpetrators themselves. The mental agony of the cow is inherited by all those who drink the polluted ama, which used to be milk; we suffer the same conditions of fear, isolation, restlessness, and melancholia. The cows' subtle memories are blackened by their captivity, directly effecting the loss of our own memories of spiritual dharmas. The plagues of hyperactivity, discombobulation, muscle pain, digestive disorders, heart disease, abdominal cramps, excess gas, constipation, bloating, and atherosclerosis in humans are the result of the Vata dosha going mad in the cow's body. Ulcerations, rashes, hives, fevers, infertility, poor absorption of nutrients, liver abscesses, and violent deaths are directly linked to the vitiated metabolic dosha of the cow.

The cow's essential nature is nurturing, solid, stoic, and providing—like a mother. As her pure Kapha nature becomes distorted, her diseases filter into the human system and create havoc. Our present epidemics of respiratory ailments, sinusitis, asthma, tonsillitis, and obesity are only some of the symptoms of the cow's betrayed Kapha condition.

The veal calf has the most cruel fate of all. It is taken within days of its birth and placed in a dark wooden stall. It cannot lie down or turn around. It is fed only iron-deficient liquid gruel and is chained to the stall to prevent it from licking its urine and excrement, which it would instinctively do to supplement its iron needs. It is slaughtered after sixteen weeks. Not surprisingly, one out of ten of these calves dies in confinement. All of this gross cruelty is inflicted in order to produce a white and lean meat. The concurrent diseases of anorexia, bulimia, and iron deficiency run parallel to the same diseased state of the veal calves. The highly carcinogenic substances used in the animals' feed have also seeped into the reproductive system of humans. Infertility and cervical cancer have increased rapidly as the atrocities of agribusiness go unquelled.

We are linked to the animals. The pain of the calves is felt through our own birthing of life. As we drink from the well of malaise, we contaminate our dhatus and feed this ama to our newborns through our breast milk. Recent studies in Britain and Australia show that the child's allergic reactions to the mother's milk relates directly to the mother's consumption of commercial quality milk. We cannot wait for scientific research to unfold these facts one at a time. We need to sit within ourselves and observe what goes against the grain of nature, see how quickly it seeps into our bodies and psyches, and know that we cannot continue to drink from this well, nor repast from this meat. We must realize that the cows' milk is the milk of the eternal mother, and that their flesh is our flesh. We have to acknowledge that the pearls of cognitive memory are held by the animals so that we may continue to develop our own stupendous potential as love embodied in a life form. We need to remember that if we allow the abuse, we are also guilty, and that if the animals lose all cognition, we will not be able to continue.

*The purified soma juices have flowed forth mixing with curds and milk. They are cleansed in the waters.*

*Rig Veda IX 1.24*

*[You] are become such as have need of milk, and not of strong meat.*

*Hebrews 5:12*

This pale and polluted fluid we call milk—steeped in human greed and ignorance and squeezed from the udders of intense anguish—is not the milk that flows from the earth's bosom. Pure unadulterated milk is the primal food of sattva, of peace and calm. It is mentioned in the Vedas as the first food, along with grains and fruits. This food is used to build the dhatus of a growing body and also to buffer the acids and hormonal activities of the mature body. The health problems caused by food in India today are due to the excessive use of milk, sugars, and oils, and to the more recent infiltration of chemical pesticides and herbicides into her livestock feed. For centuries, pure milk from healthy and happy cows was consumed in India, Europe, and Scandinavia without the present epidemic of diseases caused by the polluted milk we have been drinking for several decades.

The Vedas divide foods into three main categories for human consumption. The first consists of foods that penetrate the earth, such as plants, vegetables, fruits, roots, herbs, flowers, and so on. The second group is made up of substances such as minerals, which are derived from within the earth. The final group consists of foods that come from the animal kingdom. Milk, as well as meat and honey, belong to the animal group. Ayurveda recommends small portions of organic meat for the Vata type. The rules of hunting and killing the animal, practiced by the native peoples, were very specific and detailed. Since we are no longer observing these, I do not recommend the use of any animal meat as food, not even for the Vata types. Similarly, the milk recommended as food or medicine was organic and was produced in a manner harmonious with nature. Unless we observe the natural order of organic farming for milk, we cannot drink this food either. Of the three animal food groups, only honey has remained uncontaminated. Humans have been unable to exert power over the bees, thanks to the precocious nature of these insects, and thus the integrity of honey is protected. We do, however, misuse honey. It is a potent food, and we need only a small amount of it in our diet. It is most beneficial for Kapha and Vata types, since it is warming and cossets the cold natures of both these types. It is too strong for the Pitta type and turns to acid in the intense fire of Pitta's metabolism. Likewise, honey becomes toxic when transformed by heat. It should never be cooked.

Even though in earlier times the meat of animals was used with regard for and observation of nature's law, I believe that the time for the hunt and kill has passed. Early humans pursued the chase not only to feed themselves but also to discover their full potential. They lived among the animals, honored them, challenged and conquered them, to learn about nature and to reign supreme as a species. The meat of an animal is a highly rajasic food, a food which was used to build bulk, potency, and verve for a demanding and strenuous life. With the advent of a maturing planet and species, we have become capable of consciousness and knowledge by observation. We no longer need to hunt or to kill in order to recognize our nature.

The time and space in which we live today call for the character of sattva and not rajas. Sattva is the art of living gently on the earth. We have arrived at a time when the consequences of our collective consciousness are becoming more evident, a time for every human on the planet to raise his or her consciousness with great rapidity. For this reason, I maintain that milk—the most sattvic of foods—is very important for the planet. The quantity and quality of milk must be examined and set right. A small portion of milk goes a long way, and it must be organic milk, from happy cows and goats.

While the condition of a healthy and peaceful life depends foremost on the awareness of each person, food is necessary to help us remember our connection to every aspect of the earth. Each food serves a different purpose in the files of cognitive memory. Many nations have survived with healthy food bodies without drinking cow's milk. They have used the milk of the grains, legumes, and nuts instead. We do not have to share in the bounty of the cow's pure milk to know the scriptural dharmas and peaceful secrets of the earth or to remain free of disease. But when we do, we sustain memory, and the faculty of peace in the human heart is helped and nourished.

When we look at cultures that are presently lactose intolerant, we find two dominant factors at work. First, a nation that has not used milk as a food for many centuries, or even generations, will develop a normal intolerance to lactose. Second, it has been demonstrated that those who benefit most from a particular food will be the first to become grossly intolerant of that food if it has been tampered with. In the case of milk, it is the air and fire people who are now becoming lactose intolerant, and these are the very types who would normally fare exceedingly well with this food. This rejection is caused by the chemical poisons in milk that eventually kill the intestines' ability to produce lactose. The adverse reactions of Vata and Pitta types are experienced by their intestinal and gastric organisms, which are highly sensitive to the poisons in a food that was once vital to their health.

As we get older, our production of lactose decreases. The digestive system changes to accommodate more complex forms of food transmuted by fire. When we cease to drink milk altogether, the body decreases its production of lactose to minute percentages. When we are healthy and continue to drink good quality milk, the intestines continue to produce sufficient amounts of lactose to aid the digestion of milk.

In Ayurveda, milk is highly recommended for the Pitta, or fire type, whose natural aggression and intensity need to be soothed. A Vata, or wind type, should also use pure milk, since the wind dosha is harsh and depleting. Milk is a highly anabolic food, and Vata needs it to build body tissue, plasma, muscle, and fat, and to buffer the nervous system. On the other hand, Kapha, the water type, already has a tendency to body bulk and to respiratory vulnerabilities and thus does not need mucus-forming milk.

Kapha types, who will not generally use milk as a food, will not display a dramatic intolerance for lactose, since their organisms are not dependent on that food for their nourishment. They may demonstrate many other negative side effects, but not one of outright intolerance. Yet the Pitta types, who need milk to buffer their gastric fire and high acidity, will develop an active and positive dependency on this food, and will also react with great rapidity and despair if it becomes contaminated.

It is not unusual to find fire types who do not like to lower their level of intensity and thus will not use this sweet coolant. We can actually regulate our levels of aggression or peacefulness by the use of pure milk. It is also not unusual to find water types who choose to inundate their bodies with milk and, thus, reinforce their natural state of bulk to the point of lethargy. Every food has a quantitative and qualitative application. If we use less or more than we need, we dull our primal cognition. It is all a matter of discretion and balance. The rule of the good earth is simple. The very food which is necessary nectar to the system will turn to poison when it is polluted. Milk, like honey, has a complex energy formation. Both foods are, by nature, highly susceptible. When honey is cooked or used in excess, it becomes toxic in the body. When milk is combined with salty, pungent, or animal foods, it becomes poisonous to the system. Certainly the contaminated milk of today is one of the most damaged of all foods. The extent of disease resulting from its consumption is far more devastating than we can see.

When we question the use of pure milk as an authentic food, we must clarify the facts. The present epidemic is caused by the fact that milk has been bombarded by an artillery of contaminants. Each food has a vital memory, and its inherent DNA is connected to the earth. It transmits its quota of memory to each life that feeds on it. Every system has its grace, and when we step on it, it will bite us. In the present case of milk, we have been fatally bitten by the serpent herself.

The minds and bodies of the fire and air humans throughout the planet are well served by pure milk. But no one will be served by milk which has been poisoned. When the milk flows from the hills today, it will be because we have called for all the buckets of poisoned milk to be emptied. The call will be to free all the animals in bondage and allow them to graze peacefully for their remaining time. The call will be to free the farmers and reinstate their dignity. The call will be for compassion and fraternity in a new time when the rural and organic land rises again as animals live within their nature. Then we can hope for grace and peace within the human spirit.

## *A Healing Food*

Although I cannot give an accurate date of the first usage of milk, it appears to have preceded the Vedic period. The Upanishads and most religious scriptures on earth are replete with mention of milk as a food for humans. Because of the *sattvic* nature of milk in its original state, it has been used widely, but not wisely, through the ages. There have been many changes in our universe. As a collective species, we are no longer in the state of infancy. As a result, the use of milk has to be redefined. The Vedic guidelines advised that milk should never be used with foods such as vegetables, fish, meat, or salt, nor should it be used with meals as an accompanying beverage. The indications have also been specific: Milk is used to cool agni (fire), to calm the mind, to feed pregnant women, to offer in devotion to the Lord, and to feed babies. It helps the human system to transmute its activity and aggression into remembrances of an embryonic universe whose motion is to attain liberation and eternal love.

Milk is a potent nectar. All other milks—from grains, beans, dried or cooked fruits, and nuts—mimic the nature of this original nectar. As a teaspoon of honey is considered the healthy average per day for each person, so is a cup of pure, organic milk per day the proper amount. Milk should not be used in cooking or to make cheeses. It may be combined with dried or cooked fruits in the form of a milk drink or a sweet dessert. It should not be excessively boiled. It is a potion best drunk cool or warm, by itself. It becomes an excellent vehicle for medicines, herbs, and spices.

My reasons for defending milk as an important food are not to encourage its use in quantity, or to suggest that the gruesome liquid that is commercially available is an acceptable food. Its use should be tailored, in keeping with the original intent and according to scriptural authority.

We need the memory of milk in our bodies in order to maintain a sattvic, or peaceful, nature as humans. We therefore have to protect the animals that produce this potent food. The earth offers us *soma*, symbolic of the nectar of the gods, from the bark of the maple tree, from the coconut, from the fruit, from the grain, from the bee, from the cow, from the buffalo, from the goat, and from the tiger. We cannot serve the earth with grace and fullness if we allow the cows and other animals to become defunct. If we curtail their instincts and throw their milk away, we are aiding the demise of one of earth's natural functions.

The recipes in this book contain very small quantities of milk, mostly in the brews and beverages. If organic milk cannot be obtained, do not use commercial milk. Milk from nuts, grains, or soybeans may be substituted. I suggest the use of a small amount of ghee in cooking. It is more potent than milk because of its transmutation with fire. The recipe for ghee was handed down by the gods themselves and is mostly for medicinal use. Remember, though, that all foods in Ayurveda are considered medicinal.

Butter, known as *makhan*, should not be used for cooking. It is to be used fresh for the fortification of the dhatus during the cold or rainy seasons, and especially by Vata and Pitta types. Yogurt, known as *dadhi* or *dahi*, is the angel of health. A small quantity of it as part of a main meal activates assimilation. It encourages the growth of benign lactobacillus bacteria in the intestines and helps to destroy harmful bacteria in the system. The lactic acid content aids the digestion of calcium and phosphorus in the body. Yogurt may be sweetened for Pitta types. Vata may add appropriate spices and Kapha may use occasionally, adding herbs and diluting with water. Yogurt serves a different purpose than pure milk. It is almost fully digested in the system within an hour. We cannot blame the epidemic of yeast infections, candida, and so on, on the use of pure yogurt. The unwholesome imitations of yogurt now widely available are loaded with fillers, gels, gums, and cellulose, that destroy the original benefits of yogurt. Decades of use of these unhealthy products have created havoc in the internal bodily systems of the entire planet. Lactose malfunction and yeast malignancy are mostly due to the poisons used and to the lack of cognizance with which dairy products are cultivated and prepared. A pure organic yogurt always boasts a creamy top layer called *malai*. It is one of the most exquisite tastes a human may experience. The bulk of a cow or buffalo is evidence of milk's building capacity. The milk of the lithe and supple goat is much more pungent. That is why goat's milk is recommended for occasional use by the Kapha type.

Even the homeland of the Vedas is losing its sadhana, its wholesome connection to the knowledge of earth. Recently, India has submerged itself in the excessive use of milk in every conceivable kind of food. A potent food that is meant to remain a subtle part of our physical diet should never be abused, and milk is the most abused food in the world today. Each food has its specific quantitative use. We must seek to learn this vital secret of life. No food is meant to be used as a mono-diet—not even grains, and definitely not milk. Cheese was never part of the Vedic culture because it incorporates the use of two incompatible elements, milk and salt. The farthest acceptable departure from milk's sweet taste was found in yogurt, where a mellow sour taste was induced to help assimilate bodily minerals. Wholesome combinations and variety are the Vedic secret to good health. These healthful quantities and varieties are recommended in the Ayurvedic food energetics sections.

Milk contains the calming energies of the moon, as opposed to the nature of most foods, which bear the vivacious influence of the sun. It is meant to be used with discretion, qualitatively and quantitatively. Use only organic milk that comes from a healthy cow on a rural farm. The cow produces milk after birthing her calf in a natural cycle. She produces enough for her calf, who nurses for approximately four months, and continues to produce milk for an additional three to four months. The extra portion of milk is to be used by humans. For Pitta and Vata types, the equivalent of one glass per day is recommended. Kapha types should not use cow's milk. Pitta will mostly use cool milk during the summer season to buffer the acids produced by the heat's natural pungency. Vata types will use warm milk to build their immunity, fortify their nervous system, and build muscular and tissue strength through the depleting fall and rainy seasons. Milk may be used by mothers (all three doshas) who are breast-feeding. All children may use the equivalent of a glass of milk per day, unless the child is lactose intolerant. Be especially discerning with the use of milk if you have not used it for a long period or if your ancestors did not use it.

Because of the immense tampering with our foods, the very types who would otherwise benefit from certain foods are now becoming allergic to those foods. The excessive use of antibiotics in our culture has brought on a high incidence of candida yeast and vaginitis in many Pitta women. Thus, wheat, which is the primary grain for fire people, cannot be used by them because of the proliferation of yeast in their bodies. Similarly, the predominantly Vata and Pitta people are now the ones who—as we have said—are becoming lactose intolerant. The original intent of nature was to provide milk as a salve to regulate the digestive fires of Pitta and to boost the anabolic processing of Vata.

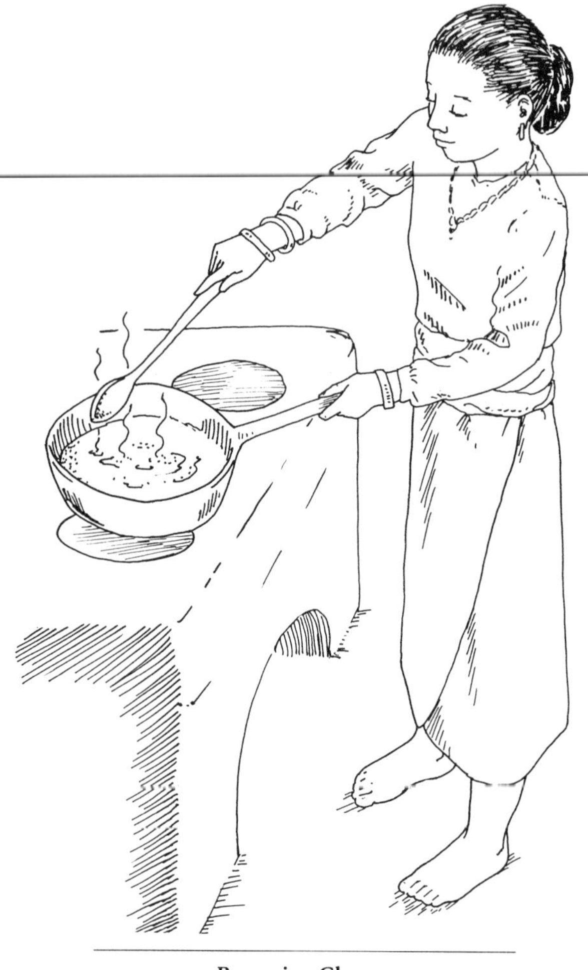

**Preparing Ghee—**
**Sadhana to Induce Sattvic Mind**

## *Milk Products Recipes*

### Ghee (ghrta, sarpi)

*It is promotive of memory, intelligence,*
*vital fire, semen, vital essence (ojas), kapha, and fat.*
*It is curative of Vata, Pitta, fever and toxins.*
*Charaka*

Ghee is one of the most ancient and sattvic foods known. Used judiciously, it is ideal for cooking as it does not burn unless heated excessively. It synergizes with the food nutrients and nourishes the bodily constituents. It also serves as a base for herbal ointments to treat burns, skin rashes, and other such conditions. Ghee is good for all doshas and is a specific for Pitta. Minimal use is recommended for Kapha types.

Ghee keeps indefinitely without refrigeration, as the elements that cause butter to spoil have been removed. Just remember to keep it covered and free from water or any other contaminants. Always dip into your ghee jar with a clean spoon.

Maintain a clean appearance and calm mind while preparing your ghee. This is one of the most healing food sadhanas when performed with grace.

**1 lb raw, unsalted organic butter**
**heavy stainless steel frying pan**
**1 stainless steel spoon**

Sterilize the storage jar, pan, and a spoon in advance by filling with (or immersing in) boiling water. Cook the butter gently over moderate heat for approximately 10 to 15 minutes. Allow the foam that surfaces during the heating process to settle on the bottom of the pan as sediment. Watch carefully to avoid burning and stir occasionally. When the ghee begins to boil silently, with only a trace of air bubbles on the surface, it is done. Allow to cool and pour ghee into a clean container, making sure that sediment remains on bottom of the saucepan.*

## Fresh Butter (makhan)

**2 quarts milk**
**1 heavy stainless steel pot**
**1 stainless steel spoon**
**1 cool clay or enamel coated cast-iron pot**

Sterilize all of the above equipment by filling with (or immersing in) boiling water. Bring milk to a boil and allow it to cool; bring it to a boil two more times. Skim cream off top and place it in a covered pot at 60 degrees for one week. (In India it is kept in an earthen pot known as a *ghara.*) Store remaining milk in a cool place.

Place cream into a large wooden or stainless steel bowl and whip briskly with a whisk until it thickens. (In India butter is whipped with several chopsticks tied together by strings.) When butter begins to emerge and separate into flakes, add two handfuls of crushed ice, which will make it lumpy. Firmly mold butter with your hands, allowing the buttermilk to separate. When no more buttermilk remains, rinse the butter with ice cold water. If you are not going to go on to make ghee, add a few pinches of fine rock salt, if desired. Garnish butter with fresh herbs, according to type, just before serving. Make fresh butter as needed, or every fortnight.

* The sediment may be taken as a snack: Vata and Pitta types may take it mixed with 1/2 teaspoon of brown sugar; Kapha types may also use it occasionally, with no sugar.

## Fresh Yogurt (dadhi)

**2 quarts milk**
**6 tbs plain (organic) yogurt (as starter)**
**2 stainless steel saucepans**
**1 long stainless steel spoon**
**thermometer**

Sterilize one heavy saucepan by filling with boiling water. Heat milk over medium-low heat until it comes to a boil. Stir constantly to avoid sticking or burning. Allow the milk to boil for 15 minutes, until it has reduced by one-eighth and is fairly thick. Set aside to cool until it reaches about 118 degrees F. on thermometer.

Sterilize second saucepan and spoon. When milk cools to 115 degrees F., pour 1 cup into newly sterilized pan. Add starter (be sure it contains acidophilus culture—Brown Cow brand is good) to 1 cup of warm milk and whip until smooth. When remaining milk has reached 112 degrees F. add it to starter mixture and blend with long spoon.

Cover pan with a clean heavy cotton cloth and quickly put yogurt in a warm place, 90 to 110 degrees F. If temperature is too warm or too cool, yogurt will not take. An oven with a gas pilot light is an ideal place; the best temperature is 100 degrees F.

Allow yogurt to sit for 6 to 7 hours. If it is not firm enough, allow to sit for a few hours more. Remove and keep in a cool place. Use yogurt within three days.

*V types: Add warming spices, such as cardamom, cinnamon, and black pepper, and dilute with water, if desired.*

*P types: Add turmeric or neem leaves, or sweeten (with fresh fruits, maple syrup, or Sucanat) or dilute with water, if desired.*

*K types: Use only occasionally, and add pinches of turmeric, black pepper, or neem and other Kapha-reducing spices.*

## Fresh Buttermilk (chaach)

When cream is churned into butter, the milky whey left in the container is buttermilk (see above). After you mold the butter, gather the buttermilk into an earthenware, stainless steel, or glass jug. Store in a cool place and use within 48 hours.

This natural buttermilk can be used as a starter to make curd cheese. Pure buttermilk is most beneficial for Vata types.

## Milk Dough (khoa)

When milk is boiled until most of its water has evaporated, the soft mass of dough that remains is called *khoa.* It is usually sweet because of the natural sugars in lactose. Often, jaggery is added to the milk when the dough is to be used to make sweets, such as peera, ladoo, and halvah.

## Curd Cheese (panir)

Authentic Vedic cheeses were made from fresh casein curds or yogurt. They were not ripened with bacteria, molds, or enzymes, nor was salt, juice, or acid added to the curd. These techniques run contrary to the sattvic quality of milk. The original curd cheese is likened to ricotta or cottage cheese in texture. (These contain, however, enzymes, salt, bacteria, and animal rennet, as do most cheeses found in the United States.)

**2 quarts whole milk**
**1/2 c cream**
**1/2 quart buttermilk**
**1 heavy stainless steel saucepan**
**thermometer**

Sterilize the saucepan. Combine the milk, cream, and buttermilk in saucepan and stir until well blended. Warm mixture over moderate heat for 45 minutes until the thermometer reads 180 degrees F. If you're using a gas stove, place pan over a flame tamer, which will cause the heat to distribute evenly. Allow the milk to simmer gently, without stirring, for 25 minutes. When the thermometer reads 195 degrees F. the curds should have a soft custard-like consistency. (For firmer curds, continue cooking an additional 30 minutes.) Line a colander with a double layer of clean cheesecloth and place over the sink. Slowly and gently pour the cheese and whey into the lined colander. Allow the curd to drain for 2 hours. Gently squeeze the remaining curd with clean hands and place in a bowl. Cover and store in a cool place. Panir should be used within 48 hours.

## CONSERVATION AND RECYCLING OF FOOD REMAINS

The one important practice that is often neglected through omission rather than violation is the sadhana of disposing of food remains after cooking a meal. From the perspective of sadhanas, how we dispose of the unusable reflects our knowledge of actions that are harmonious to the environment, and our reverence for the planet.

According to Ayurvedic thinking, the question is not how much we need to recycle, but how little we need to use of that which cannot dissolve naturally back into the earth. The following methods of preservation can help prevent the generation of unnecessary and irreverent waste products.

1. Use cotton kitchen towels and dinner napkins, which may be washed and reused. Refrain from using paper towels and napkins (or paper plates and cups).
2. Reuse plastic and paper shopping bags from the market as containers for inorganic garbage. These may then be disposed of through recycling centers, if available.
3. Refrain from purchasing plastic products, such as garbage bags, plastic wrap or baggies, and plastic utensils. You may reuse the clear plastic fruit and vegetable bags from the store for your various wrapping needs. Understandably a certain amount of plastic will be necessary for the present-day mode of living—the option is to

minimize the usage. In sum, continue to use what you own, but do not support the production of more paper or plastic.

4. Minimize the use of aluminum foil and containers made of foil, such as baking pans. Instead use pans and containers that can be washed and reused for all of your cooking needs.
5. If possible, create a compost pile for the vegetables, fruits, grain, dhals, and spices that remain after meal preparation. In this way, the unusable remains of foods are returned naturally to their source, Mother Earth, along with the used portions. Speak to the proprietor of your neighborhood gardening supply store to learn how to create and maintain a compost pile.
6. Be especially alert to preparing only the quantity of food needed for your meals. Avoid generating any excess that will then have to be thrown away. If there is excess, feed it to the animals, or compost it.
7. Collect the stems, stones, and husks remaining from your grain cleaning in a small container. Make a weekly or biweekly visit to the earth to dispose of your collection.

## A SMALL PLOT OF LAND

The need for small community food gardens is imperative. Whether we reside in urban or rural areas, the plan for a small plot of earth where people share the work and the crops is a vital necessity for our preservation. The best response to the paucity of clean foods is to create our own supply and augment it from the organic produce of other farmers. We cannot depend solely on the health food market or the many small organic farms. The deepest change will come when we contribute to the health and longevity of nature with our own hands and heart.

Each year, nearly three billion tons of topsoil is eroded from the croplands of this country. The soil is being killed by chemical fertilizers and depleted of its natural minerals by repeated planting of the same crops on the same acres of land. Over the last forty years of mono-cropping, the United States has incurred a devastating loss of farmland. We cannot rebuild this land. More than half of our water supply throughout the country is contaminated with the chemical pesticides used in farming. Our bodies are made of soil and water. These elements are the foundation of plant life and other organisms upon which our lives depend. We are burning up more fossil fuel to produce chemical and synthetic fertilizers than to cultivate and harvest all the crops in the United States. The use of human energy used in the farming of our croplands is becoming extinct.

The Environmental Protection Agency of the United States considers 90 percent of all fungicides, 60 percent of all herbicides, and 30 percent of all insecticides to be carcinogenic. Pesticides are implicated in the cause of cancer, birth defects, nerve damage, and genetic mutations. The remaining percentages of these chemicals contribute to the devastating transmutation of our internal systems. The more our food sources, soil, and water are tampered with, the less linkage we are able to maintain with memory of the earth and nature. Unless we maintain our memory

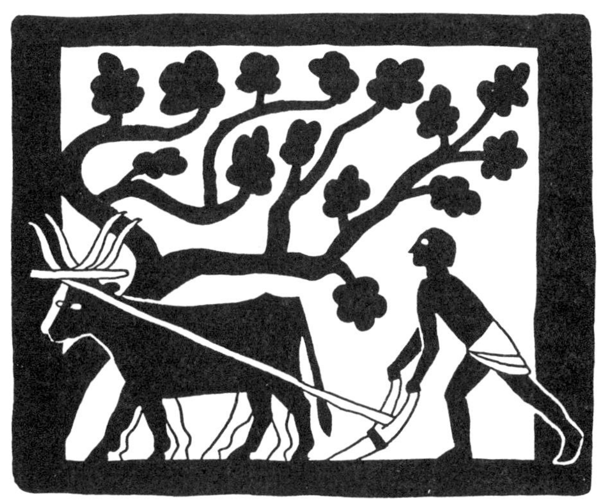

**Man and Oxen Ploughing the Land. From Egyptian relief, 2,000 B.C.**

base through the use of earth's plants and organisms, we cannot continue to develop as a species.

Each sense organ links us to the beginning of time, connecting us to the past in order that we may chart the future. Water is the sole contributor to taste. The most important of the five senses, taste directly melds us with our food bodies, the earth, and the universe. With the present tasteless and taste-distorted fare of chemical-fed foods, we slip deeper and deeper into cosmic amnesia.

One acre of land can produce forty thousand pounds of potatoes, thirty thousand pounds of carrots, forty thousand pounds of onions, and sixty thousand pounds of celery every year. The same acre of land used to raise cattle produces fifty pounds of meat per year.

### *Companion Planting*

A small garden plot divided into three separate divisions will generate nearly thirty different crops. The following recommendations highlight the plants that will exist happily together. Companion planting is necessary to protect the soil's minerals and to minimize infestation by insects, worms, and so forth. Caring for the plants requires attention, water, and good natural mulching of the soil. Occasionally bean powder may also be used to protect leafy vegetables from worms and other pests.

In the rows of the first division, the bushy plants are grown. From May until the end of the vegetation period, runner beans, cucumbers, cabbage, broad beans, potatoes, and early peas are planted. Each item is planted in a row of its own, with rows approximately two feet apart.

In the rows of the second division, two full crops may be harvested in the first and second half of the growing season. Leeks, onions, black salsify, daikon, cauliflower, celery, kidney beans, spring greens, (collards, kale, mustard greens, lettuces, arugula, and other leafy greens), beets, parsnips, and burdock are planted in separate rows, with rows approximately two feet apart.

In the rows of the third division, the plants that have a short growing season and low growth are sown. Early carrots, bib lettuce, late carrots, onion sets raised from seeds, red lettuce, endive, kohlrabi, fennel, parsnips, and leeks are planted in separate rows, with rows one foot apart.

Around the perimeters of all three divisions, annual and perennial herbs may be planted. Basil, dill, chives, parsley, mint, cilantro, rosemary, tarragon, oregano, thyme, chili, and black pepper are just a few of the herb varieties you may choose to plant. You may also plant the roots of ginger, licorice, and lotus. If you are living in a warm climate, you may import neem seeds from India and plant the bush in your first division of companion planting. Apart from their essential features in Vedic cuisine and Ayurvedic pharmacology, neem leaves are a natural pesticide, protecting the whole garden from most bugs, insects, and worms.

The sadhana of gardening is one of the richest experiences a person can enjoy. Nature plants her luxuriant gardens throughout the earth. All we need to do is observe the dynamics of the plants that live together, their seasons and conditions, and mimic this process in our little plots of land.

I recommend an excellent book called *Companion Planting* by Gertrud Franck. This book has been a tremendous help to me in my own efforts at companion planting. Gertrud Franck's method of gardening is very close to the ancient systems of farming and to the natural order of the land.

## DAILY ROUTINES

These routines exemplify the way we should spend our time according to the Ayurvedic ideal. If you are working a typical nine-to-five job, which does not permit much flexibility, then practice these sadhanas to the best of your ability in the time that is available to you. For example, you can observe the morning and evening sadhanas in full. You may also observe these sadhanas fully during your days off.

## *Daily Vata Sadhana*

### Times of Increased Pressure

2:00–6:00 A.M. and P.M.
September, October, and November
Old age
Rainy, damp weather

### Ideal Routine

| | |
|---|---|
| Morning | Rise promptly on awakening<br>Engage in calming activities |
| 6:00–7:00 A.M. | Perform a gentle dry-brush body scrub twice a week |
| | Take a warm bath with bath oils |
| | Massage body gently with sesame oil or natural body lotion |
| | Perform morning pranayama and gentle yoga asanas |
| 7:00–8:00 A.M. | Have breakfast |
| 10:00 A.M.–2:00 P.M. | Activity and work time |
| | Attend meetings and communicate with others in general |
| | Do chores and errands of the day |
| 12:00–1:00 P.M. | Lunch peacefully and calmly: eat slowly and enjoy your food |
| 2:00–4:00 P.M. | Rest; enjoy the stillness and pleasant sounds |
| | Take a nap |
| | Do gentle yoga stretches |
| | Meditate or chant |
| | Garner thoughts in stillness |
| | Listen to nature's sounds (rivers, brooks, wind, leaves) or to beautiful music |
| 4:00–4:30 P.M. | Tea time |
| 5:00–6:00 P.M. | Time to reflect on the day, wind down; plan ahead |
| | Continue work activities |
| 6:00–7:00 P.M. | Have dinner with friends or family |
| 7:00–7:30 P.M. | Take a nurturing evening brew |
| 7:00–10:00 P.M. | Wind down |
| | Take gentle after-dinner walks or perform other relaxing activity |
| | Do evening pranayama |
| | Meditate or do aromatherapy* |
| 10:00 P.M. | Retire |

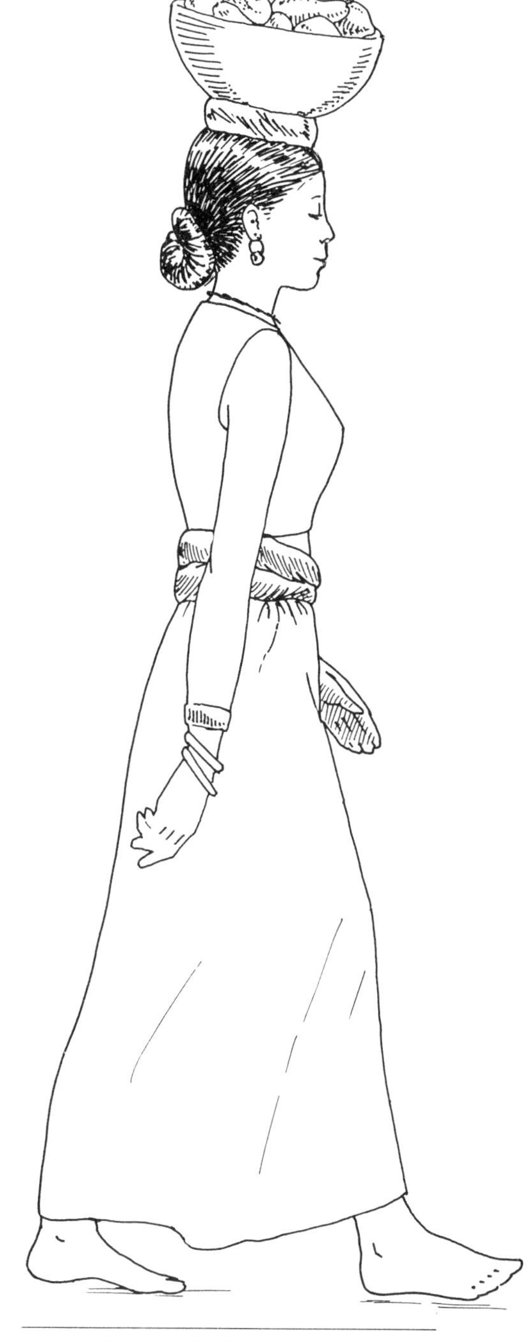

**Carrying Basket of Food—Sadhana to Invite Clarity**

Note: During weekends, include the practice of your food sadhanas and sadhana of the land. Also, during the fall, rise an hour later and be especially sensitive to your needs for quiet and focused thinking and activities.

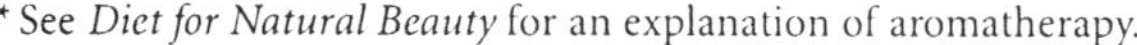

* See *Diet for Natural Beauty* for an explanation of aromatherapy.

## *Daily Pitta Sadhana*

### Times of Increased Pressure

12:00–2:00 A.M. and P.M.
Mid-April, May, June, July, and August
Mid-life
Hot, humid weather

### Ideal Routine

| | |
|---|---|
| Morning | Arise promptly on awakening |
| 6:00–8:00 A.M. | Engage in calming activities: |
| | Perform a gentle dry-brush body scrub three times a week |
| | Take a cool shower or bath |
| | Apply mild natural lotions and sandhalwood powder to body |
| | Perform morning pranayama and meditation |
| | Do yoga asanas or run |
| 7:00–8:00 A.M. | Breakfast |
| 9:00–10:00 A.M. | Engage in work-related activities, communication, etc. |
| 10:00 A.M.–2:00 P.M. | Engage in contemplative activities; remain calm and alert |
| | Perform even-tempered workout |
| | Do creative, nonstressful work (artwork and other visual activities are generally calming) |
| | Exercise care and sensitivity while dealing with others during this time |
| 12:00–1:00 P.M. | Have a peaceful and quiet lunch |
| 2:00–4:00 P.M. | Engage in work details, communication, meetings |
| | Present ideas and proposals during this time |
| 3:00–4:00 P.M. | Break for tea or snack |
| 4:00–4:30 P.M. | Regroup; sit back and assess your success or lack of success (very important for Pittas). Hold the reins of your fire close to your chest at this time |
| 5:00–6:00 P.M. | Time to reflect on the day, wind down; plan ahead |
| 6:00–7:00 P.M. | Have dinner with family or friends |
| | Take a long walk, engage in soothing activities |
| 7:00–9:00 P.M. | Reduce activities: reading/work preparation |
| 8:00–8:30 P.M. | Take a nurturing evening brew |
| 9:00–10:00 P.M. | Perform bedtime pranayama and meditation or aromatherapy |
| | Do evening yoga asanas |
| 10:00–10:30 P.M. | Retire |

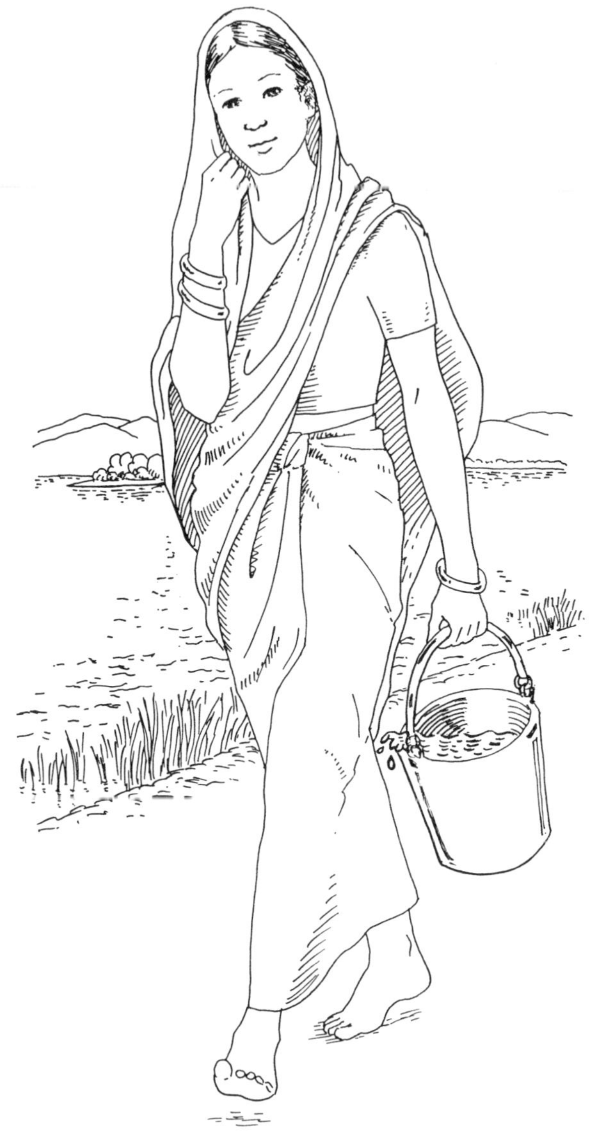

**Carrying Water from the Well—
Sadhana to Invite New Life and Cleansing**

Note: During weekends, include the kitchen sadhanas (grains, spices, etc.) and sadhana of the land. Also, in the summer be especially attentive to cooling down your activities and to regrouping and engaging in calm contemplation.

## *Daily Kapha Sadhana*

### Times of Increased Pressure

6:00–10:00 A.M. and P.M.
December, January, February, March, mid-April
Childhood, youth
Cold, damp weather

### Ideal Routine

| | |
|---|---|
| Morning | Rise promptly on awakening |
| 6:00–8:00 A.M. | Engage in vital activities: |
| | Perform a vigorous dry-brush body scrub daily |
| | Take a warm shower |
| | Massage body with a mild natural body lotion |
| | Perform morning pranayama |
| | Do 30 minutes of yoga asanas or run or do some active sports (do something stimulating first thing each day) |
| 8:00–9:00 A.M. | Light breakfast |
| 9:00 A.M.–2:00 P.M. | Engage in normal work activities of the day |

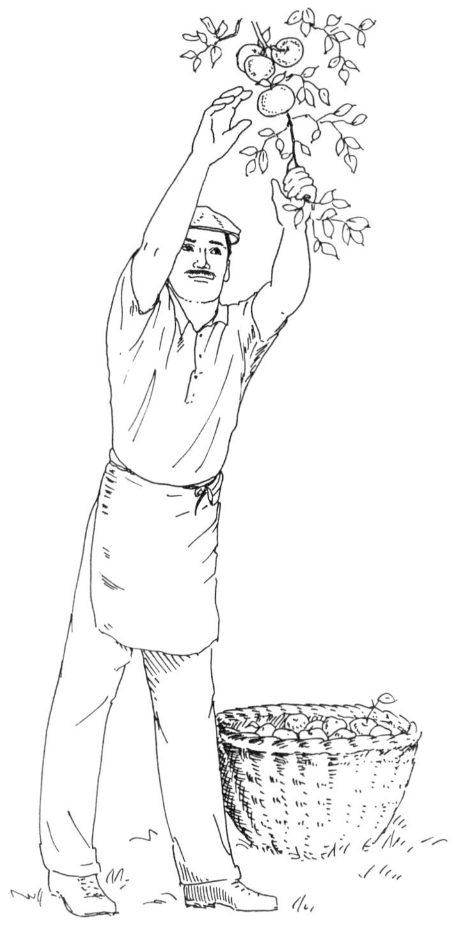

Picking Fruit—Sadhana for Celebration

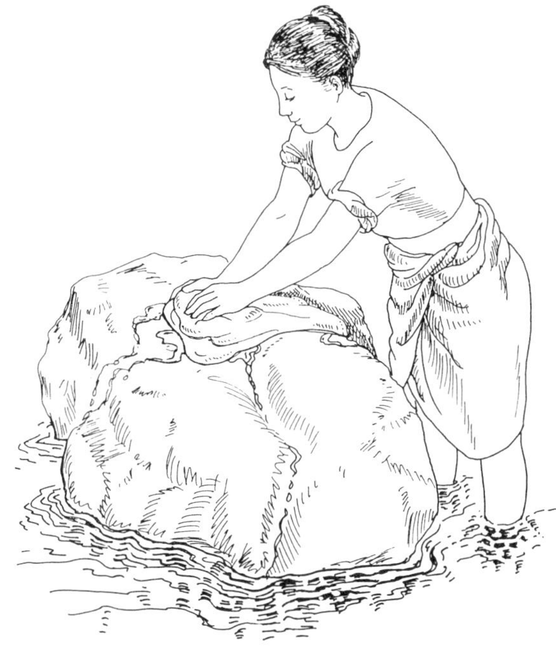

Washing Clothes in the River—Sadhana for Contemplation

| | |
|---|---|
| 1:00–2:00 P.M. | Have a hearty meal |
| 3:00–6:00 P.M. | Perform normal activities of the day |
| 4:00–4:30 P.M. | Afternoon tea |
| 6:00–7:00 P.M. | Light dinner with family |
| 7:00–9:00 P.M. | Participate in a consistent evening program outside of the home (do not nap or watch TV during or after dinner) |
| | Join yoga groups and engage in stimulating lectures or events |
| 9:00–10:00 P.M. | Wind down |
| | Perform evening pranayama |
| | Meditate or pray |

Note: During weekends, include the kitchen sadhanas (grains, spices, etc.), the preparation of condiments, chutneys, and pickles, and the sadhanas of the land.

Be especially alert and active during winter and early spring.

PART THREE

# Universal Recipes for Each Body Type

# INTRODUCTION TO THE RECIPES

*The intelligent person, remembering the pain of diseases,*
*should take food which is suitable to him, and*
*according to proper quantity and timing.*
*Charaka*

I wish it were possible for me to scan the entire world and all its cultures to evaluate the Ayurvedic energetics of all of God's foods. Ayurvedic cooking is not modern Indian cooking. Ayurveda is a living ideal with universal principles that embrace all cultures, all living entities. In keeping with this line of thought, in this book I have evaluated Ayurvedically a wide variety of food staples including many foods traditionally found in a macrobiotic diet. This should help you—the consumers—to determine which foods are suitable for your constitutional type. For some body types, Oriental foods can be too salty, too sour, and/or too fermented.

The handling of foods is a most important aspect of cooking. Approach the kitchen with a prayerful attitude. Wash all grains and vegetables properly. Be sure your cooking utensils are clean and preferably made from stainless steel, cast iron, or clay. Avoid Teflon, aluminum, electric cookware, and microwave ovens. Microwaves are a natural enemy to the harmonious energies of food. Gas stoves and open fires provide the best energy for cooking. Pressure cookers are imperative for the cooking of grains and beans. Minimize the use of all electrical appliances. Refrigerators encourage us to use stale and frozen foods and to store leftovers. Purchase fresh vegetables daily, if possible.

When the term "natural" appears before a food item, the food should be purchased in a natural foods store. Each recipe is prefaced by a symbol noting the season during which it is best eaten

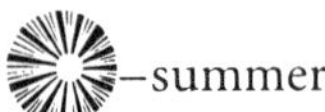

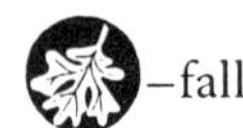

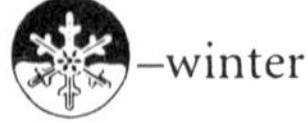

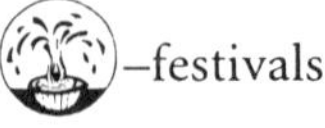


and by letters indicating the body types that can eat it. Substitutions, when recommended, appear below the ingredient list. Some recipes appropriate for your body type may contain small amounts of an ingredient that is not recommended by the food charts. Small amounts of these foods will not hinder the overall dosha-benefiting aspects of that dish. When the term "occasionally" appears after a list of types (such as V, VK, KP) it applies to the types listed in that line. Some recipes end with the statement "Serve with appropriate grain, sauce"; this refers to a grain or sauce appropriate to your body type. A minimum of oil is used in these recipes; you may increase this amount slightly (but not too much, or it will throw off the balance of the recipe). The letters PC after a recipe title alert you to the need for a pressure cooker. While there is a simplicity to all of the recipes in this book, some of the equipment and techniques that are called for may be unfamiliar. The following glossary should provide you with the practical information you need to put these tools and methods to use.

## EQUIPMENT AND TOOLS

### *Bamboo mat*

Rather than a lid, the bamboo mat allows the food to breathe and remain fresh long after it has been cooked. Bamboo mats are available in most Japanese and Oriental grocery stores.

### *Cookware*

If your kitchen is equipped with varying sizes of stainless steel pans, a regular skillet, and a few cast-iron skillets of varying sizes, you should be able to prepare the recipes in this book. A cast-iron skillet is used mostly for roasting (dry or with oil), as well as for dishes with short cooking times. Stainless-steel pans are used mainly for dishes with long cooking times, such as curries and soups.

A pressure cooker is invaluable for cooking grains. I strongly urge you to use one for all "long cooking" grains and beans. It produces a much more nutritious and tasty meal. However, if you do not have one on hand, grains may also be cooked in a clay pot, enamel coated cast-iron pot, or a heavy stainless steel pot.

Although the recipes call predominantly for stainless steel and cast-iron cookware, it is a good idea to vary your cooking utensils. Use copper, glass, and occasionally earthenware for a variety of benefits.

### *Ceramic and Earthenware Pots*

These pots maintain Earth's energy in the food and are available through most health food stores, gourmet utensil and equipment stores, and Oriental grocery stores.

### *Ceramic Hand Grater*

This ideal tool for grating ginger or nutmeg can be found in natural food stores.

### *Cheesecloth*

The use of paper products inhibits the development of natural sadhana instincts and is discouraged. Cheesecloth is suggested as an alternative to paper towels in this book.

### *Electric Blender, Grinder, and Juicer*

When there are no other options, you may resort to these appliances. Be sure to use sparingly. The hand grinders and mortar and pestle are far more conducive to the practice of sadhana and should be used as much as possible for grinding and puréeing needs.

### *Hand Grinders*

These provide a wonderful form of kitchen sadhana. The small version (#2, which is 4" in diameter) may be used instead of a mortar and pestle or Japanese suribachi for grinding spices, nuts, and seeds. The larger versions (#2, at 6" in diameter, and #4, at 8" in diameter) are used for grinding wet dhals and grains for idli and dosa. They may also be used for puréeing vegetables and soups and for pulping fruits. See Appendix for suppliers.

### *Hand Stone (as Mallet) and Grinding Stone*

See Sadhanas of Spices, chapter 8.

### *Idli Steamer*

Resembling an egg poaching pan, the idli steamer consists of three or four tiered trays containing three or four molds each. The molds are perforated, which allows the steam to escape. To prepare, with steamer trays disassembled, lightly oil each mold. Or you may lightly oil small pieces of cheesecloth and place in each mold; this allows for easy removal. Pour batter into each tray. When all trays are filled, assemble steamer. Idli steamers are available at Indian grocery stores.

### *Karai*

This forerunner to the Chinese wok is available in many sizes through Indian food stores. To prevent rusting, the iron karai pans must be seasoned after use.

### *Suribachi*

Japanese mortar and pestle.

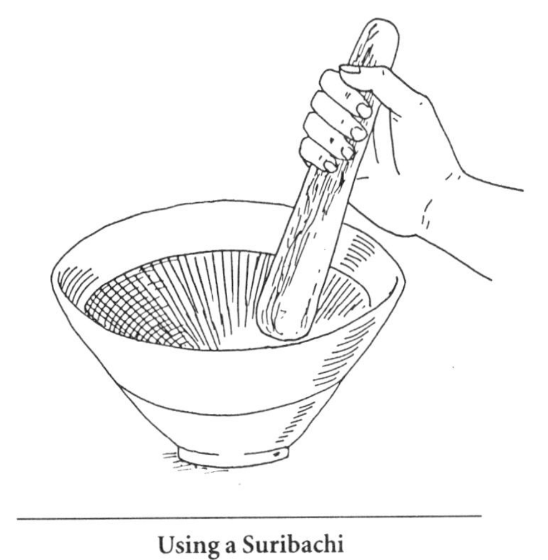

**Using a Suribachi**

### *Tava*

Native to India, this slightly concave iron skillet is preferred over flat skillets for making chapatis, rotis, and dosas. Lighter than cast-iron, the tava heats faster and reduces cooking time.

## TECHNIQUES

### *Grinding Wet Grains and Dhals*

Use a large hand grinder that clamps onto counter or kitchen table. Place approximately 1 cup of wet grains or dhals into mouth of grinder. Place a bowl under the spout and turn the handle. If a fine smooth consistency is needed, regrind the dhals or grains once more. Using this method, it takes about 30 minutes to grind 2 to 3 pounds of wet dhal or grain. Wet dhals and grains may also be ground in a very large mortar with pestle.

### *Juicing Fresh Ginger*

If you have a ceramic hand grater and plump, fresh green ginger, you can do this by hand. Peel 1/2 a finger length of fresh ginger and grate to a fine pulp with a ceramic grater. Wash your hands and, placing the grated ginger in you stronger hand, squeeze the pulp firmly over a small bowl. Use the pulp to cook with or to make fresh ginger tea. Half a finger length of ginger will make approximately two tablespoons of juice.

If fresh young ginger is not available, grate 1/4 finger's length of dried ginger with a ceramic grater. Use 2 teaspoons of this grated ginger in recipes that call for 2 tablespoons of ginger juice.

### *Making Fresh Coconut Milk*

Select a fresh coconut: shake it to be sure there is water inside. The coconut should be heavier than it looks. Preheat oven to 400 degrees F. Using a sharp knife or ice pick, pierce two of the eyes and drain the coconut water. (The coconut water may be used to drink or mix with the grated coconut to form the coconut milk, below.) Place coconut in heated oven for 15 minutes, until the shell begins to crack. Open the coconut with a hammer and allow to cool for 10 minutes. Pry nut pieces away from the shell using a small knife, and scrape off thin brown film. Using a hand grinder, grate the coconut pieces; place 1 cup of grated coconut in a stainless steel bowl with 2 cups of water (coconut or spring water) for 30 minutes. With a slotted spoon, gather the grated coconut and place in the center of a clean cloth over the bowl. Wrap the cloth tightly around the coconut and twist both ends in opposite directions; squeeze until remaining milk is released into bowl with soaking water.

Alternately, combine 2 cups of water with 1 cup fresh coconut pieces in a blender and purée for 3 to 5 minutes, until all the coconut has been dissolved and the milk is smooth.

Pour coconut milk into a jar and use fresh. Use less water for a thicker milk.

### *Making Fresh Almond Milk*

In a large bowl, combine 4 cups of hot water and 1 cup whole almonds and allow to sit for 30 minutes, until skins loosen. Slip skins off with your fingers and discard, along with soaking water. Place skinned almonds and 2 cups of cold water in a blender and purée for 3 to 5 minutes, until the nuts are completely dissolved and the milky liquid is smooth. Pour into a jar and use right away. Use less water for a thicker milk.

### *Grilling Eggplant*

Wash the eggplant, keeping its stem intact. Using either an open grill or a gas stove burner, place the eggplant over a direct flame until the skin becomes charred. If using a gas burner, place a metal bread rack, about 8-10" in diameter and 1" in height, to rest directly over the burner and grill the eggplant over a low flame.

Turn occasionally with metal prongs to ensure even roasting. When cooked, using the prongs, place the eggplant in a metal colander over the sink for 5 minutes to cool. Run cool water over the skin as you peel the charred skin off with your fingers. Place the skinned eggplant on a cutting board and remove the stem with a knife.

### *Sprouting Beans*

In India, sprouted beans are called *ugadela kathar.* The following instructions are for mung, the most commonly used dhal for sprouting. Wash beans well with cold water. In a bowl, combine 4 parts warm water (70–80 degrees F.) with 1 part dhal. Cover with a plastic wrap, securely fastened, and allow to sit overnight. Drain well and divide among several clean quart jars, putting about 1/4 cup of soaked dhal in each. Place a double thickness of cheesecloth around rim and secure with a rubber band. Keep jars in a warm, dark place. Twice a day, fill jars with tepid water and shake gently to water all legumes. Through the cheesecloth, drain and return jars to their resting place. Continue this process for 3 to 5 days, until beans produce sprouts of desired length. (In India, legumes are usually only sprouted until a very small white shoot appears. In these recipes, however, you may allow the sprout to grow to whatever length you desire.)

### *Making Tamarind Paste from Dried Tamarind Slab*

Cut a 2-inch piece of dried tamarind and place in 2 cups of boiling water. Remove from heat and allow to soak for 4 hours. Remove softened tamarind from the water and squeeze it with clean fingers into a fine sieve with a bowl underneath, releasing the pulp from the fibers. Mash the fibers inside the sieve and scrape additional pulp off the bottom of the sieve into the bowl. It is best to prepare tamarind just before serving, allowing sufficient time for preparation. The roughage is a good addition to dhals and soups; it should be removed and discarded before serving the dishes.

## PREPARING THE VEGETABLES

The ancient Vedic cultures approached food and the preparation of food with great reverence. The handling of each food completely reflects its vital power and taste. Unruly scrambling, tossing, or throwing does not lend itself to a splendid meal.

Approach each vegetable with a respect for the universal intelligence. The natural grain of each vegetable will tell you how it is to be cleaned and cut.

Vegetables that grow on a stalk, such as broccoli and celery, should be first cut lengthwise and then, if smaller pieces are needed, horizontally. Leafy greens are to be cut along the grains of the leaves; their stems may be diced horizontally. Avoid using the coarse or purplish parts of the stems. Elongated root vegetables, such as carrots, daikon, and parsnips, may be cut in many ways. The initial cut needs to be a horizontal one, on a slant, as each cut of the root vegetable should incorporate the air/space (top) energy, the earth/water (bottom) energy, and the fire (middle) energy. Round root vegetables, such as rutabagas, potatoes, and onions, have a grain that runs along their center length. Onions and potatoes in particular endure the most unjust handling—they are generally cut opposite their grain (people seem fascinated by the circular rings rather than the proper lengthy slices). Incidentally, when cut correctly they taste much sweeter.

To observe foods closely and to work with them thoughtfully and harmoniously is truly a marvel. Doing so adds joy to cooking and strengthens our link to the universe.

## *Cutting Techniques*

### Cabbage

***Shredding:*** Cut cabbage in half, lengthwise, along center grain, and then again in quarters. Remove core from all four quarters. Place each quarter lengthwise on cutting board and slice thinly along the grain.

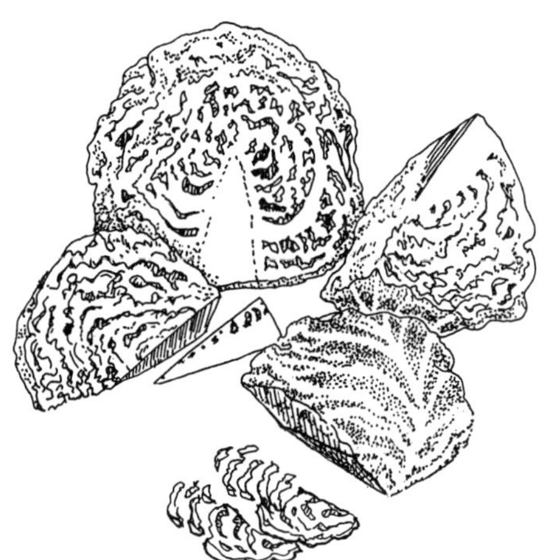

***Matchsticks:*** Cut cabbage cores in pieces 1/4" thick. Place pieces in stacks 1" high and cross-cut at a thickness of 1/16" to produce matchsticks.

### Large Leafy Greens

***Diagonal slice:*** Fold each leaf lengthwise along its spine and cut off the stem. Open the leaves and stack them 12 pieces high. Fold the stack over along the spine and slice thinly on the diagonal, along leaf grain. Gather the stems and cut finely on the diagonal.

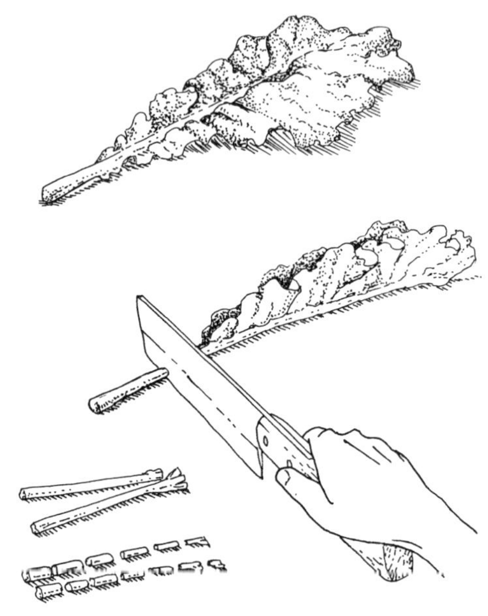

### Broccoli/Cauliflower

***Florets:*** Cut below the flower and hold flower face down on cutting board. Cut into the stem toward the flower (do not cut through flower). Gently pull flowers apart with your hands.

***Half-moon stems:*** Always use your broccoli and cauliflower stems. Peel stems of broccoli if skins are thick. Cut lengthwise down the center of stems. Place center face down on cutting board. Cut on the diagonal or in half-moons 1/4" thick.

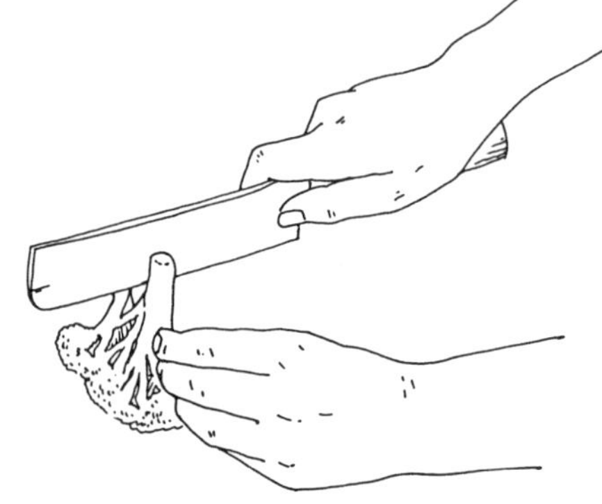

## Long Root Vegetables

***Shavings:*** Hold root vegetable in your hand, away from your body. Shave the vegetable by chipping away in thin or thick shavings.

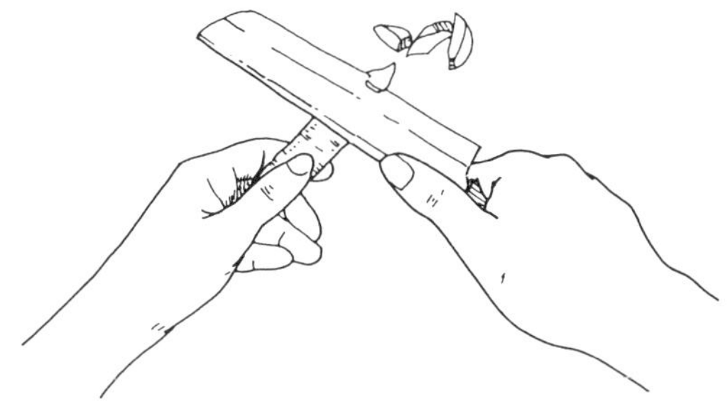

***Matchsticks:*** Slice root vegetable on the diagonal, 1/8" thick. Place the slices in stacks 1" high and cross-cut at a thickness of 1/16" to produce matchsticks.

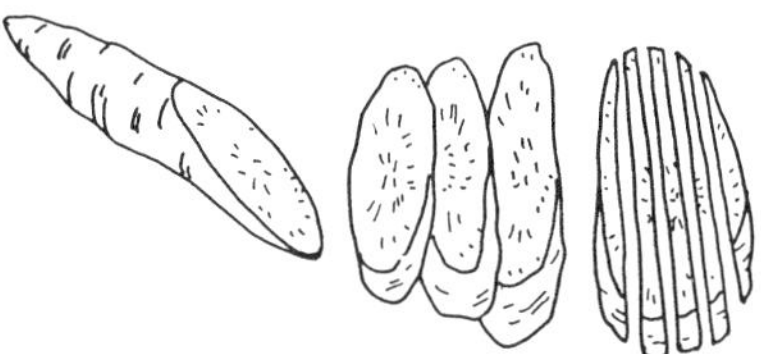

***Half-rounds:*** Slice root vegetable in half lengthwise. Place center down on cutting board. Cross-cut in half-rounds to desired thickness.

***Quarter-rounds:*** Slice root vegetable in half, then again in quarters, lengthwise. Place center down on cutting board. Cross-cut in quarter-rounds to desired thickness.

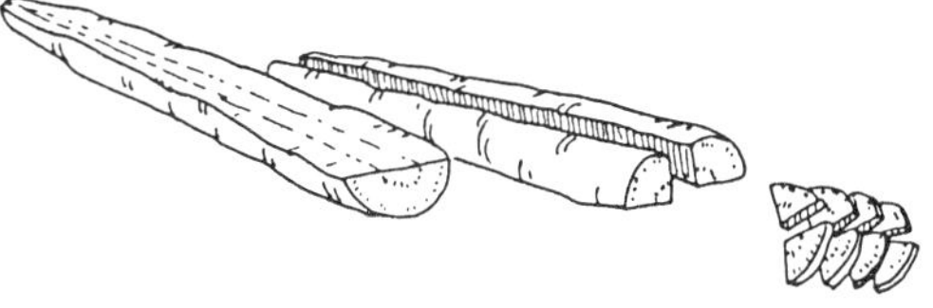

***Log-cut:*** Cut root vegetable in pieces 2" long. Cut each piece into vertical slabs. Slice each slab lengthwise at a thickness of 1/4–1/2".

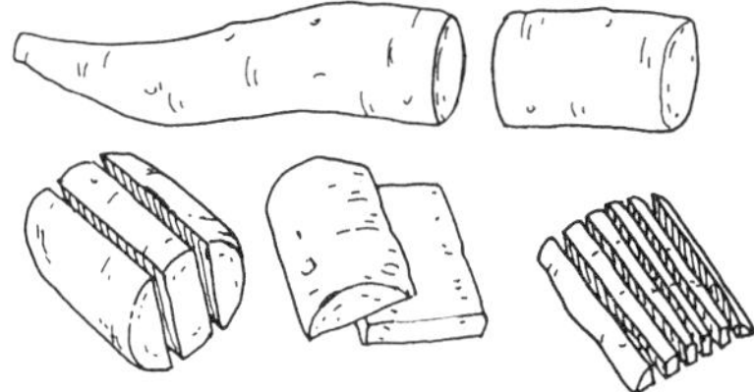

***Roll-cut:*** Cut root vegetable once on the diagonal at a thickness of 1". Roll vegetable 90 degrees away from you and cut again. Continue rolling vegetable back and forth, repeating process until the whole vegetable is cut.

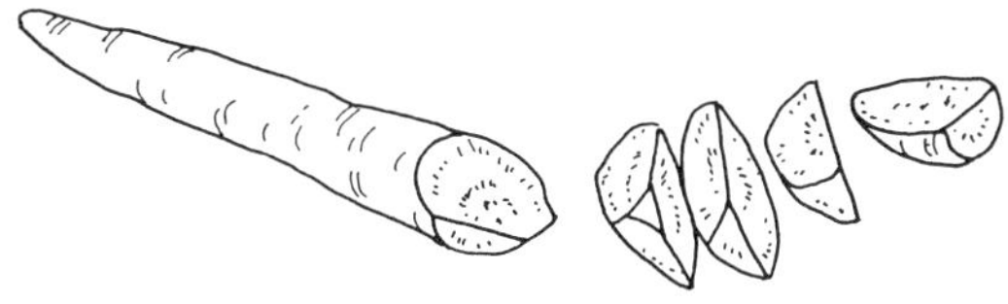

## Small Round Vegetables

***Cubes:*** Slice vegetable into three vertical slabs. Slice each slab into vertical logs. Cross-cut in cubes of desired size.

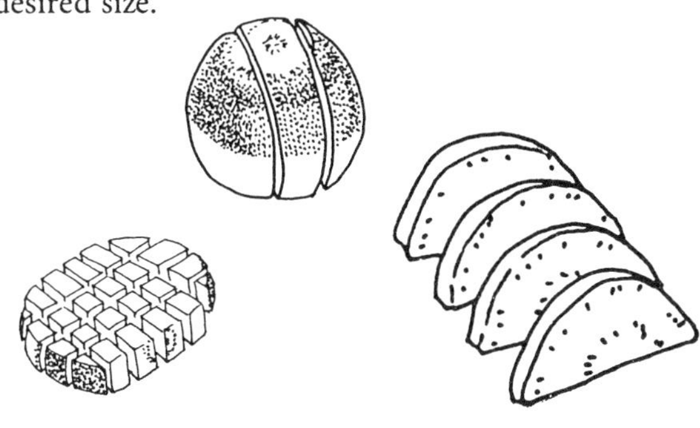

## Onions

***Crescents:*** Cut onion in half, lengthwise, along center grain. Place each half face down on cutting board. Slice lengthwise along the grain in crescents of desired thickness.

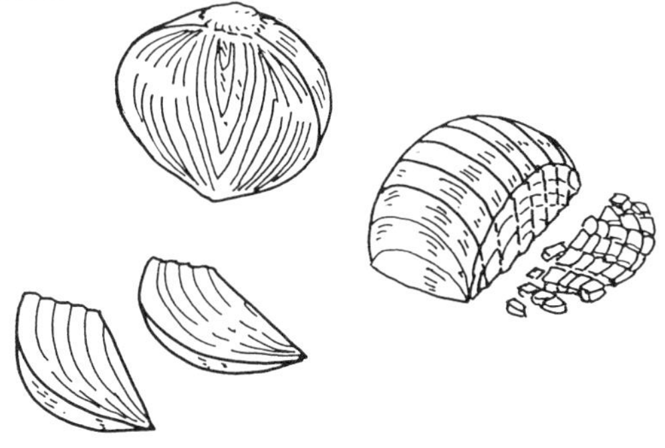

***Minced:*** Cut onion in half, lengthwise, along center grain. Place each half face down on cutting board. Slice lengthwise along the grain, then turn the cutting board and cross-cut against the grain to desired size.

### Squash

***Halves:*** Remove stem with a paring knife and cut squash in half, lengthwise, along center grain. Remove fibrous innards and seeds with a spoon.

***Chunks:*** Remove stem with a paring knife and cut squash in half, lengthwise, along center grain. Place halves face down on cutting board. Cut each half lengthwise down the center in two pieces. Turn cutting board and cross-cut against the grain to desired size.

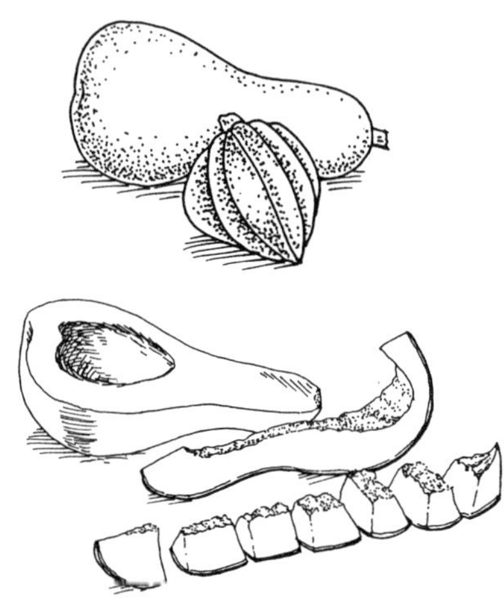

## COOKING METHODS

### *Chaunking*

In Vedic times, all spices were roasted in ghee or oil before being added to a dish. This process, called *chaunking,* is one that continues in India today. It serves to readily seal the spices while at the same time opening their flavor and energies. Traditionally seeds, such as cumin, coriander, and mustard, are chaunked together with various seasonings, such as freshly ground ginger root, minced or whole chilies, and chana or urad dhal in a heavy cast-iron skillet. The seeds may be whole, crushed, or powdered before chaunking. Chaunks may be added at the beginning or end of a dish; in the case of kichadi (a dhal and rice combination), the chaunk is added toward the end. For the sake of simplicity, in the recipes in this book I have used the term *roast* or *sauté* when referring to chaunking.

### *Dry-roasting*

In this book, parching, toasting, and dry roasting refer to the same procedure.

Known as *bhona* in Sanskrit, dry roasting is done in the same manner as chaunking, except without the use of ghee or oils. In today's world, we find chaunking being displaced by dry roasting. Powdered or crushed spices that are more than one week old can be enlivened by the dry-roasting process. Sometimes spices and crushed or whole seeds, along with other seasonings, are dry roasted in a heavy skillet with chickpea flour *(besan).*

Heat a heavy stainless steel frying pan or cast-iron skillet over medium heat. Wash all seeds in a colander and allow them to drain completely. Add seeds to the hot pan and stir frequently with a wooden spoon to prevent them from sticking together. Lower the heat and allow the seeds to roast for 10 minutes. Stir occasionally while roasting. When they are golden brown, or crisp enough to snap between your fingers, transfer seeds to a bowl and serve while hot and crunchy, or use in recipe.

If salt and powdered spices are to be added to the seeds, use the same skillet to roast them over low heat for 2 minutes. Then combine the roasted salt and spices with the seeds before serving. A good ratio of these ingredients would be 1 cup seeds, 1/2 teaspoon salt, and 1/2 teaspoon powdered spices.

If tamari is to be added, dilute it with an equal amount of water and pour over the seeds during the last 3 minutes of the roasting process. Mix thoroughly. A good ratio of these ingredients would be 1 cup seeds, 1 tablespoon each tamari and water.

### *Steaming*

This is an excellent method for preserving the freshness and vital minerals in foods. In India this procedure, known as *bhap dayana,* is generally used in the spring and summer. Although it may be done throughout the year, steaming is not advisable in the cold seasons since heat is not retained in the food.

Steamers—both of bamboo and stainless steel—are available with anywhere from one to four tiers. Place a small amount of water in the bottom of a pan that has a tight-fitting lid; the water level should remain below the lowest steam basket. Add the steamer, filled with uncooked vegetables, to the pan and cover. Maintain a medium-high heat to keep the water boiling.

The cooking time varies from 7 to 45 minutes depending on the soft or firm qualities of the vegetables, the cutting styles used, and the desired result.

Leafy greens and watery vegetables take about 10 minutes to steam; stalk vegetables, such as broccoli, cauliflower, and Brussels sprouts, take about 15 to 20 minutes, as do soft root vegetables, such as daikon. Hard root vegetables, such as carrots, burdock, and potato chunks, require a deeper pot and more water; they take about 30 to 35 minutes to steam. With leafy greens, be careful not to oversteam; ideally, the cooked leaf should be a vibrant green. Vegetables are best cooked just until fairly crisp, or al dente.

### *Sautéing*

This method, lightly cooking a food in a small amount of oil, is ideal for most vegetables. The freshness and vital minerals are maintained in the vegetables, while the rich accent of oil adds to the flavor of the food. Sautéing requires much less oil than frying—a mere 2 teaspoons of oil being enough to sauté a handful of vegetables. The addition of a few teaspoons of water extends the effects of the oil on the food. Vegetables may also be sautéed in a few tablespoons of water, instead of oil. If spices are called for, they may be sautéed in the oil before the vegetables are added. Either a heavy stainless steel frying pan or a cast-iron skillet, both with a tight-fitting lid, is required for sautéing.

Moderate heat is best for sautéing. The cooking time varies from 5 to 25 minutes depending on the soft or firm qualities of the vegetables, the cutting styles used, and the desired result.

Place the oil in the skillet and allow to warm over medium heat. Add the spices (if called for) and sauté for 2 minutes. Add the vegetables and water equal to the amount of oil used and cook until done. Vata types: use 1 tablespoon oil to 1 handful of vegetables; Pitta types: use 2 teaspoons of oil to 1 handful of vegetables; Kapha types: use 1 tablespoon of oil to 1 handful of vegetables.

# TRADITIONAL GROUND DHALS AND GRAINS

In India, dhals and grains are freshly ground into various textures, such as flours and wet-pastes, for daily use. Once broken, the grains and seeds begin to lose their vital energy. The longer the time between the processing and use of ground dhal and grain, the more depleted their energy. Freshly ground flours and pastes produce the most nutritive and wholesome results. The grinding processes are very simple (see page 194). Once you incorporate them into your daily cooking routines, you'll find it difficult to revert to cooking with lifeless flour.

*Vadai* and *amavadai* are deep-fried patties made from ground dhal that have been spiced and soaked in yogurt. Traditional to South India, the vadai are made with urad dhal and the amavadai are made with toor or chana dhal. They are often served at religious ceremonies and wedding festivities.

*Adai* and *othappam* are also traditional to South India. Adai is made from freshly ground mung dhal and basmati rice, and othappam is made from urad dhal and rice. The dhals and rice are soaked and ground separately and then combined. The adai batter is used immediately, whereas the othappam usually ferments for one day before use.

Othappam is also known as dosa, or Indian pancakes. This traditional food is made from a batter of freshly ground grains and dhals. Dosa batters are usually fermented, but this step is not required. To ensure maximum nutrition, a ratio of approximately 2.5 parts grain to 1 part dhal (beans, dried peas, lentils) is used. A combination of different dhals may also be used with the grain.

Traditionally, the grain used for making dosas is rice; during the last half of this century, processed white rice has been commonly used. Except for white basmati rice, I do not recommend the use of processed white rice; nor do I recommend the use of parboiled rice. In the recipes that follow, each body type may substitute the appropriate grain and dhal. Also, V types may add a pinch of asafoetida,

K types 1/4 teaspoon of fenugreek seeds, and P types 1/4 teaspoon of cinnamon or coriander.

Perhaps the king of fresh grain and bean foods is *rice idli*—a dome-shaped steamed patty made from a slightly fermented ground rice and dhal batter. A traditional breakfast food of South India, idli is usually served with sambar (a spicy vegetable-dhal soup) or chutney. *Uppama,* the classic breakfast cereal of South India, is made from cracked wheat; roasted dhals, vegetables, and spices are added to create a wheat pilaf, which is usually served with a coconut chutney.

*Vada* is a festive food of both North and South India made from freshly ground urad dhal mixed with the customary freshly ground condiments and spices, such as coconut, ginger, and onions, and formed into small balls that are then deep-fried and served with chutneys.

*Chapatis* are the original unleavened bread. From primordial time, bread has been an important part of humankind's daily sustenance. From the "breaking of bread" to the "daily bread," bread has been the symbol of serving, reaping, and sharing. The original chapati was made into a dough from whole wheat and then buried under coals in a baking hole dug into the earth. Over the centuries, thousands of variations upon this primal theme have been developed. In northern India, wheat in its freshly ground form, used in the preparation of chapatis, is more common than either wheat berries or rice.

*Roti,* or *paratha,* is another form of unleavened flat bread. These are usually thicker than chapati.

The deep-fried preparations presented on the pages that follow are for occasional use only. K types need to be especially wary of all richly oiled and salted foods, and use them sparingly. Vadas, pakoras, and bondis may be baked instead of deep-fried. Also, rye, millet, and barley are best substituted for rice in the following recipes for K types. P types may omit the heat-producing spices such as chilis and ginger; reduce the quantity of mustard seeds; add the P type balancing spices, such as coriander, cumin, and cardamom; and use barley and wheat instead of rice. The deep-frying method may be used by V and P types, but all excess oil should be thoroughly drained off. Grated daikon should be served with all fried and oily foods for all types. Daikon helps the body break down and remove excess oil which would normally be stored in the tissues as fat.

## Vadai

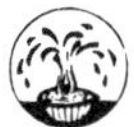

**ALL TYPES**
**Serves 2 (makes 6 patties)**

**1 c split urad dhal, without skins**
**1 tbs rice flour**
**1/4 tsp minced ginger**
**Pinch of asafoetida**
**Pinch of sea salt**
**1 c sunflower oil (for deep frying)**
**2 c fresh plain yogurt (for soaking)**

*V and K types: add 1/4 teaspoon minced red chili peppers.*

*P types: use a pinch of ginger and black pepper instead of asafoetida.*

Wash urad dhal until water runs clear. Soak in 6 cups cold water for about 6 hours. Drain and grind wet dhal into a fine, stiff paste using a hand grinder, large mortar and pestle, or blender. Add a few tablespoons of water as needed. Mix in the rice flour, ginger, asafoetida, and salt.

Heat oil in a small, deep pan. Lightly oil your hands and make 6 flat patties, 3" in diameter. Make a hole in the center of each patty with your finger, like a doughnut. When the oil is very hot, fry three vadai at a time; cook evenly for about 3 minutes on each side. Place two layers of cheesecloth in a colander over the sink. Remove vadai from pan with a spatula and drain in colander for 10 to 15 minutes. Remove and soak in yogurt for half an hour before serving.

## Amavadai

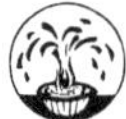

ALL TYPES
Serves 2 (makes 6 patties)

**1 c toor dhal**
**1 tbs rice flour**
**$^1/_4$ tsp sea salt**
**$^1/_2$ tsp fine black pepper**
**1 c sunflower oil (for deep-frying)**
**2 c fresh plain yogurt (for soaking)**

***V and K types: add $^1/_4$ teaspoon minced red chili peppers and/or any other V and K spices.***

Wash toor dhal until water runs clear. Soak in 3 cups of cold water for about 6 hours. Drain and grind to a fine paste using a hand grinder, large mortar and pestle, or blender. Add a few tablespoons of water as necessary. Stir in rice flour, salt, and pepper and mix into a stiff batter.

Heat oil in a small, deep pan. Lightly oil your hands and shape dough into 6 flat patties, 3" in diameter. Make a hole in center of the patty, if desired. When the oil is very hot, fry three amavadai at a time; cook evenly for about 3 minutes on each side. Place two layers of cheesecloth in a colander over the sink. Remove amavadai from pan with a spatula and drain in colander for 10 to 15 minutes. Remove and soak in yogurt for half an hour before serving.

## Adai

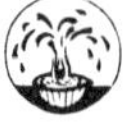

ALL TYPES
Serves 4

**2 c split mung dhal**
**$^1/_2$ c brown basmati rice**
**3 dried curry leaves**
**$^1/_8$ c minced fresh cilantro**
**$^1/_4$ tsp sea salt**
**2 tbs sunflower oil**
**Spiced yogurt or chutney**

***V and K types: add $^1/_2$ teaspoon minced fresh ginger and $^1/_2$ teaspoon minced green chili peppers.***
***K types: substitute $^1/_2$ cup rye or millet for the brown basmati.***

Wash mung dhal and rice separately until water runs clear. Soak each separately in enough cold water to cover by at least 2" for about 6 hours in a cool place.

Rinse and drain dhal; grind it, along with curry leaves, into a somewhat coarse paste using a hand grinder, large mortar and pestle, or blender. Add a few tablespoons of water, if needed. Separately drain and grind the rice to a similar consistency. Combine the two mixtures and add cilantro, salt, and 1 tablespoon of the oil. Add a few tablespoons of water, if needed. The batter should be thick and coarse.

Lightly coat a preheated griddle with remaining oil. Spread batter with a spatula on the griddle and shape into $^1/_4$" thick patties, 4" in diameter. Cook thoroughly, 3 or 4 minutes on each side, maintaining an even medium heat. Serve with spiced yogurt or chutney for an occasional festive breakfast.

## Othappam

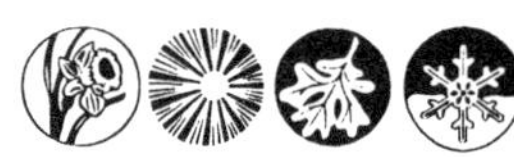

ALL TYPES
Serves 2

**1 c brown basmati rice**
**$^3/_8$ c split urad dhal, without skins**
**$^1/_2$ c minced onion**
**$^1/_4$ tsp minced ginger**
**$^1/_2$ c minced fresh cilantro**
**$^1/_4$ tsp sea salt**
**1 tbs sunflower oil**
**Assorted chutneys**

***V and K types: add $^1/_4$ teaspoon red chili pepper.***

***P types: omit ginger.***

***K types: substitute 1 cup millet for rice.***

Wash rice and urad dhal separately until water runs clear. Soak each separately in enough cold water to cover by at least 2" for 8 hours; rinse and drain. Grind together using a hand grinder, large mortar and pestle, or blender and place in a bowl. Cover with a damp cotton cloth, and store in a warm place for 12 hours.

After fermenting, add onion, ginger, cilantro, salt, and enough water to mix into a thin pancake batter. Lightly oil a preheated griddle. Pour batter about 1/8" thick in center of griddle. With the back of a spoon, use a clockwise motion to spread the batter until it forms a circle about 8" to 10" in diameter. Cook each side thoroughly. Serve hot with appropriate chutneys for each type.

## Plain Dosa

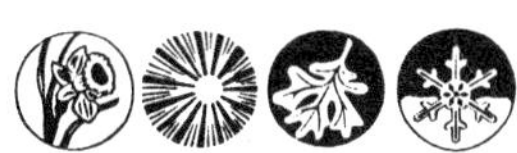

ALL TYPES
Serves 2

**1 c short-grain brown rice**
**3/8 c split urad dhal, without skins**
**1 tbs sunflower oil**
**Pinch of sea salt**
**Assorted chutneys**

***K types: substitute 1 cup millet or rye for brown rice.***

Wash rice and urad dhal separately until water runs clear. Soak each separately in enough cold water to cover by at least 2" for 8 hours; rinse and drain. Combine and grind using a hand grinder, large mortar and pestle, or blender, adding a little water as needed; place in a bowl. Cover with a damp cotton cloth, and allow to sit in a warm place for 8 hours.

Lightly coat a preheated griddle evenly with oil. Just before cooking, add salt and enough water to make a thin batter. Place two spoonfuls of batter about 1/8" thick in center of griddle. With back of the spoon, use a clockwise motion to spread the batter until it becomes paper thin. Cook dosa 1 minute per side, carefully flipping with a spatula. Serve with appropriate chutney for each type.

## Urad, Mung, and Rice Dosa

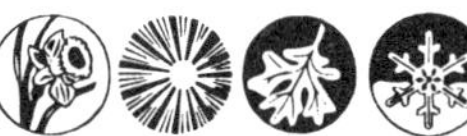

ALL TYPES
Serves 4

**1/4 c split urad dhal, without skins**
**1/4 c yellow split peas**
**1/8 c split mung dhal**
**1/8 c masoor dhal**
**2 1/2 c long-grain brown rice**
**1 tbs sunflower oil**
**1/2 tsp sea salt**
**Assorted chutneys**

Combine and wash the four dhals until water runs clear. Do same with the rice. Soak rice and dhals separately overnight in enough cold water to cover by at least 2". (Dhals are soaked together.) Grind both mixtures to a fine paste using a hand grinder, large mortar and pestle, or blender, adding a little water as needed. Combine the two batters, cover with a damp cotton cloth, and allow to sit in a warm place for 2 1/2 hours.

Lightly coat a preheated griddle evenly with oil. Add salt to mixture just before cooking. Place two spoonfuls of batter in center of the griddle. With back of the spoon, use a clockwise motion to spread the batter until it becomes paper thin. Cook dosa 1 minute per side, carefully flipping with a spatula. Serve with appropriate chutney for each type.

## Rye and Urad Dosa

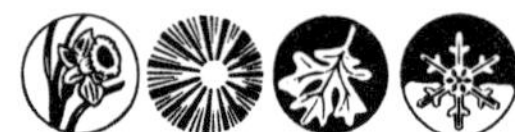

K, KV, KP
Serves 4

**2½ c rye kernels**
**1 c split urad dhal, without skins**
**1 tsp fenugreek seeds, roasted**
**¼ tsp sea salt**
**½ tbs sunflower oil**
**Assorted chutneys**

Wash rye kernels and dhal separately until water runs clear. Soak separately overnight in enough cold water to cover by at least 2". Drain and grind each into a fine paste using a hand grinder, large mortar and pestle, or blender. Combine the two mixtures and allow to sit in a warm place for 3½ hours. Add roasted fenugreek and salt.

Lightly coat a preheated griddle evenly with oil. Add salt to mixture just before cooking. Place two spoonfuls of batter in center of the griddle. With back of the spoon, use a clockwise motion to spread the batter until it becomes paper thin. Cook dosa 1 minute per side, carefully flipping with a spatula. Serve with appropriate chutney for each type.

## Wheat and Split Pea Dosa

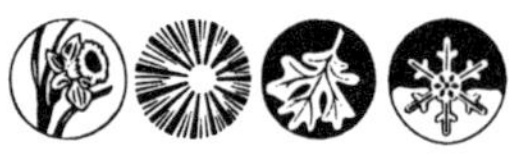

V, VP, VK, P, PV, PK
Serves 4

**2½ c wheat berries**
**1 c yellow split peas**
**1 tsp freshly ground coriander seeds**
**1 tbs coconut oil**
**½ tsp sea salt**
**Assorted chutneys**

Wash wheat berries and split peas separately until water runs clear. Soak separately overnight in enough cold water to cover by at least 2". Drain and grind each into a fine paste using a hand grinder, large mortar and pestle, or blender, adding a little water as needed. Combine the two mixtures and allow to sit in a warm place for 3½ hours. Add coriander seeds.

Lightly coat a preheated griddle evenly with oil. Add salt to mixture just before cooking. Place two spoonfuls of batter in center of the griddle. With back of the spoon, use a clockwise motion to spread the batter until paper thin. Cook dosa 1 minute per side, carefully flipping with a spatula. Serve with appropriate chutney for each type.

## Masala Dosa (Filling)

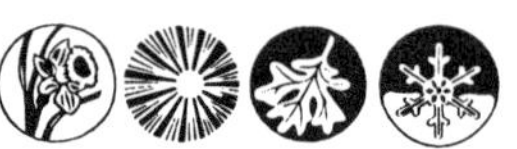

ALL TYPES
Serves 4 (fills 6 dosas)

**Filling for the appropriate dosa recipe, according to type**
**4 large potatoes**
**1 tbs sunflower oil**
**¼ tsp black mustard seeds**
**½ c minced onion**
**¼ tsp turmeric**
**2 tbs minced fresh cilantro**
**½ tsp sea salt**
**½ tsp lemon juice**

*V types: use 4 parsnips, 3 sweet potatoes, or 1 small buttercup squash instead of white potatoes.*
*P types: use ¼ teaspoon orange rind instead of lemon juice.*
*K types: use pinch of salt and ½ teaspoon oil only; add 1 green chili pepper.*

Scrub the potatoes, cut into large pieces, and boil for 25 minutes. When cooled, peel and cut into 1" cubes; set aside. In a large skillet, heat oil and sauté mustard seeds until they pop; add onion, turmeric, and cilantro and continue to sauté an additional 4 minutes. Stir in potatoes and salt. Cover and simmer over low heat for 8 minutes. Add lemon juice just before filling dosa. Place 3 tablespoons of potato filling in center of each dosa and fold over both edges.

## Rice Idli

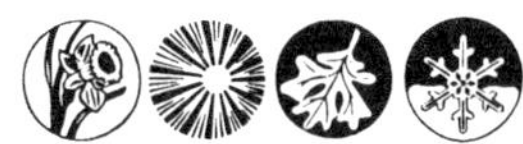

V, VK, VP
Serves 2

1 c split urad dhal, without skins
2 c brown (or white) basmati rice
1/4 tsp sea salt
2 tbs sesame oil
1/2 tbs lemon juice
Sambar or chutney

*Batter Preparation:*
Wash urad dhal and rice separately, until water runs clear. Soak each in separate bowls with enough cold water to cover by at least 2" for about 6 hours. Rinse and drain each. Adding a small amount of water, grind dhal and rice separately using a hand grinder, large mortar and pestle, or blender, so that each forms a fine paste. Combine the two batters, cover with a damp cotton cloth, and let sit for 8 hours in a warm place to mildly ferment. Add salt, oil, and lemon juice immediately before steaming.

*Steaming Procedure:*
Fill molds of an idli steamer (see Equipment and Tools, page 194). Place steamer in a large, deep pot containing 2" of boiling water. Make sure water bubbles are below the bottom of the steamer tray. Keep water boiling rapidly. Cover and steam for 20 minutes, or until a fork comes out clean. Uncover and allow trays to cool for 3 minutes before disassembling. Scoop the idlis out with a rounded soup spoon. Serve hot with sambar or chutney of your choice.

## Peppered Barley Idli

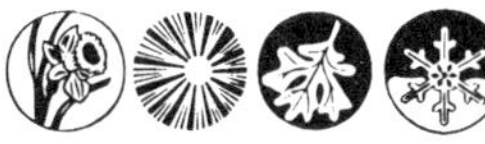

K, KV, KP
Serves 4

2 c split urad dhal, without skins
1 c pearled barley
1 tsp sunflower oil
1/2 tsp coarse black pepper
1 tsp lemon juice
Pinch of lemon rind
Pinch of sea salt
Sambar

Wash urad dhal until water runs clear. Soak dhal and barley separately in enough water to cover by at least 2" for about 2 hours. Rinse and drain separately. Grind each into a fine paste using a hand grinder, large mortar and pestle, or blender. Add water as needed. Combine the two batters, cover with a damp cotton cloth, and allow to sit for 6 hours in a warm place.

Heat oil in a skillet and stir-fry black pepper for 2 minutes. Add the pepper-oil mixture to the batter, along with lemon juice, rind, and salt. Fill molds of idli steamer (see Rice Idli recipe) and steam for 20 minutes. Serve alone or with sambar.

## Wheat and Cinnamon Idli

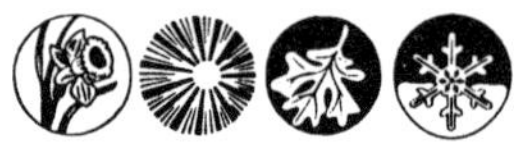

V, VP, VK, P, PV, PK
Serves 4

1 c split urad dhal, without skins
2 c bulgur
1/4 tsp cinnamon powder
1 tbs walnut oil
1/4 tsp sea salt
1/4 tsp orange rind
Orange and Cherry Chutney or Coconut Chutney

Wash urad dhal until water runs clear. Soak dhal in 3 cups of cold water for about 2 hours; rinse and drain. Wet bulgur. Grind each separately into a fine paste using a hand grinder, large mortar and pestle, or blender. Add water as needed. Combine the two batters and mix in walnut oil. Cover with a damp cotton cloth, and allow to sit for 6 hours in a warm place. Add cinnamon, salt, and rind. Fill idli steamer (see Rice Idli recipe) and steam for 20 minutes. Serve warm or cool, with Orange and Cherry Chutney or Coconut Chutney.

## Spiced Wheat Uppama

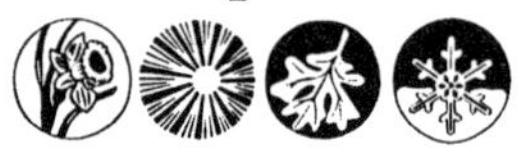

V, VP, VK, P, PV, PK
Serves 2

1 c cracked wheat
1/2 tsp black mustard seeds
1 tsp split urad dhal, without skins
1 tsp sunflower oil
6 curry leaves, preferably fresh
1/4 tsp coriander powder
2 tbs minced fresh cilantro
1 1/2 c boiling water

Dry-roast cracked wheat in a cast-iron skillet over medium heat until golden brown. Remove and, in the same skillet, heat mustard seeds and urad dhal in hot oil until seeds pop. Add curry leaves, coriander powder, and cilantro, and sauté for 30 seconds. Add roasted wheat and sauté a few minutes. Transfer mixture to a stainless steel pan containing boiling water. Stir, cover, and simmer over very low heat for 25 minutes. Toss and serve for breakfast.

## Vegetable Uppama

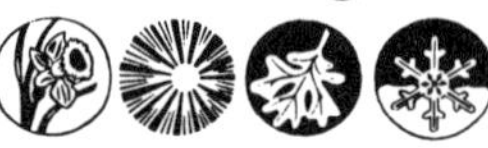

V, VP, VK
Serves 2

1 c short-grain brown rice
2 tbs light sesame oil
1/2 tsp black mustard seeds
2 tsp split urad dhal, without skins
1 tsp yellow split peas
1 dried whole red chili pepper
1/4 c minced onion
1/4 c diced carrots
2 tbs minced fresh Italian parsley
1/2 tsp minced ginger
Pinch of asafoetida
1/2 tsp sea salt
1 1/2 c boiling water

Dry-roast rice in a large cast-iron skillet until golden brown. Crack rice in a blender until each kernel is in 4 or 5 pieces; set aside. In the same skillet, heat the oil and pop the mustard seeds; add the dhals and chili pepper and brown for a few minutes. Remove spice mixture and place in a bowl. Use the same skillet to sauté onion, carrots, parsley, ginger, asafoetida, and salt. Cover and simmer over low heat for 3 minutes. Transfer both mixtures to a pot and top with the roasted cracked rice. Add the boiling water; cover and simmer over low heat for 40 minutes. Serve hot.

## Vada

ALL TYPES
Serves 2 (makes 8 balls)

1 c split urad dhal, without skins
2 tbs water
2 tbs minced onion
1/4 tsp turmeric
1/4 tsp sea salt
1/2 c sunflower oil

*V and K types: serve with Hot Chili Pepper Chutney.*
*K types: bake at 350 degrees F. instead of frying.*

Wash urad dhal until water runs clear. Soak for 1 hour in 3 cups of cold water; rinse and drain. Grind into a coarse paste using a hand grinder, large mortar and pestle, or blender, adding water as needed. Allow to sit for 2 hours in a warm place to mildly ferment. Add onion, turmeric, and salt. Shape into 8 small balls, 1" in diameter, and deep-fry as in Vadai recipe (page 201).

## Dahi Vada

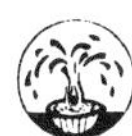

V, VP, VK
Serves 2 (makes 8 balls)

1 c split urad dhal, without skins
1 tsp minced ginger
2 minced green chili peppers
1 tsp coconut oil
3/4 c fresh plain yogurt
1/2 c water
2 tbs minced fresh cilantro
1/2 tsp sea salt
Pinch of asafoetida

Wash urad dhal until water runs clear. Soak for 1 hour in 3 cups of cold water; rinse and drain. In a skillet, sauté ginger and chili peppers in the oil for a few minutes. Add drained dhal and combine well. Remove from pan and grind into a coarse paste using a hand grinder, large mortar and pestle, or blender. Shape into 8 balls, 1" in diameter, and deep-fry as in Vadai recipe (page 201).

Pour yogurt into a bowl and whip with an eggbeater until smooth. Slowly add water, cilantro, salt, and asafoetida. Continue to beat until smooth and fluid. Soak the fried vadas in the yogurt mixture in a cool place for 30 minutes Serve with basmati rice for a festive lunch. Prepare only the amount needed for one meal.

## Chapati

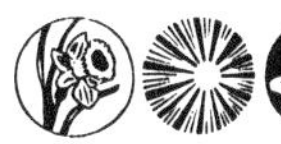 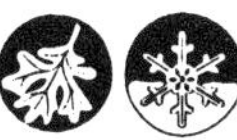

ALL TYPES
Serves 4

2 c whole wheat flour, or atta
1/4 tsp sea salt
1 tbs sunflower oil
3/4 c water

*K types: substitute 2 cups either barley or rye flour for whole wheat flour; use only 1 teaspoon oil.*

Use freshly ground flour whenever possible. Combine flour and salt; add oil and work it with your fingertips into the flour. Add half the water and knead the dough for 5 minutes. Add the remaining water and knead for an additional 5 minutes. Cover with a damp cotton cloth and allow to sit for 2 hours. Divide dough into 12 small pieces.

Lightly flour a clean table surface and roll out each piece into a thin patty using a rolling pin. (Instead, you may use your hands to press dough pieces into patties and toss into the air to enlarge.)

Preheat a griddle and cook the chapati for 30 seconds on each side over medium heat. Remove gently with tongs. If you have a gas stove, wave the chapati over an open flame for a few seconds until it puffs up. (If you do not have a gas stove, ignore this step.) Serve hot.

## Oil Roti

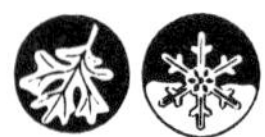

V, VP, VK, P, PV, PK
Serves 4 (makes 12 roti)

1 c whole wheat flour, or atta
1 c unbleached white flour
1/4 cup wheat bran
Pinch of sea salt
1 tbs sunflower oil
3/4 c water

Prepare the dough as instructed in Chapati recipe (page 207). Divide dough into 12 small pieces. Roll each piece to a 1/2" thick patty, 4" in diameter. Rub 1/4 teaspoon oil on top of each patty. Fold the sides of each patty inward to form square envelopes. Cover with a damp cotton towel and allow dough to sit for 15 minutes.

Roll each piece into a 1/4" thick square, approximately 8" by 8", and dust with flour. Lightly oil a preheated griddle and cook on each side for 30 seconds. After turning patty once, apply a light coat of oil to each side, using a muslin cloth; roti will bubble. Remove from griddle and, with a clean towel in your hands, slap roti back and forth. This will keep the roti soft.

## Potato Roti

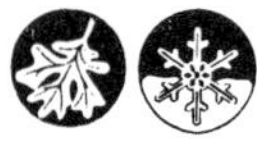

V, VP, VK, P, PV, PK
Serves 4

Follow instructions for preparing Oil Roti, but add the following potato filling instead of oil before folding into envelopes. Do not slap the roti between your hands after cooking.

*Potato Filling:*
1 large potato
1/4 c minced onion
1/2 tsp ghee
Pinch of sea salt

Scrub, wash, and cut potato into quarters. Boil until soft, then remove skin. Sauté onion in ghee for 4 minutes. Combine with boiled potatoes and lightly mash until lumpy (not smooth). Add salt and place 3 tablespoons of filling in each roti.

## Cumin and Basmati Rice

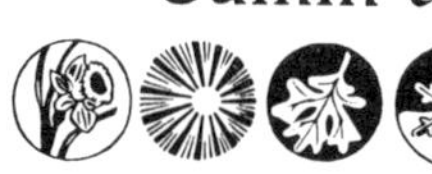

ALL TYPES (K TYPES, SPARINGLY)
Serves 4

1 tbs cumin seeds
2 c white basmati rice
3 c boiling water
Pinch of sea salt
1 tsp ghee

Dry-roast cumin seeds in small cast-iron pan until golden. Wash rice until water runs clear; drain. Add boiling water, roasted seeds, and salt to rice. Cover and simmer over medium-low heat for 20 to 25 minutes until rice fluffs. Remove from heat and stir in ghee. Serve hot.

## Rye and Corn

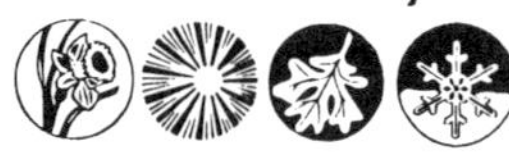

K, KV, KP
Serves 2

1 c rye berries
3 1/2 c water
1/2 c fresh corn kernels
1 tbs freshly ground chili powder
Pinch of salt

Wash rye berries until water runs clear. Soak in 3 cups of cold water for 1 hour. Drain, rinse, and boil in water for 35 minutes. Add corn, chili powder, and salt. Cover and simmer over medium heat for an additional 25 minutes. Serve hot.

## Millet and Cauliflower

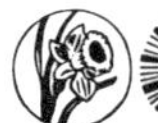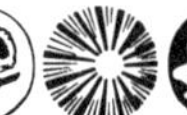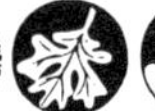

P, PV, PK, K, KV, KP
Serves 4

1 c cauliflower florets
1/2 c diced onion
2 c hulled millet
4 1/2 c water
Pinch of turmeric
Pinch of sea salt

Place cauliflower florets and onion in a pot. Wash the millet thoroughly and place on top of vegetables. Add water, turmeric, and salt and bring to a boil. Reduce heat to low, cover, and simmer for 25 minutes. Serve hot. This dish may be lightly mashed and served to children.

## Bulgur and Peas

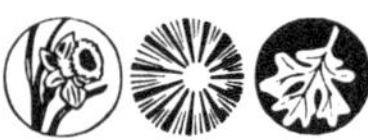

V, VP, VK, P, PV, PK
Serves 4

3 c water
2 c bulgur
1 1/2 c fresh peas
Pinch of salt
2 tbs orange juice
2 sprigs minced cilantro

*V and VP: substitute 1 1/2 cups diced carrots for peas.*

In a medium pan, bring water to a boil. Add bulgur, peas, and salt. Cover and simmer over low heat for 20 minutes. In a small pan or large spoon, heat orange juice and minced cilantro for 30 seconds. Stir into bulgur. Serve hot.

## Millet and Corn

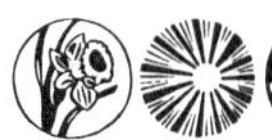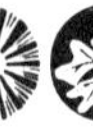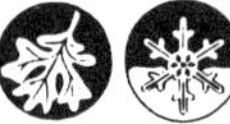

P, PV, PK, K, KV, KP
*V types may use occasionally because this dish is moist and sweet.*
Serves 4

2 c hulled millet
4 c boiling water
1 c fresh corn kernels
Pinch each of salt, turmeric, black pepper

Wash millet thoroughly. Add to boiling water. Cover and simmer for 15 minutes over low heat. Add corn and spices; cook over low heat for an additional 10 minutes. Serve warm.

## Saffron Rice and Corn (PC)

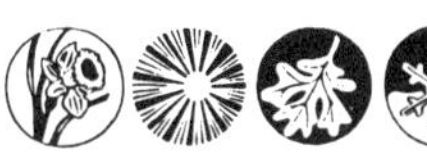

V, VP, VK
P, PV, PK OCCASIONALLY
Serves 4

2 c short-grain brown rice
4 c boiling water
Pinch of salt
1 c fresh corn kernels
8 strands saffron

Wash rice until water runs clear. Drain and add to boiling water in a pressure cooker. Add salt. Lock, cover, and bring to pressure over high heat. Cook gently over medium-low heat for 35 minutes. Allow pressure to fall naturally, about 15 minutes. (For conventional cooking, add rice to 5 cups boiling water. Cover and cook over medium heat for 45 minutes.) Mix corn and saffron into the rice. Cover without locking and continue to simmer an additional 15 minutes. Remove from heat and serve.

## Soft Rice

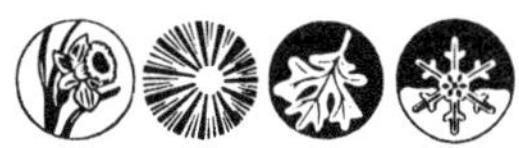

V, VP, VK
P, PV, PK OCCASIONALLY
Serves 2

**1" square of kombu seaweed**
**1 c short-grain brown rice**
**5 c water**
**Gomasio**

Place kombu in a small bowl of water and rub gently to remove salt. Wash rice until water runs clear; drain. Combine rice, water, and washed kombu in a medium saucepan and bring to a boil. Cover and simmer over low heat for 1 hour. The rice should be creamy, with a few whole kernels. Serve warm with gomasio.

## Fried Rice

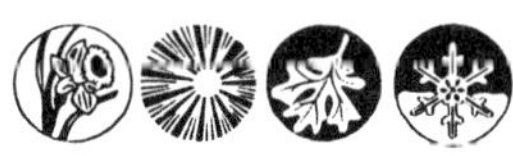

V, VP, VK
Serves 6

**1 tbs sesame oil**
**1 c thinly sliced carrots**
**1 c small broccoli florets and peeled stem pieces**
**1 c finely chopped onion**
**3 c short-grain brown rice, cooked**
**1/2 tsp tamari**
**1/2 tsp ginger juice (see page 194)**
**1/4 c water**
*K and KV: use millet instead of rice.*

Heat oil in a large skillet. Add carrots and simmer, covered, over low heat for 5 minutes. Add broccoli and simmer an additional 5 minutes. Stir in onion and simmer 3 minutes more. Place cooked rice on top of vegetables. Dilute tamari and ginger juice in water. Add to rice and vegetables and mix together. Cover and simmer entire mixture over low heat for 5 minutes. Serve hot.

## Soft Fried Rice

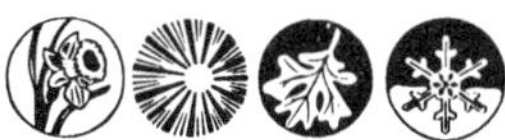

V, VP, VK
P, PV, PK OCCASIONALLY
Serves 6

**1 1/2 tsp sunflower oil**
**1 c thinly sliced okra pods**
**1 c finely minced onion**
**1 c thinly sliced zucchini**
**1/2 bunch watercress**
**1/4 tsp turmeric**
**1/4 tsp sea salt**
**3 c long-grain brown rice, cooked**
***K, KV, and KP: substitute 3 cups cooked millet for rice.***

Heat oil in a large skillet. Add okra, onion, and zucchini. Cover and simmer over low heat for 10 minutes. In a small pan, lightly boil watercress in 1/2 cup of water for 3 minutes and set aside. Remove watercress and set aside for garnish. Dilute turmeric and salt in the watercress water.

Place cooked rice on top of vegetables. Add spiced water; cover and simmer over low heat for an additional 5 minutes. Mix together; place watercress on top of rice and serve.

## Wheat Berries and Cloves (PC)

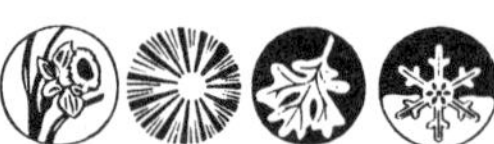

V, VP, VK
P, PV, PK
Serves 4

**2 c wheat berries**
**1/2 c aduki beans**
**8 whole cloves**
**Pinch of sea salt**
**4 cups water**
**1/4 tsp coarse black pepper**
**1 tsp sunflower oil**

Wash wheat berries until water runs clear. Soak in 4 cups of cold water for 5 hours. Rinse and drain. Put wheat berries, beans, cloves, salt, and water in pressure cooker. Cover without locking lid and bring to a boil. Lock cover and bring to pressure. Simmer over medium heat for 45 minutes. Remove from heat and allow pressure to fall naturally. (For conventional cooking, add wheat berries to 7 cups boiling water. Cover and cook over medium heat for 50 to 55 minutes.)

Sauté black pepper in oil for 2 minutes. Add to wheat mixture. Cover again without locking lid and simmer for an additional 15 minutes. Serve warm.

## Whole Oats and Corn (PC)

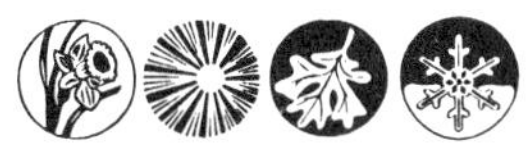

P, PV, PK
V, VP, VK OCCASIONALLY
Serves 4

2 c whole oats
2 ears corn, husked
Pinch of sea salt
2" cinnamon stick (broken into pieces)
4 c water
1 tbs caraway seeds

Soak oats in 4 cups of cold water for 3 hours. Strip corn from the ears. Place oats, salt, cinnamon stick, stripped cobs, and water in pressure cooker. Cover without locking and bring to a boil. Lock cover and bring to pressure. Cook over medium heat 50 minutes. Remove from heat and allow pressure to fall naturally.

Dry-roast caraway seeds in a small cast-iron pan until golden. Add seeds and corn kernels to oats; remove the cobs and discard. Cover again without locking lid and allow to simmer for an additional 10 to 15 minutes.(For conventionsl cooking, add whole oats to 7 cups boiling water. Cover and cook over medium heat for 40 minutes to 1 hour.) Remove cinnamon pieces and serve dish warm or cool.

## Buckwheat and Peas

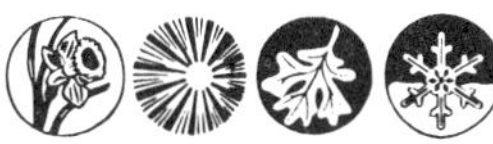

K, KV, KP
Serves 4

2 c buckwheat groats
$3^1/_2$ c boiling water
$^1/_4$ tsp turmeric
$^1/_4$ tsp chili powder
Pinch of sea salt
$^1/_2$ tsp cumin seeds
$^1/_2$ c fresh peas

Wash buckwheat groats and add to boiling water along with turmeric, chili powder, and salt. Cover and simmer over medium heat for 25 minutes. Dry-roast cumin seeds in a small cast-iron skillet for 2 minutes; add roasted seeds and peas to buckwheat. Continue simmering over low heat an additional 15 minutes. Serve hot.

## Cumin Millet

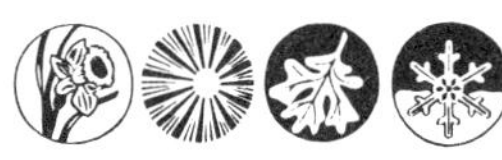

K, KV, KP
Serves 4

$^1/_2$ cup split mung dhal (optional)
2 c hulled millet
3 c boiling water
Pinch of sea salt
Touch of ghee
1 tbs cumin or caraway seeds

Wash mung and millet thoroughly. Dry-roast millet in a large cast-iron skillet over low heat, stirring or shaking constantly until dry and golden. Add to boiling water along with salt and ghee, and mung (if desired). Cover and simmer over medium-low heat for 15 minutes.

Dry-roast seeds in a small cast-iron pan until golden. Add to millet and cook an additional 10 minutes. Serve hot.

## Caraway Rice

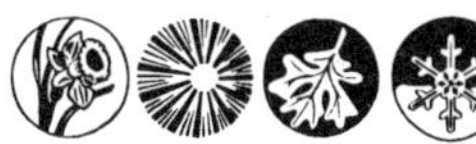

V, VP, VK
P, PV, PK OCCASIONALLY
Serves 4

1/2 c whole mung dhal
2 c long-grain brown rice
3 1/2 c boiling water
1/4 c minced onion
1/2 tsp dark sesame oil
Pinch of sea salt
2 tsp caraway seeds

Wash mung dhal until water runs clear. Soak in 2 cups of cold water for 8 hours or overnight; rinse and drain. Wash rice until water runs clear and add, along with mung, to boiling water. Sauté onion in oil until translucent and add to rice and mung. Add salt. Cover and simmer over medium-low heat for 25 minutes.

Dry-roast caraway seeds in a small cast-iron pan until golden. Add to rice mixture and cook an additional 5 minutes. Serve warm.

## Cumin Quinoa

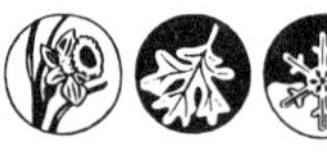

V, VP, VK, K, KV, KP
Serves 4

2 c quinoa
2 3/4 c boiling water
Pinch of sea salt
1 tbs cumin seeds
Pinch of turmeric

Wash quinoa until water runs clear. Add to boiling water with salt and simmer, covered, over medium-low heat for 7 minutes. Dry-roast cumin seeds with turmeric in a small cast-iron pan for 2 minutes. Add seeds to quinoa. Continue to simmer an additional 7 minutes. Serve hot.

## Saffron Basmati Rice

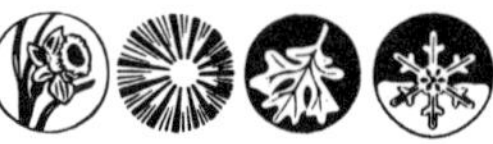

ALL TYPES (K TYPES, SPARINGLY)
Serves 4

2 c brown basmati rice
3 1/2 c boiling water
12 strands saffron
Pinch of sea salt
1 tsp ghee

Wash rice until water runs clear, drain, and add to boiling water along with saffron and salt. Cover and simmer over medium-low heat for 35 to 40 minutes until rice fluffs. Remove from heat; mix in ghee. Serve hot.

## Sweet Spiced Pullau

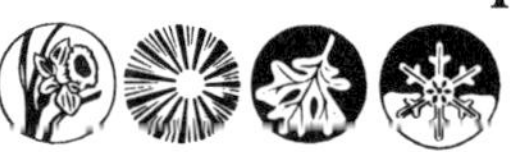

V, VP, VK, P, PV, PK
Serves 4

1/8 c diced onion
1/4 c ghee
2 c bulgur
4 c water
4 whole cloves
8 coarsely crushed cardamom seeds
2" cinnamon stick (broken into pieces)
1/2 tbs unrefined brown sugar
1/2 tsp sea salt

In a medium saucepan, sauté onion in ghee for a few minutes. Stir in bulgur and sauté over medium heat until golden brown. Boil water in a small saucepan and add cloves, cardamom, cinnamon, and sugar; stir in bulgur mixture and salt. Cover and simmer over low heat for 35 minutes. Remove cloves and cinnamon. Serve warm or cool.

## Quinoa and Carrots

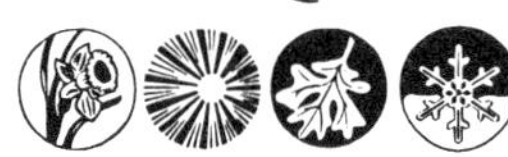

ALL TYPES
Serves 2

1 c quinoa
$1^1/_2$ c water
$^1/_2$ c diced carrots
1 tsp roasted caraway seeds

*P types: substitute 1 cup couscous for quinoa.*

Wash quinoa until water runs clear. Place in water, along with carrots, and bring to a boil. Add roasted caraway seeds. Cover and simmer over low heat for 15 minutes. Serve hot.

## Yogurt Rice

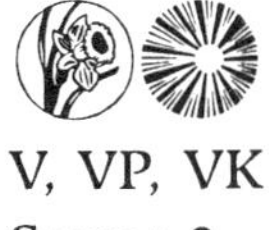

V, VP, VK
Serves 2

1 c white basmati rice
3 c water
1 tsp split urad dhal, without skins
1 tsp black mustard seeds
1 tsp sesame oil
$^1/_2$ tsp minced ginger
2 minced green chili peppers
2 tbs minced fresh cilantro
1 c fresh plain yogurt
$^1/_4$ tsp sea salt

Wash rice until water runs clear; drain. Combine with water and bring to a boil; simmer over medium heat for 25 minutes until well cooked. Allow to cool.

In a preheated griddle, roast urad dhal and mustard seeds in oil until the dhal is light brown and the seeds begin to pop. Remove dhal and seeds from the griddle and add ginger and chili peppers Sauté for 4 minutes over low heat; add cilantro during the last minute. Pour yogurt into a large wooden bowl and mix in the dhal, seeds, herbs, and salt. Add the rice and combine well. Serve warm for lunch.

## Tamarind Rice

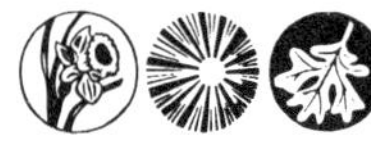

V, VK
Serves 2

1 c long-grain brown rice*
$2^1/_2$ c boiling water
$^1/_4$ tsp sea salt
Pinch of turmeric
2 tbs light sesame oil
2 tbs yellow split peas
1 tbs split urad dhal, without skins
2 dried whole red chili peppers
$^1/_8$ c cashew pieces
1 tsp coriander seeds
1 tsp black mustard seeds
Pinch of asafoetida
1 tsp tamarind pulp
$^1/_2$ c warm water

**White or short-grain brown rice can also be used.*
*K and KV: substitute 1 cup millet for brown rice.*

Wash rice until water runs clear; drain and add to boiling water with salt and turmeric. Cover and simmer over medium heat for 30 to 35 minutes, until rice is well-cooked but kernels separate easily. In a large skillet, heat 1 tablespoon of the oil and lightly brown yellow split peas, urad dhal, chili peppers, and cashew pieces. Remove from pan. Gently sauté coriander and mustard seeds until seeds begin to pop. Combine sautéed condiments; add asafoetida and set aside.

In a small pan, dilute tamarind pulp in warm water. Add remaining tablespoon of oil and gently boil for 2 minutes. Pour over sautéed condiments and mix with your hands to make a smooth, fluid paste. Spread rice evenly on the bottom of a large serving dish. Pour tamarind mixture over rice and daub with hands until each grain is coated. Serve warm.

## Mola Hora

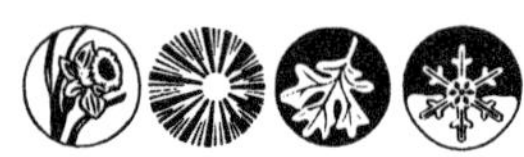

ALL TYPES
Serves 2

1 c long-grain brown rice
3 c boiling water
Pinch of sea salt
2 tbs ghee
1 tsp coarse black pepper
Pinch of asafoetida

*P types: substitute either 1 cup barley or wheat for brown rice; use 1 tablespoon ghee.*

*K types: substitute 1 cup millet for brown rice; use 1 teaspoon ghee.*

Wash rice until water runs clear, drain, and add to boiling water with salt. Cover and simmer over medium heat for 30 minutes. In a small skillet, heat ghee. Add black pepper and sauté for 2 minutes. Add asafoetida and spice mixture to cooked rice. Serve hot.

## Coconut Rice

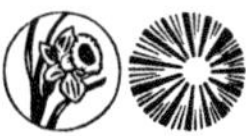

V, VP, VK, P, PV, PK
Serves 4

2 c medium-grain arborio rice
4 c water
1/4 tsp sea salt
2 tbs coconut oil
1/2 tsp black mustard seeds
1 tbs yellow split peas
1 tsp split urad dhal, without skins
2 curry leaves, preferably fresh
1/2 c finely grated fresh coconut

*Garnish:*
1/8 c roasted sunflower seeds

*All types: substitute 2 cups bulgur for arborio rice, if desired (same amount of water and same cooking time).*

Wash rice until water runs clear. Drain and combine with water and salt. Bring to a boil and simmer over medium heat for 25 minutes.

In a large skillet, heat oil and sauté mustard seeds until they pop. Add yellow split peas and dhal and sauté until light brown. Add curry leaves and grated coconut and continue to sauté for 4 minutes over low heat, until coconut turns golden. Combine the sautéed ingredients and mix into the cooked rice. Garnish with roasted sunflower seeds and serve warm.

## Sesame Rice

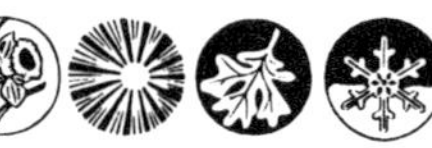

V, VP, VK
Serves 2

1 c medium-grain brown rice
2 1/2 c boiling water
1/2 tsp sea salt
1/8 c sesame seeds
1 tbs sesame oil
1/4 c toor dhal
2 dried whole red chili peppers
1/4 tsp asafoetida

*Garnish:*
Roasted sesame seeds

Wash rice until water runs clear. Drain and add to boiling water with salt. Cover and bring to a boil; simmer over medium-low heat for 30 minutes. Wash sesame seeds and dry-roast in a cast-iron skillet over low heat until they are crunchy to the touch. Remove from skillet and set aside.

Add 1 teaspoon oil to the skillet and sauté toor dhal over low heat for 8 minutes until evenly brown. Grind dhal and chili peppers into a fine paste using a hand grinder, mortar and pestle, or blender. Allow rice to cool for 10 minutes. Stir dhal paste and asafoetida into rice. Garnish with roasted sesame seeds and serve warm.

## Cracked Rice Uppama

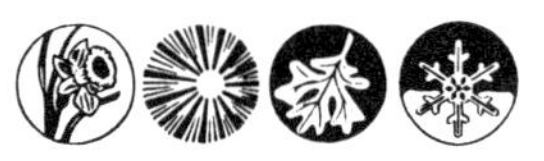

V, VP, VK, P, PV, PK
Serves 2

1 c short-grain brown rice
1 tsp olive oil
1/2 tsp black mustard seeds
1/2 tsp minced ginger
2 minced green chili peppers
3 crushed dried curry leaves
1/4 tsp sea salt
2 c boiling water

*P types: omit chili peppers and ginger and use 1 teaspoon coriander seeds instead.*

Wash rice until water runs clear. Air-dry and toast in a large cast-iron skillet over low heat until rice is golden. Pound in a suribachi or grind with a hand grinder very coarsely. Return to skillet and set aside.

In a small skillet, heat oil and roast mustard seeds until they pop and turn grey. Mix in ginger, chili peppers, and curry leaves and continue to cook 3 minutes. Add to cracked rice. Place salt in boiling water and pour over rice mixture; cover and simmer over medium heat for 15 minutes. Serve warm.

## Cinnamon Spiced Wheat (PC)

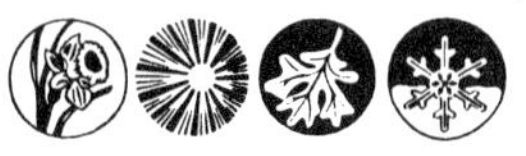

V, VP, VK, P, PV, PK
Serves 2

1/2 c wheat berries
4 c boiling water
4 whole cloves
1 small piece cinnamon stick
2 dried curry leaves
2 tsp walnut oil
1 tbs yellow split peas
1 tsp coriander seeds
1/2 tsp poppy seeds
1/4 tsp sea salt

*Garnish:*
Minced fresh parsley

Soak wheat berries in 2 cups of cold water for 5 hours. Rinse and add to boiling water in pressure cooker with cloves, cinnamon, and curry leaves. Lock cover and bring to pressure. Cook over medium heat for 35 minutes. Remove from heat and allow pressure to fall naturally. Allow to cool for 15 minutes. (For conventional cooking, add wheat berries to 5 cups boiling water. Cover and cook over medium heat for 55 to 60 minutes.)

In a small skillet, heat oil and lightly brown peas and coriander seeds; add poppy seeds and salt toward the end. Grind into a fine paste and mix into wheat berries. Garnish with fresh parsley and serve warm.

## Spiced Rice and Millet

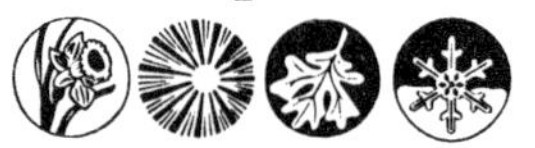

V, VP, VK, K, KV, KP
Serves 2

**1 c millet hulled**
**1/2 c long-grain brown rice**
**1/4 cup split urad dhal, without skins**
**1/2 tsp black mustard seeds**
**1/2 tsp coriander seeds**
**1 minced green chili pepper**
**2 crushed dried curry leaves**
**Pinch of asafoetida**
**Pinch of sea salt**
**3 1/2 c boiling water**

*Garnish:*
**Lemon slices and fresh parsley**

*V types: roast spices in 2 teaspoons sesame oil.*

Wash millet and rice until water runs clear. Air-dry and toast in large cast-iron skillet until evenly golden. In a small skillet, dry-roast dhal, mustard and coriander seeds, chili pepper, and curry leaves for a few minutes. Add asafoetida and salt during last 30 seconds of roasting. Stir into grains. Pour boiling water over grain mixture; cover and simmer over medium-low heat for 35 minutes. Garnish with lemon slices and fresh parsley. Serve warm.

## GRAIN BALLS AND ROLLS

Nori are thin dark purple sheets of dried seaweed. Nori balls and rolls are just a small part of the majestic tradition of Japanese food culture. Both are compact, lend strength to the body, and require no refrigeration—a perfect food for traveling. Seaweeds are very high in calcium and minerals. Nori is considered the most delicious among the various types of seaweed. Although it is not customary in the Japanese tradition to use other than refined rice, macrobiotics has introduced the more nutritive brown rice in these rolls and balls.

Rice is best for predominant Vata types, and occasionally for predominant Pitta types. Couscous, a whole wheat flour product, is a good occasional alternative for both Vata and Pitta types. Predominant Kapha types should use millet instead of rice and wasabi mustard instead of umeboshi plum. Since seaweeds are naturally salty, both Pitta and Kapha should eat these items only occasionally.

## Rice Nori Balls

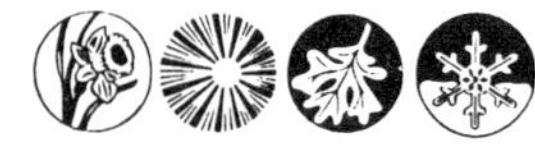

V, VP, VK
Makes 2 balls

**1 sheet nori seaweed**
**1 c sushi rice, cooked**
**1/2 umeboshi plum, pitted and halved again**

If you have a gas stove, toast nori by slowly waving it over a medium flame; otherwise use sheet untoasted. Fold and tear sheet into four equal pieces. With wet hands, mold half of the rice into a ball. Press a hole in the center of rice ball and insert one piece of umeboshi plum. Pack the ball again to close the hole.

Place one piece of nori on top of ball and fold down the points. Turn the ball over and add a second piece of nori to fit in between the points of the first piece and cover all the rice. Mold the ball again between your palms. Repeat process with remaining 1/2 cup rice and 2 nori pieces for second ball. Serve at room temperature.

## Millet Nori Balls

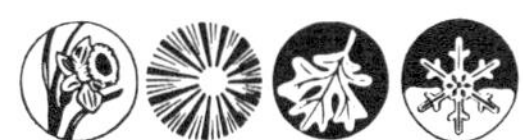

K, KV, KP
Makes 2 balls

**1 sheet nori seaweed**
**1/2 tsp wasabi mustard**
**1 c millet, well cooked (see page 170)**

If you have a gas stove, toast nori by slowly waving it over a medium flame; otherwise use sheet untoasted. Fold and tear sheet into four equal pieces. Add a few drops of water to wasabi mustard to dilute into a thin paste. With wet hands, mold half of the millet into a ball. Press a hole in the center of millet ball and insert half the wasabi paste. Pack the ball again to close the hole.

Place one piece of nori on top of ball and fold down the points. Turn the ball over and add a second piece of nori to fit in between the points of the first piece and cover all the millet. Mold the ball again between your palms. Repeat process with remaining 1/2 cup millet and 2 nori pieces for second ball. Serve at room temperature.

## Rice Nori Rolls

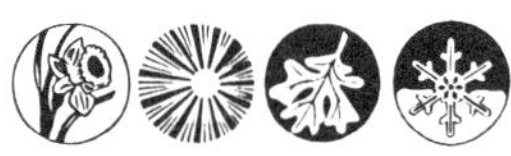

ALL TYPES
Makes about 8 roll pieces, 2" wide

**2 sheets nori seaweed**
**1 c short-grain brown rice, cooked and sticky**
**1/4 c carrot strips, boiled (al dente)**
**2 long scallion greens**
**1/2 tsp umeboshi paste**

If you have a gas stove, toast nori by slowly waving it over a medium flame; otherwise use sheet untoasted. Place nori on a bamboo sushi mat. Spread half of rice evenly over a nori sheet, leaving a 1/2" space at either end. Lay half of carrots and scallions parallel to and about 1" from bottom of sheet (the end closest to you). Spread a thin layer of umeboshi paste on the bottom edge of rice.

Lightly moisten top edge of nori and, pressing the bamboo mat firmly against nori and rice, roll the mat and its contents, continuing to press firmly while rolling. Pull mat back while rolling so it doesn't get rolled into the nori. The moistened top edge will seal nori together, preventing the roll from falling apart. Wet a sharp knife and slice the roll into four 2" pieces. Repeat procedure for second roll. Serve at room temperature.

Alternative fillings: strips of cucumber, avocado, cooked burdock, watercress, firmly cooked squash.

## Millet Nori Rolls

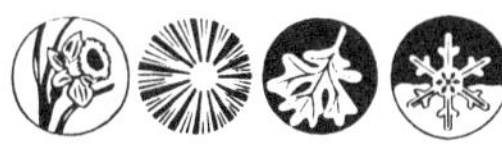

K, KV, KP
Serves 2

Makes 16 small roll pieces

**2 sheets nori seaweed**
**1 c millet, cooked and sticky (see page 170)**
**2 leaves mustard greens, steamed**
**1 carrot, cut into strips and boiled (al dente)**
**1/2 tsp wasabi mustard**

If you have a gas stove, toast nori by slowly waving it over a medium flame; otherwise use sheet untoasted. Place nori on a bamboo sushi mat. Spread half of millet evenly over nori sheet, leaving a 1/2" space at either end. Place half of mustard greens over the millet and top with half of carrots.

Moisten the wasabi with drops of water and spread a thin layer on the bottom edge of rice. See the preceding recipe for Rice Nori Rolls for instructions on rolling. Repeat procedure for second roll. Wet a sharp knife and slice each roll into eight 1" pieces. Serve at room temperature.

## Collard Nori Rolls

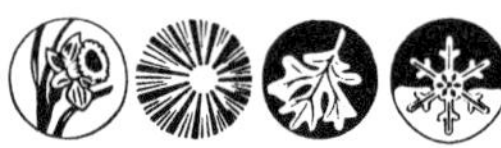

ALL TYPES
Serves 2

Makes 8 roll pieces, 2" wide

2 sheets nori seaweed
Rice vinegar
1 c white sushi rice, cooked
1 steamed collard leaf, cut in half
1/4 c carrot strips, boiled (al dente)
1/2 tsp umeboshi paste

If you have a gas stove, toast nori by slowly waving it over a medium flame; otherwise use sheet untoasted. Add a touch of vinegar to the cooked sushi rice. Place nori on a bamboo sushi mat, leaving 1/2" space at either end. Top the rice with half a collard leaf; place a line of carrot strips parallel to the edge, about 1" from the bottom edge (the end closest to you).

Spread a thin layer of umeboshi paste along the bottom edge of rice. See Rice Nori Rolls, page 217, for instruction on rolling. Repeat procedure for second roll. Wet a sharp knife and slice each roll into four 2" pieces. Serve at room temperature.

## South Indian Steamed Rice Balls

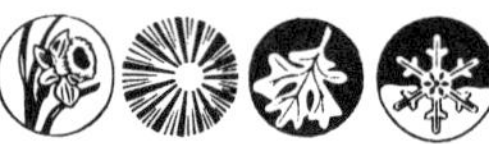

V, VP, VK
Serves 2

1/2 c short-grain brown rice
1 tbs split urad dhal, without skins
2 tsp black mustard seeds
2 dried curry leaves
2 minced green chili peppers
1 tbs sunflower oil
1 tbs lemon juice
1 tbs sesame oil
Pinch of salt
1 1/2 c water
Pan of boiling water

Roast rice in a large skillet over medium heat for 7 minutes. In another pan, sauté urad dhal, mustard seeds, curry leaves, and chili peppers in hot oil until mustard seeds pop. Using a hand grinder or a large mortar and pestle, grind roasted rice into a coarse flour and add to sautéed mixture along with lemon juice, sesame oil, and salt. Add 1 1/2 cups water and simmer, covered, over low heat for 15 minutes. Remove mixture from heat and allow to cool.

Knead into a dough and with lightly oiled hands, roll dough into 12 small balls. Insert a steamer or a colander with legs into a pan of boiling water. (Keep water level below bottom of the steamer.) Add rice balls and cover; steam over low heat for 15 minutes. Cool and serve with dhal and vegetables.

## South Indian Wheat Balls

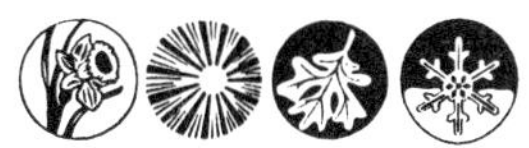

V, P, PV, PK
Serves 2

**1/2 c bulgur**
**1 tbs walnut oil**
**1 tbs split urad dhal, without skins**
**3 crushed dried curry leaves**
**1 tsp coriander seeds**
**1 tsp cumin seeds**
**1 tbs orange juice**
**1/2 tsp orange rind**
**1/2 tsp cardamom powder**
**1/4 tsp turmeric**
**1/4 tsp sea salt**
**1 1/2 c water**
***Garnish:***
**2 tbs minced fresh cilantro**

Dry-roast bulgur in a cast-iron skillet over medium heat for 7 minutes. Using a hand grinder or large mortar and pestle, grind roasted bulgur into a coarse flour. Heat oil in a skillet and brown urad, curry leaves, and coriander and cumin seeds. Add bulgur flour, orange juice, orange rind, cardamom powder, turmeric, salt, and water. Mix, cover, and simmer over low heat for 15 minutes. Remove from skillet and allow to cool.

Knead into a dough and with lightly oiled hands, roll into 12 small balls. Steam, as in South Indian Steamed Rice Balls, page 218. Garnish with cilantro and cool. Serve with dhal and vegetables.

## South Indian Millet Balls

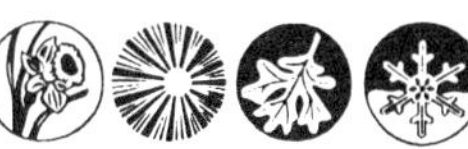

K, KV
Serves 2

**1/2 c millet**
**1 tbs split urad dhal, without skins**
**2 minced green chili peppers**
**3 dried curry leaves**
**1 tbs black mustard seeds**
**1/2 tsp dried fenugreek leaves**
**1 tsp lemon juice**
**1 1/2 c water**
**Pinch of salt**
**2 tbs minced fresh parsley**

Dry-roast millet in a cast-iron skillet over medium heat for 7 minutes. Using a hand grinder or large mortar and pestle, grind roasted millet into a coarse flour. In a cast-iron skillet, dry-roast urad dhal, chili peppers, curry leaves, mustard seeds, and fenugreek for a few minutes. Add millet flour, lemon juice, water, salt, and parsley. Mix, cover, and simmer over low heat for 10 minutes. Remove mixture from skillet and allow to cool.

Knead into a dough and with lightly oiled hands, roll into 12 small balls. Steam as in South Indian Steamed Rice Balls, page 218. Cool and serve with dhal and vegetables.

# BREAKFAST GRAINS

## Cream of Wheat Porridge

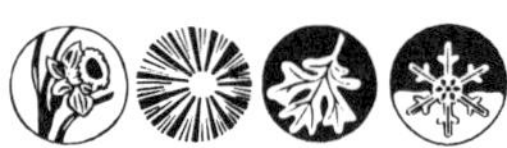

V, VP, P, PV, PK
Serves 1

1/4 c water
1/2 c certified raw cow's milk
1/4 c cream of wheat
2 tbs raisins
1/2 tsp ghee
1/2 tsp unrefined brown sugar

In a small saucepan, bring water and milk to boil. Add cream of wheat, raisins, ghee, and brown sugar and stir. Simmer uncovered over low heat for 10 minutes. Serve hot.

## Soft Breakfast Rice

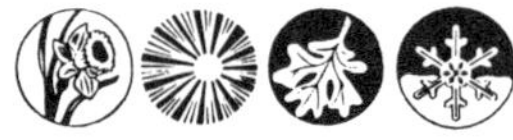

ALL TYPES
Serves 2

3 c water
1/2 c short-grain brown rice
1/2 tsp ghee
1/4 tsp sea salt
Gomasio

In a medium saucepan, bring water to boil. Add rice, ghee, and salt. Cover and allow to simmer over medium-low heat for 1 1/2 hours. Serve warm with gomasio.

## Eggless French Toast

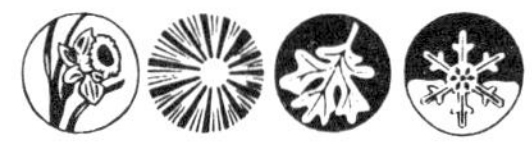

V, VP, VK, P, PV, PK
Serves 2

4 slices of fresh whole wheat bread

*Batter:*
1 tsp kudzu (or arrowroot)
1/4 c cold water
1/2 c soy, almond, or cow's milk
1/4 tsp turmeric
2 tbs maple syrup or unrefined brown sugar
1/4 tsp cinnamon
1 tsp rose water
1/4 tsp rock salt

*PK: use soy milk.*

Dilute kudzu in 1/4 cup of cold water and set aside. Mix remaining ingredients together in a saucepan and bring to boil over medium heat; add kudzu. When batter begins to gel, remove from heat.

Toast bread in well-seasoned cast-iron skillet over low heat. Pour batter over toast and continue to cook over medium heat about 3 minutes on each side. Serve warm.

## Couscous and Carrots

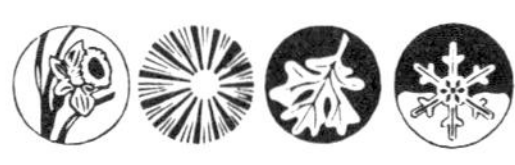

V, VP, P, PV, PK
Serves 2

2 1/2 c water
1 c couscous
1/2 c finely diced carrots

*Garnish:*
Fresh cilantro or roasted cumin seeds

Bring water to boil; add couscous and carrots. Cover and simmer over medium heat for 5 to 8 minutes. Garnish with fresh cilantro or roasted cumin seeds. Serve wam.

## Millet Croquettes

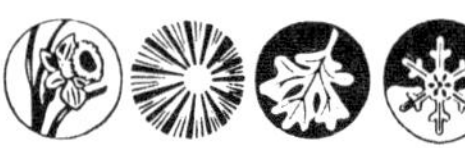

K, KV, KP
Serves 2

1/2 tsp sunflower oil
1/4 c diced carrots
1/4 c diced onions
1/2 c millet, cooked (see page 170)
Pinch of salt
Pinch of coarse black pepper

Heat oil in a preheated skillet and sauté carrots and onions over medium heat for 3 minutes. Add millet, salt, and pepper. Stir together and allow to cool. Dampen hands and shape mixture into 6 palm-sized patties. Clean skillet and dry-roast patties over low heat to desired crispness.

## Soft Millet and Carrots

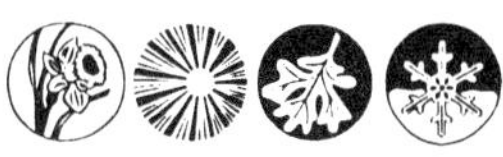

P, PK, K, KV, KP
Serves 2

1 c millet
4 c water
1/2 c diced carrots
1/2 tsp sea salt

Wash millet until water runs clear; drain. Parch over medium heat until dry in a large cast-iron skillet. Bring water to boil in a saucepan. Add millet, carrots, and salt. Cover and simmer over medium heat for 40 minutes. Add water to soften further, if necessary. Serve hot.

## Roasted Breakfast Grain

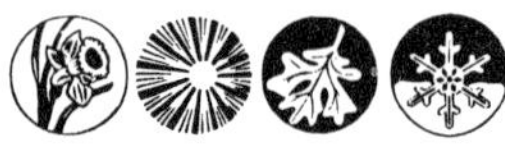

P, PK, K, KV, KP
Serves 2

Add water to moisten any leftover grain. Knead into a bulky dough. Heat skillet. Using a rolling pin, roll out the grain dough on a clean surface and parch in skillet over medium-low heat for 15 minutes until crisp. Serve with dry or wet chutneys.

## Crisp Cooked Millet

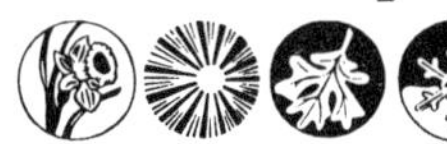

K, KV, KP
Serves 4

2 c soft cooked millet (see page 170)
1/4 c minced onions
1/4 tsp sea salt

Mix all ingredients together. Heat a flat cast-iron skillet or a thin chapati skillet. Spread a 1/2" layer of millet mixture onto skillet. Allow to parch over low heat for about 35 minutes. Remove from skillet and serve warm with chutney and vegetables.

## Cooked Wheat Berries

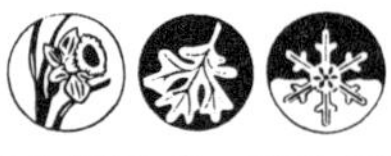

V, VP, P, PV, PK
Serves 2

6 c water
1 c wheat berries
1/4 tsp salt

In a medium saucepan, bring water to boil. Add wheat berries and salt. Cover and simmer over medium-low heat for 3 hours. Drain and serve warm.

## White Basmati and Millet

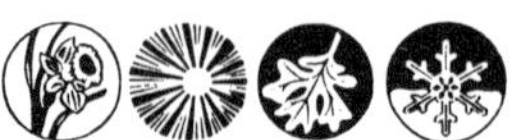

ALL TYPES
Serves 2

1/2 c white basmati rice
1/2 c millet
3 c water
6 curry leaves, preferably fresh
Pinch of sea salt

Wash grains until water runs clear. Bring water to boil in a saucepan; add grains, curry leaves, and salt. Cover and simmer for 20 minutes, until grains swell. Remove from heat and serve.

## Coconut Oatmeal Porridge

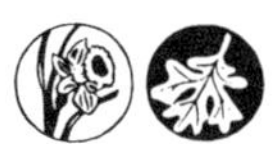

V, VP, P, PV, PK
Serves 2

1/4 c shredded coconut (fresh or dried)
1 c soy milk
1 c water
1/2 c rolled oats
Pinch of cinnamon
Pinch of rock salt
Maple syrup to taste (optional)

Roast coconut in a skillet over medium heat until edges brown. In a saucepan, bring milk and water to boil; add oats and roasted coconut. Simmer for 5 minutes; add cinnamon and salt. Sweeten with maple syrup, if desired.

# UNIVERSAL VEGETABLE DISHES

## Spinach Masala

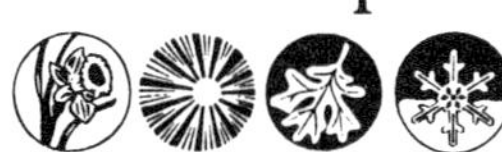

V, VK, K, KV
Serves 2

1 large bunch spinach
2 tsp sunflower oil
1 tbs split urad dhal, without skins
1/2 tsp minced ginger
1 minced fresh red chili pepper
Pinch of turmeric
Pinch of asafoetida
Pinch of sea salt

Clean spinach thoroughly and cut into small pieces.

In a large skillet, heat oil and brown urad dhal, ginger, and chili pepper. Stir in turmeric, asafoetida, and salt and lightly roast for a few minutes. Add spinach and a few drops of water. Cover and simmer over low heat for 5 minutes. Serve with appropriate grain.

## Spicy Home Fries

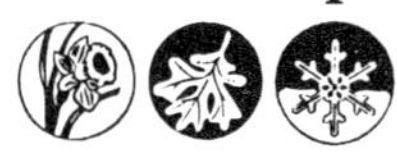

V, VP, P, PV, PK
Serves 2

2 large sweet potatoes
1 tbs sunflower oil
1 tbs ghee
1/4 c diced onion
1/2 tsp fine black pepper
1/2 tsp sea salt

*V types: add 1/2 teaspoon of minced fresh green chili pepper.*

Scrub potatoes and cut into 1/2" cubes. Heat the oil and ghee in a cast-iron skillet. Add potatoes, onion, black pepper, and salt (V types add chili pepper here). Cover and fry over medium heat for 15 minutes. Stir occasionally to prevent sticking.

## Dill and Parsley Potatoes

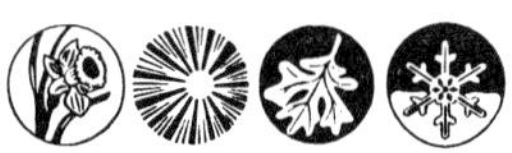

V, VK, K, KV
Serves 4

**4 medium white potatoes**
**1 tsp sunflower oil**
**2 tsp cumin seeds**
**1 minced green chili pepper**
**1/4 c diced onion**
**1/4 tsp cayenne**
**1/2 c water**
**1 tbs minced fresh dill**
**3 tbs minced fresh parsley**

Scrub potatoes and cut into 1" pieces.

In a large skillet, heat oil and brown the cumin seeds, chili peppers, and onion for 4 minutes. Add cayenne and potatoes. Stir, cover, and simmer for a few minutes. Add water, lower heat, and simmer 10 minutes more. Add a few drops of water and stir occasionally to loosen potatoes from pan. Cook for 30 minutes. Sprinkle with fresh parsley and dill.

## Spinach and Tofu Curry

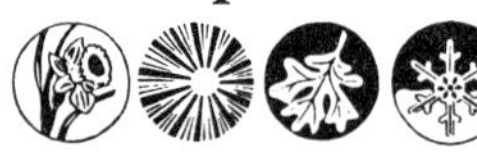

ALL TYPES
Serves 2

**Pinch of salt**
**1/4 tsp fine black pepper**
**1/2 tsp coriander powder**
**1/2 lb firm tofu, cubed**
**1 tsp ghee**
**1 large bunch spinach**
**1/2 c water**
**1/4 tsp turmeric**
**1/4 cup minced fresh cilantro**
**2 tbs garam masala**

*P and K types: use 1 cup of green peas instead of spinach.*

Put salt, black pepper, and coriander in a small paper bag; add cubed tofu and shake. In a large skillet, heat ghee and seasoned tofu mixture; pan fry, turning tofu to cook on each side.

Wash spinach thoroughly and cut into small pieces. Add to tofu along with water and turmeric. Cover and simmer over medium heat for 10 minutes. Add fresh cilantro and garam masala and stir. Cover and simmer for additional 10 minutes over very low heat. Serve with appropriate dhal and grain.

## Eggplant and Potato Curry

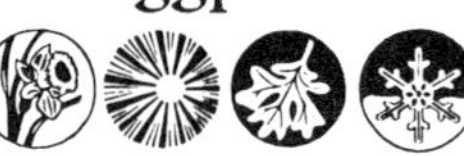

K, KV, KP
Serves 2

**2 medium white potatoes**
**1 medium eggplant**
**2 tsp sunflower oil**
**1 tsp cumin seeds**
**1/2 tsp dried fenugreek leaves**
**2 minced green chili peppers**
**1 minced garlic clove**
**1/4 c diced onion**
**1/2 tsp cayenne**
**1 tbs curry powder**
**1/4 tsp lemon juice**
**3 organic dried tomatoes, sliced**
**1 c water**

Scrub potatoes and eggplant and cut into 1/2" cubes.

In a large skillet, heat oil and roast cumin seeds and fenugreek for a few minutes. Add chili peppers, garlic, and onion, and sauté for 3 minutes. Add cayenne, curry, and lemon juice. Add potatoes, eggplant, and tomatoes and stir until well coated with spices. Add 1/2 cup water. Cover and simmer for 15 minutes. Add remaining water and cook over medium-low heat for 25 minutes. Serve over millet.

## Dried Masala Okra

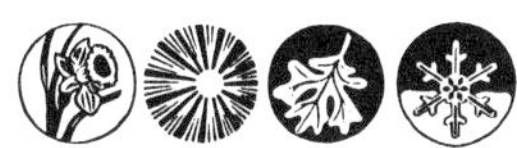

ALL TYPES
Serves 2

1 lb okra pods
1 tbs sunflower oil
1/4 c diced onion
1/4 tsp black mustard seeds
1/4 tsp turmeric
1/4 tsp garam masala
Pinch of sea salt
1/4 c water

*Garnish:*
1 tbs minced fresh cilantro

*P types: omit black mustard seeds.*
*K types: use 1/2 teaspoon oil.*

Wash okra pods, cut off ends, and slice into thin rounds.

In a large skillet, heat oil and sauté onion and mustard seeds for a few minutes. Add turmeric, garam masala, and salt and lightly brown. Add okra and 1/4 cup of water. Cover and simmer over low heat for 2 to 5 minutes. Uncover and continue to cook over very low heat for 15 minutes; stir occasionally. Cook until okra pods are crisp but not burned. Garnish with cilantro and serve with appropriate dhal and grain.

## Cauliflower and Potato Soufflé

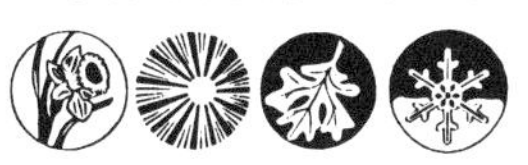

P, PV, PK, K, KV, KP
Serves 2

3 large white potatoes
2 1/2 c water
1 head of cauliflower
1 tbs coarse black pepper
1 tbs ghee
Pinch of salt

*K type: use only 1 teaspoon ghee.*

Scrub potatoes and cut into large chunks; boil in water for 15 minutes. Cut cauliflower into chunks and add to potatoes; boil for an additional 10 minutes. Preheat oven to 450 degrees F. Peel skin from potato pieces and discard. Using a potato masher, purée potato with cauliflower.

Sauté pepper in ghee for a minute and mix into soufflé with salt. Place soufflé in baking dish and bake for 7 minutes to brown the top. Serve hot.

## Cauliflower and Potato Masala

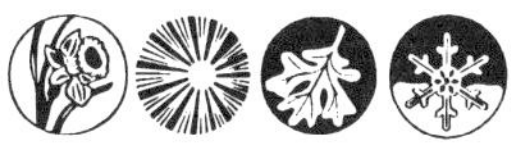

P, PV, PK, K, KV, KP
Serves 4

1 medium cauliflower
2 medium potatoes
2 tsp sunflower oil
1 tsp fennel seeds
1 tsp cumin seeds
1 tsp coriander seeds
1/4 tsp coarse black pepper
2 dried red chili peppers
1/2 tsp turmeric
1 tsp garam masala
1/4 tsp dried fenugreek leaves
Pinch of sea salt
1/4 c water

*P types: omit fenugreek and chili peppers.*

Cut cauliflower into florets and small stem pieces. Scrub potatoes and cut into 1" cubes.

In a large skillet, heat oil and brown seeds, black pepper, and chili peppers. Add cauliflower and potatoes. Cover and simmer for 5 minutes. Stir in turmeric, garam masala, fenugreek, and salt. Add half of the water. Cover and simmer over medium-low heat until dry. Add remaining water and turn heat to low. Cover and simmer for an additional 10 minutes. Serve with appropriate grain and a pressed salad (see pages 270–272).

## Squash and Potato Soufflé

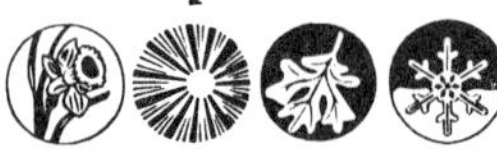

ALL TYPES, OCCASIONALLY
Serves 4

1 butternut squash
3 white potatoes
2 tbs fresh plain yogurt
1 tbs umeboshi paste
1/4 tsp salt

Scrub squash and potatoes. Cut into large chunks and boil for 25 minutes until soft. Preheat oven to 450 degrees F. Peel squash skin and peel potato pieces. Discard skins and mix pulp with clean hands in a bowl. Add yogurt, umeboshi paste, and salt.

Place soufflé in baking dish and bake for 7 minutes to brown the top. Serve hot.

## Brussels Sprouts and Pepper Rings

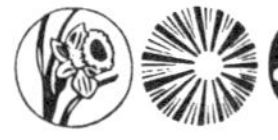
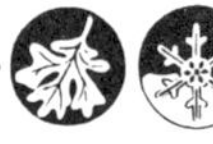

P, PK, K, KP
Serves 2

2 red bell peppers
1/4 c water
1/2 tsp rice vinegar
1/2 tsp orange juice
Pinch of turmeric
Pinch of salt
2 c small Brussels sprouts

*P types: add a touch of oil to marinating mixture.*

Slice peppers into rings and marinate in water, rice vinegar, orange juice, turmeric, and salt for three hours. Cook Brussels sprouts in boiling water, covered, for 5 minutes. Serve with the marinated pepper rings.

## Karikai (Eggplant and Potatoes)

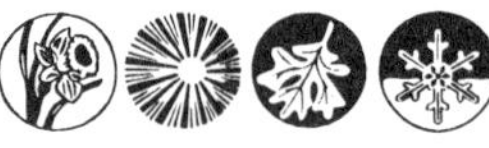

K, KV, KP
Serves 2

1 c cubed (1/2") potatoes
1/2 c boiling water
1 tsp sunflower oil
1 tsp black mustard seeds
1/8 c toor dhal
3 dried red chili peppers
1/4 tsp minced ginger
2 whole garlic cloves
1 c cubed (1/2") eggplant
Pinch of sea salt
1/2 tsp turmeric
2 tbs minced fresh parsley

Place potatoes in boiling water and cook for 15 minutes.

In a large skillet, heat oil and add mustard seeds, toor dhal, and chili peppers, sautéing until dhal turns light brown. Add ginger and garlic cloves. Sauté for a few minutes. Add cubed eggplant, salt, turmeric, parsley, and 4 tablespoons of the water. Drain potatoes and add to eggplant mixture with remaining water. Cover and simmer over medium heat for 12 minutes. Serve with millet.

## Karikai (Carrots and Plantain)

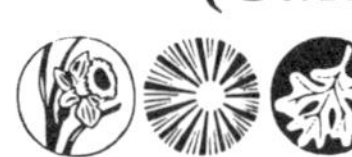
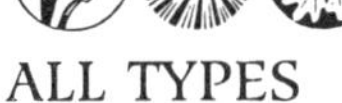

ALL TYPES
Serves 2

1 c 1/2" carrot pieces, cut on a slant
1 c 1/2" peeled green plantain pieces, cut on a slant
1 c boiling water
2 tsp sunflower oil
1 tsp split urad dhal, without skins
1/8 c toor dhal
1/2 tsp coriander seeds

1/4 tsp black mustard seeds
1/2 tsp turmeric
1/4 tsp sea salt

*Garnish:*
2 tbs minced fresh cilantro

Add prepared carrots and plantain to boiling water and cook for 8 minutes. Drain, reserving cooking water.

In a large skillet, heat the oil and lightly roast the dhals for a few minutes until evenly browned. Add the seeds. When mustard seeds begin to pop, add the drained carrots and plantains. Sprinkle with turmeric and salt. Cover and simmer for 3 minutes. Add one quarter of the vegetable water. Cover and simmer over medium heat for 7 minutes, until dhals are well cooked. Garnish with cilantro and serve with appropriate grain.

## Karikai (Squash Curry)

*Karikai is a thick stew-like curry.*

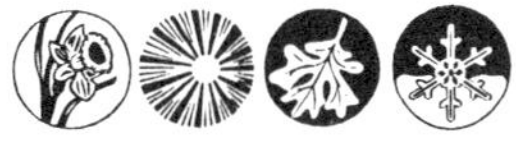

V, VP, P, PV,
Serves 2

2 c peeled, cubed (1/2") butternut squash
1/4 tsp sea salt
1/2 tsp turmeric
1 c boiling water
2 tbs ghee
1 tsp split urad dhal, without skins
2 dried red chili peppers
1/2 tsp black mustard seeds
1/4 c freshly grated coconut

*P types: omit chili peppers and reduce ghee to 1 tablespoon.*

Add squash cubes, salt, and turmeric to boiling water. Cover and simmer for 10 minutes. Drain squash water and use in soup or salad dressing.

In a large skillet, heat ghee and lightly roast urad dhal, chili peppers, and mustard seeds until seeds begin to pop. Add coconut and sauté for a few minutes. Add squash to sautéed spices and allow to simmer for 2 minutes. Remove from heat. Serve with appropriate grain and toor dhal.

## Karikai (Daikon and Sweet Potatoes)

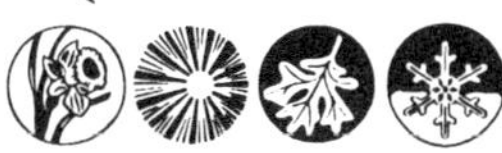

V, VP, VK
Serves 2

1 c cubed (1/2") sweet potatoes
1 c boiling water
1 c cubed (1/2") daikon
2 tbs ghee
1 tsp black mustard seeds
1/2 tsp coriander seeds
3 dried red chili peppers
1 tsp split urad dhal
1/4 c freshly grated coconut
1/2 tsp turmeric
1/2 tsp sea salt
Pinch of asafoetida

Place potatoes in boiling water and cook for 7 minutes. Add daikon and continue cooking for another 5 minutes. Drain water and use in soup or salad dressing.

In a large skillet, heat ghee and lightly roast mustard and coriander seeds, chili peppers, and dhal until dhal turns light brown. Add coconut and sauté for a few minutes. Add drained daikon and sweet potatoes to sautéed spices. Sprinkle with turmeric, salt, and asafoetida. Mix, cover, and simmer for 3 minutes. Serve with appropriate grain and toor dhal.

## Rutabaga Stew with Dumplings

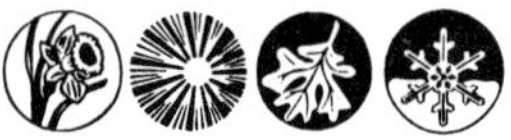

V, VP, VK, P, PV, PK
Serves 2

*Dumpling Batter:*
1/4 c cornmeal
1/4 c whole wheat flour
1/4 c soy milk
Pinch of salt
Water, as needed

Mix ingredients together. Add enough water to make a pancake-like batter. Cover bowl with thin damp cotton cloth; let sit for 30 minutes.

*Stew:*
1 tbs avocado oil
1 c onion chunks
8 black olives, pitted and halved
8 okra pods, halved lengthwise
1/4 tsp salt
1/2 tsp cumin powder
1/4 tsp ginger powder
1/4 tsp coriander powder
Dash of asafoetida
1/2 rutabaga, cut in 1" chunks
4 c water
8 thinly sliced collard leaves
1/2 c water

*V types: add a touch of rice vinegar to the collards, if desired.*

In a large skillet, heat oil and sauté onion, black olives, okra pods, salt, and spices for 3 minutes. Set aside. In a large pot, boil rutabaga in 4 cups of water for 25 minutes. Add dumpling batter, one tablespoonful at a time, to the boiling water; cover and allow to simmer over medium heat for 5 minutes. Add sautéed vegetable mixture and continue to simmer over low heat until okra pods are tender.

In a separate pot, boil collards in a half cup of water for a few minutes until tender (do not overcook). Pour collard water into stew. Serve stew over appropriate grain and garnish with the cooked collards.

## Shepherd's Pie (PC)

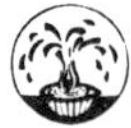

V, VP, P, PV
KV, KP OCCASIONALLY
Serves 8

1 c wheat berries
4 large white potatoes
4 sweet potatoes
2 broccoli stalks with florets
2 tsp sunflower oil
1/2 c minced onion
1/2 c grated carrots
1 whole red bell pepper (cut in thin lengths)
1/2 lb minced soft tofu
1/2 tsp cumin powder
1/2 tsp coriander powder
1/2 tsp curry powder
Pinch of turmeric
1/4 c apple cider
1/2 c soy milk
2 tbs unsalted butter
1/4 tsp salt

*K types: omit sweet potatoes and butter.*

Place wheat berries and 2 1/2 cups of water in a pressure cooker. Cover without locking and bring to a boil. Lock cover and bring to pressure. Cook over medium heat for 45 minutes. Remove from heat and allow pressure to fall naturally. (For conventional cooking, bring wheat berries to boil in 4 1/2 cups of water. Cover and cook over medium heat for 2 hours.)

Scrub both kinds of potatoes and cut into large chunks. Boil for 20 minutes until soft. Drain, reserving the water, and remove skins. Cut broccoli florets and peeled stems into large pieces and boil in potato water for 5 minutes.

In a cast-iron skillet, heat oil and sauté onion, carrots, bell pepper, and tofu. Add salt and spices; cover and simmer over low heat for 5 minutes. Preheat oven to 400 degrees F.

In a large mixing bowl, combine the cooked wheat berries, broccoli, and sautéed mixture. Add cider. Mix thoroughly with clean hands. Place in eight individual baking bowls. Add soy milk, butter, and salt to potatoes, and mash with a potato masher until creamy. Top the bowls with a layer of mashed potatoes. Place in preheated oven and bake for 20 minutes, until the edges of potatoes are browned.

## Ratatouille

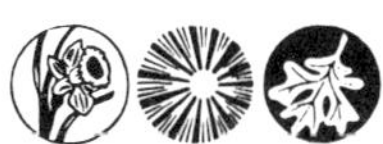

ALL TYPES
Serves 2

**6 zucchini**
**1 tsp sunflower oil**
**1/2 c minced onion**
**1/2 tsp cayenne pepper**
**Pinch of salt**
**1/4 c water**

Slice zucchini diagonally into 1/4" pieces. Heat oil in frying pan and add onion, cayenne, and salt. Stir for a few minutes over high heat and then add zucchini. Add water; cover and simmer over low heat for 10 minutes. Serve with appropriate grain.

## Spinach "Soufflé"

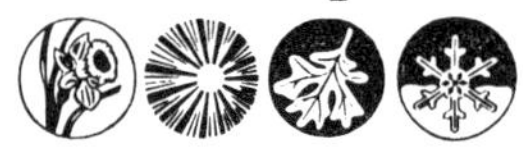

ALL TYPES
Serves 2

**1 lb spinach**
**2 tbs chopped fresh parsley**
**3 tsp olive oil**
**1/4 c water**
**1 tsp fine black pepper**
**1/2 tsp black mustard seeds**
**1/2 tsp red chili powder**
**Pinch of salt**
**3 tbs pine nuts**

***P, PV, and PK types: omit red chili powder and parsley.***

***K, KV, and KP types: substitute 1 teaspoon sunflower oil for olive oil.***

Wash and chop spinach. In a large saucepan, cook spinach and parsley in 1 teaspoon oil and water for 5 minutes, covered. Drain. Purée with a hand grinder.

Preheat a cast-iron skillet and sauté spices, salt, and nuts in remaining oil for a few minutes. Add puréed greens to mixture. Serve warm.

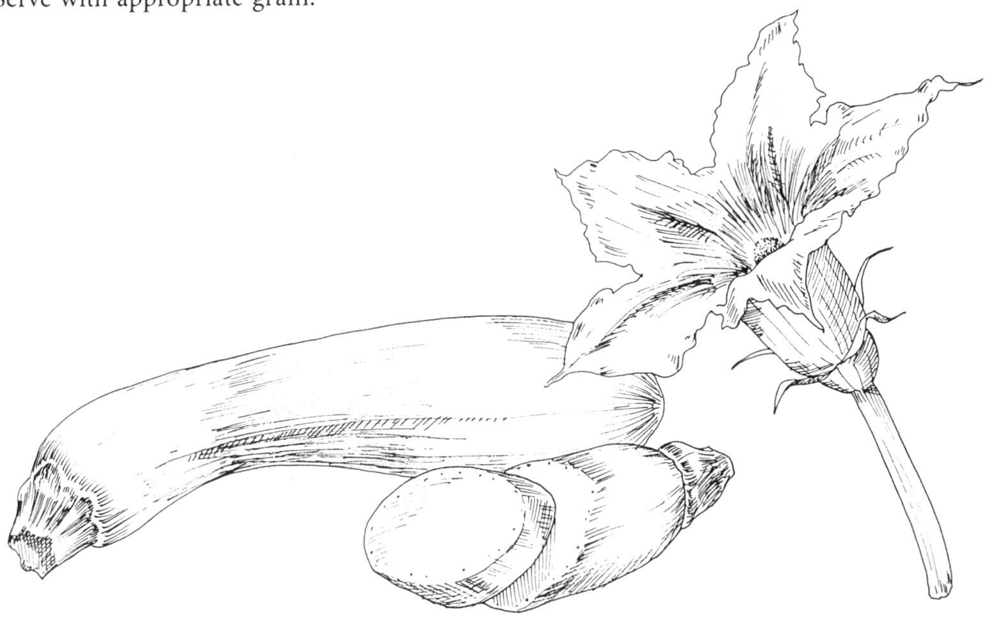

Zucchini Vegetable and Flower

## Fennel-Roasted Eggplant

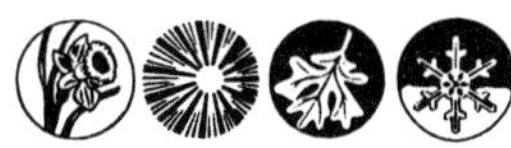

P, PV, PK, K, KV, KP
Serves 2

2 eggplants
1/4 c coconut milk
1/2 tsp roasted fennel seeds
1/2 tsp roasted coriander seeds
1 tsp chopped parsley
1 tsp olive oil
Pinch of salt

Place grate or metal bread rack over a low flame or an open fire. Roast eggplants with skins on. Turn frequently to cook evenly. The roasting process usually takes about 15 minutes. Remove eggplant from heat and separate pulp from the charred skins and stems. Allow to cool and with clean hands mix pulp with coconut milk, roasted seeds, parsley, oil, and salt. Serve warm as a side dish.

## Peppered Corn on the Cob

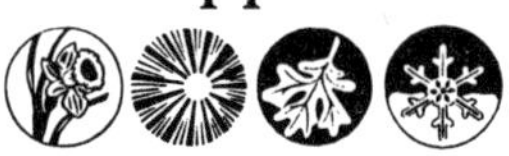

ALL TYPES
Serves 3

6 ears corn
2 tbs whole peppercorns
3 tbs ghee

*K types: use 1/4 teaspoon ghee per ear.*

Pull husks back but do not detach. Remove silk and pull husks up again; twist or tie closed. Boil corn ears in husks for 10 minutes; remove from water immediately. Grind peppercorn coarsely and heat in ghee for 2 minutes. Peel corn and brush with peppered ghee. Serve hot.

## Vegetable Stir-Fry

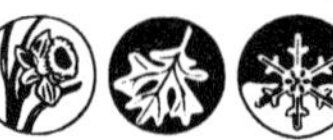

ALL TYPES
Serves 6

1/4 c sunflower oil
1/2 c chopped onion
1/4 tsp turmeric
1/2 tsp sea salt
1/4 tsp fine black pepper
1 c carrots, cut into matchsticks
1 c cauliflower florets
2 c fresh spinach leaves, chopped
1 small thinly sliced cabbage
1 c mung sprouts

*V types: substitute 1 cup each of snow peas and broccoli florets for cabbage and cauliflower.*

In a large karai, heat the oil and add onion, turmeric, salt, and pepper. Fry over medium heat for 2 minutes. Add carrots and cauliflower pieces and stir. Cover and simmer over medium heat for 4 minutes.

Add the spinach, cabbage, and mung sprouts. Lower heat slightly. Cover and cook for an additional 3 minutes. Remove karai from heat and serve with mild tamari sauce.

## Carrot and Burdock Kimpira

*Kimpira refers to a Japanese method of sautéing matchstick-size root vegetables in oil.*

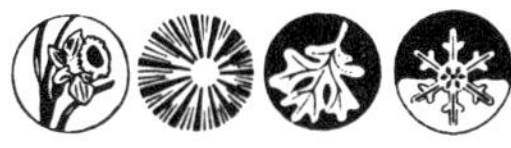

ALL TYPES
Serves 2

3 carrots
2 burdock roots
1 tsp light sesame oil
3 tbs water
1 tsp mirin
Pinch of salt

*P and K types: substitute 1/2 teaspoon walnut oil and almond oil, respectively, for sesame oil.*

Scrub carrots and burdock roots; cut into matchsticks. Heat oil in stainless-steel pan and sauté vegetables over medium heat until cooked but still crisp. Add water and cover. Simmer over low heat a few minutes. Add mirin and salt; continue to simmer for another 5 minutes.

For other vegetable combinations (see below), cut root vegetables into matchsticks, and cut all other vegetables into long slivers. Leave corn kernels whole.

*Other vegetable combinations:*
P, PK, K, KP: winter squash/rutabagas
All types: winter squash/daikon; green beans/fresh corn; snow peas/fresh bamboo shoots

## Steamed Broccoli, Cauliflower, and Carrots

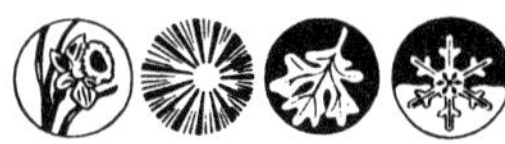

ALL TYPES
Serves 2

1 bunch broccoli
1 head cauliflower
3 carrots

Wash broccoli and cut into long, thin spears. Wash cauliflower and cut into florets. Scrub carrots and quarter into 4" strips. Place with small amount of water in a steamer and steam for 10 minutes. Arrange on plate, alternating the broccoli and carrot strips. Place cauliflower pieces across the top. Serve with an appropriate sauce (see pages 276–280).

## Spicy Roasted Eggplant

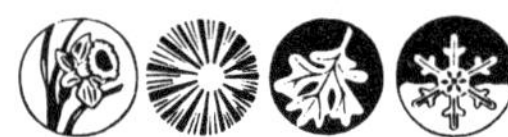

K, KV, KP
Serves 2

2 eggplants
1/4 c minced onion
1/4 tsp minced garlic
1 tsp sunflower oil
Pinch of salt

Place grate or metal bread rack over a low flame or an open fire. Roast eggplants with skins on. Turn frequently to cook evenly. The roasting process usually takes about 15 minutes. Remove eggplant from heat and separate pulp from the charred skins and stems. Allow to cool and with clean hands, mix pulp with the raw onion, garlic, oil, and salt. Serve warm as a side dish.

## Sweet and Sour Vegetables

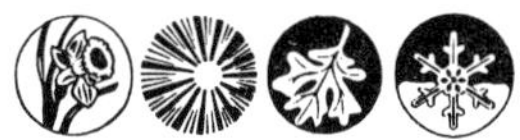

V, VP, VK
Serves 2

6 pearl onions
4 large carrots
1/2 rutabaga
1 daikon radish
1/4 lb fresh pineapple, peeled
2 tsp walnut oil
1 tbs tamarind paste
1/4 c warm water
1 tbs kudzu (or arrowroot)
1/4 c warm water
1/2 c pineapple juice
1 minced garlic clove
1 tsp umeboshi vinegar
Pinch of asafoetida

To peel pearl onions, boil for 1 minute then place in cold water. Trim ends and slip off skins. Cut carrots, rutabaga, daikon, and pineapple into 1/2" cubes. In a large skillet, heat oil and add prepared vegetables and pineapple. Sauté over medium heat for 5 minutes; cover and simmer for 3 minutes.

Dilute tamarind paste in 1/4 cup warm water. Dilute kudzu in 1/4 cup cold water. Add diluted tamarind, pineapple juice, garlic, vinegar, and asafoetida to vegetables. Cover and simmer over low heat for 20 minutes until vegetables are tender. Stir in diluted kudzu. Serve hot over appropriate grain.

## Steamed Snow Peas and Acorn Squash

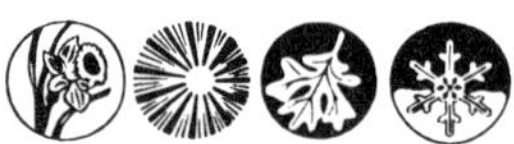

ALL TYPES
Serves 2

1 acorn squash
1 handful snow peas

*V and P types: garnish with black olive halves and olive oil.*

*K types: garnish with half a red bell pepper marinated in 1/2 teaspoon of rice vinegar for 15 minutes.*

Scrub squash and cut into thin lengths along indentations. Steam for 20 minutes until firm but tender. Add snow peas to steamer during the last 3 minutes.

## Yellow Squash and Baby Onions

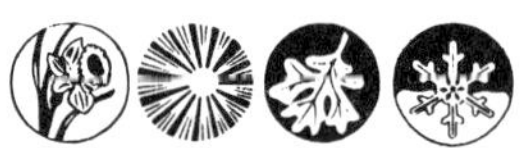

ALL TYPES
Serves 2

6 peeled pearl onions
3 yellow crookneck squash
1 tbs sunflower oil
Pinch of sea salt
Pinch of turmeric
3 tbs water

*V, VP, and VK types: substitute 1 tablespoon sesame oil instead of sunflower oil; add 1 tablespoon light mugi miso (diluted in 3 tablespoons water) during the last 3 minutes of cooking.*

To peel pearl onions, boil for 1 minute then place in cold water. Trim ends and slip off skins. Cut squash on a slant into 1/4" pieces. In a preheated skillet, sauté pearl onions in oil over medium heat for 3 minutes. Add squash, salt, turmeric, and water. Cover and simmer for another 10 minutes.

## Shiitake and Onions

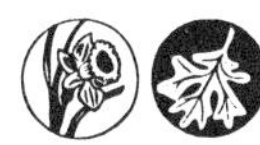

P, PV, PK, K, KV, KP
Serves 2

**6 fresh shiitake mushrooms**
**1/4 c sliced onion**
**1 tsp sunflower oil**
**2 tbs water**
**1/2 tsp tamari**

Remove stems and slice mushrooms into thin pieces; finely chop the stems. Sauté together with onion in oil over low heat for 5 minutes. Add water and cover with a tight-fitting lid. Remove from heat and stir in tamari. Serve warm.

## Broccoli and Shiitake

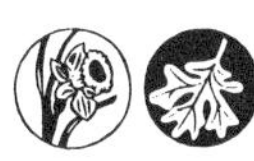

P, PV, PK, K, KV, KP
Serves 2

**6 dried shiitake mushrooms**
**1/2 tbs sunflower oil**
**2 broccoli stalks with florets**
**1/4 c broccoli cooking water**
**Pinch of salt**
**1 tbs mirin**
**1/4 c roasted sunflower seeds**
**Pinch of turmeric**

Soak mushrooms in water to cover for a few minutes. Slice thinly and sauté in oil over medium heat for 3 minutes. Cut broccoli florets and peeled stems into small pieces. Boil for 4 minutes. Add 1/4 cup broccoli cooking water, salt, mirin, and broccoli to shiitakes. Wash sunflower seeds and dry-roast in a cast-iron skillet over low heat until dry and golden. Sprinkle turmeric over broccoli and shiitake mixture.

## Stuffed Mushrooms (Rye Bread Crumbs)

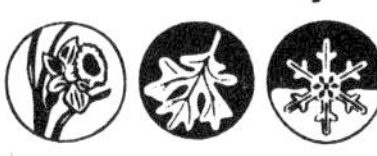

P, PV, PK
Serves 2

**1/8 c minced onion**
**3 tbs minced fresh parsley**
**Pinch of asafoetida**
**1 tsp olive oil**
**3 tbs finely chopped walnuts**
**1/2 c stale, unyeasted rye bread crumbs**
**10 large mushrooms, stems removed**

Preheat oven to 350 degrees F. Sauté onion, parsley, and asafoetida in oil over medium heat for a few minutes. In another pan, toast walnuts and bread crumbs for 3 minutes until crisp and add to mixture. Lightly grease baking pan with oil. Fill cavity of each mushroom with 1 tablespoon of stuffing; pack firmly. Bake for 15 minutes.

## Stuffed Mushrooms (Wheat Bread Crumbs)

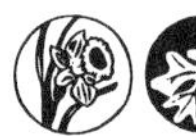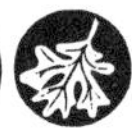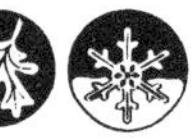

P, PV, PK
Serves 2

**1/4 c minced onion**
**2 tbs minced fresh parsley**
**2 tbs minced fresh cilantro**
**1 tsp coriander powder**
**1/2 tbs olive oil**
**1/2 c stale, whole wheat bread crumbs**
**3 tbs finely chopped walnuts**
**1 tbs water**
**12 large mushrooms, stems removed and caps cleaned**

Preheat oven to 350 degrees F. Sauté onion, parsley, cilantro, and coriander powder in oil over medium heat for a few minutes. In a frying pan, toast walnuts and bread crumbs for a few minutes until crisp. Add, along with a tablespoon of water to spice mixture and stir. Lightly grease baking pan with oil. Fill cavity of each mushroom with 1 tablespoon of stuffing; pack firmly. Arrange in pan and bake for 15 minutes.

## Landcress and Chestnuts

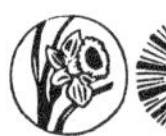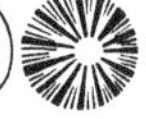

ALL TYPES
Serves 2

**1/2 lb landcress**
**8 peeled water chestnuts**
**1 tsp sunflower oil**
**1/2 tsp mirin**

Wash landcress and boil for 3 minutes. Set aside. In water to cover, boil and mince the water chestnuts. In a skillet, sauté chestnuts in hot oil with mirin over medium heat for 3 minutes. Remove landcress from water and add to chestnut mixture. Serve hot.

## Mustard Greens and Asparagus with Hollandaise Sauce

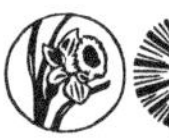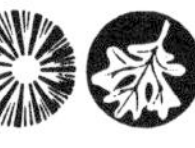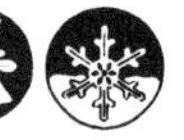

ALL TYPES
Serves 6

**3 dozen asparagus spears**
**12 large, whole mustard green leaves, stems removed**
***Garnish:***
**12 red radishes**

Make Hollandaise Sauce (see page 279).

Wash and trim vegetables. Boil asparagus for 5 minutes. Using asparagus water, steam mustard greens for 3 minutes. Place 3 asparagus spears in the center of each mustard leaf. Drizzle 1/4 cup of Hollandaise sauce onto the asparagus, zigzagging along the center spear. Place one radish at the base of each leaf to garnish.

## Broccoli Rabe with Lemon

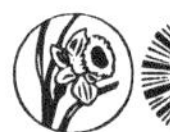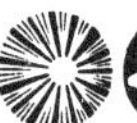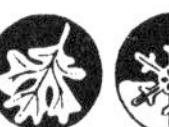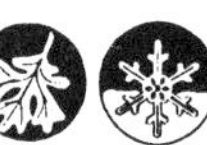

ALL TYPES
Serves 2

**1 bunch broccoli rabe**
**1/2 c water**
**1/2 tbs lemon juice**

Wash broccoli rabe and trim 1/2" from stems; cut lengthwise into long spears. Boil in water for 3 minutes. Drain and add lemon juice and serve.

## Sautéed Asparagus

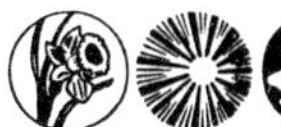
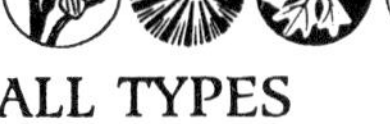

ALL TYPES
Serves 2

1 lb fresh asparagus
1/4 tsp coarse black pepper
1 tsp ghee

Trim 1/2" from ends of asparagus stalks and boil asparagus until cooked but firm. In a medium-sized frying pan, sauté black pepper in ghee for 2 minutes; add asparagus. Serve hot.

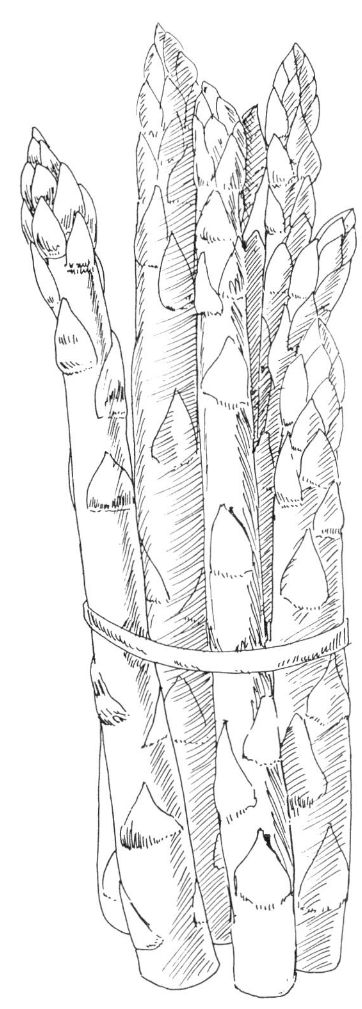

Asparagus

## Watercress with Sesame Seeds

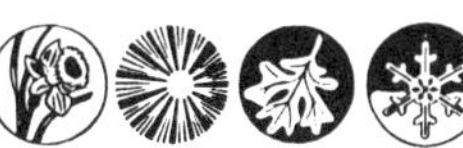

ALL TYPES
Serves 2

1 bunch watercress
2 tbs black sesame seeds
1/2 tsp walnut oil
1 tsp mirin

*P, PV, and PK: use 2 tablespoons sunflower seeds instead of sesame seeds.*
*K, KV, and KP: use 1/2 teaspoon almond oil and 2 tablespoons sunflower seeds.*

Wash watercress and trim off 1/2" from stems; boil for 1 minute and strain. In a cast-iron skillet, sauté seeds in oil for 1 minute. Add mirin. Add watercress to seed mixture. Stir for a few minutes and serve.

## Sweet and Sour Landcress

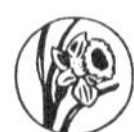
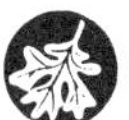
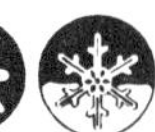

V, VP, VK
Serves 2

1/2 lb landcress
2 tbs sesame seeds
1/2 tsp walnut oil
1/2 tsp tamarind paste
2 tbs water
1 tsp mirin

*P, PV, and PK: use 2 tablespoons sunflower seeds instead of sesame seeds.*
*K, KV, and KP: use 1/2 teaspoon almond oil and 2 tablespoons sunflower seeds.*

Wash landcress and boil for 3 minutes. In a cast-iron skillet, roast seeds in oil over medium heat for 5 minutes. Dilute tamarind paste in 2 tablespoons of water and add mirin. Add tamarind mixture to seeds. Remove greens from water and brush with tamarind mixture with a small natural bristle brush. Serve hot.

## Green Beans and Almonds with Oil and Vinegar Dressing

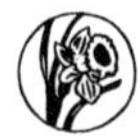 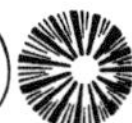 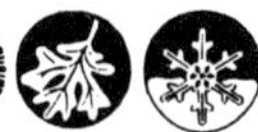

V, VP, VK
Serves 2

1 oz blanched almonds
1/2 lb green beans

Blanch almonds by soaking in cold water for 8 hours. (If time does not permit, you may use the fast method: place almonds in boiling water for 1 minute.) Trim ends of beans and leave whole. Boil beans for 5 minutes. Peel blanched almonds and sliver. Drain beans and toss with nuts.

*Oil and Vinegar Dressing:*
1/2 minced garlic clove
5 tbs olive oil
1 tbs black mustard seeds
1/2 tbs rice vinegar

In a small frying pan, lightly sauté the garlic in 1 tablespoon of oil; add mustard seeds and roast until they pop. Stir in rice vinegar and pour over the beans and almonds.

## Zucchini and Cucumber with Oil and Vinegar Dressing

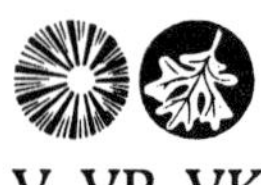

V, VP, VK
Serves 2

1 large cucumber
1 large zucchini
Oil and Vinegar Dressing

Peel cucumber and zucchini and cut each in half; remove seeds with an apple corer. Slice into 1/4" half-rounds. Blanch cucumber pieces in hot water for 30 seconds. Lightly boil zucchini pieces for 4 minutes. Combine and serve warm topped with oil and vinegar dressing (see preceding recipe).

## Glazed Carrots

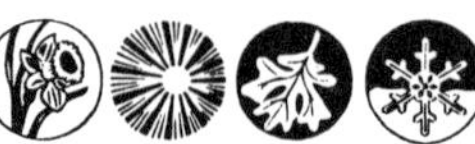

ALL TYPES (K OCCASIONALLY)
Serves 2

1 lb baby carrots, whole
1 tbs sunflower oil
2 tbs rice syrup
Pinch of turmeric
Pinch of salt
1/4 c carrot cooking water

Boil carrots until cooked but firm. Remove carrots and reserve cooking water. In a medium-sized frying pan, heat oil and sauté carrots for 30 seconds. Dilute rice syrup, turmeric, and salt in 1/4 cup carrot cooking water; add to carrots. Heat and serve.

## Escarole and Garlic

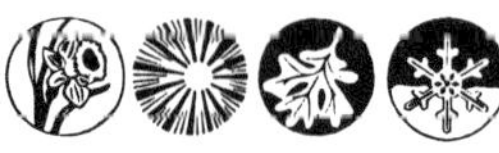

V, VK, K, KV, KP
Serves 2

1/2 lb escarole
1 c boiling water
1/2 tbs olive oil
1 minced garlic clove
Pinch of sea salt

Wash escarole and cut into small pieces. Add to boiling water for 3 minutes. In a small skillet, heat oil and sauté garlic until golden brown. Drain escarole and add, along with salt, to cooked garlic. Serve hot.

## Corn Balls and Red Peppers

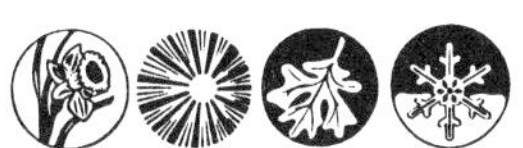

K, KV, KP

Serves 2 (Makes 12 balls)

4 ears corn, husked
1/4 c toasted cornmeal
2 c boiling water
1/4 tsp turmeric
1/4 tsp coarse black pepper
Pinch of salt
1 red bell pepper
3 tbs sunflower oil

Using a hand grater, grate kernels from each ear of corn and mix into toasted cornmeal. Place the stripped cobs in boiling water for 15 minutes. Add 1/4 cup of resulting corn water to corn mixture. Add spices and salt.

Cut red pepper into thin strips. Add 1 tablespoon oil to a preheated pan and sauté peppers for 3 minutes; remove from pan. Roll the corn mixture between your palms to form small balls 1" in diameter. Lightly pan-fry in remaining oil over low heat in a covered skillet for 5 minutes; remove from skillet. Garnish with cooked peppers. Serve hot.

## Creamed Squash

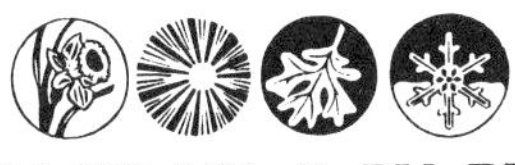

V, VP, VK, P, PV, PK

Serves 2

1 medium buttercup squash
3 c boiling water
1/2 c toasted soy flour
1 tbs minced fresh cilantro
1/2 tbs minced fresh basil
1/2 tsp cardamom powder
1/2 tsp coarse black pepper
1 tbs ghee

*Garnish:*
3 sprigs fresh mint

Wash, cut in half lengthwise, and core squash. Add to boiling water for 18 minutes; reserve 1/4 cup of cooking water. Preheat oven to 500 degrees F.

Remove skin from squash. Using a fork, mash squash and toasted flour. Sauté herbs and spices in ghee over medium heat for 30 seconds. Stir into squash mixture. Add reserved cooking water, stir, and place into a baking dish. Bake uncovered for 5 minutes. Garnish with whole sprigs of mint.

## Okra and Onions

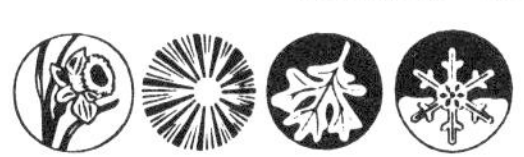

V, VP, VK, K, KV, KP

Serves 2

12 okra pods
1/2 tbs sunflower oil
1 tsp black mustard seeds
1/2 tsp fenugreek powder
1 large white onion, sliced lengthwise
1 tsp chili powder
1/2 c water

*V types: add 1/2 teaspoon sea salt.*

Cut off hard ends from okra pods. Cut diagonally into 1/4" slices. Heat oil in a medium skillet and sauté mustard seeds, fenugreek, onion, and chili powder for 3 minutes. Add okra and water. Cover and simmer over low heat for 20 minutes. Serve hot.

## Sautéed Red Cabbage

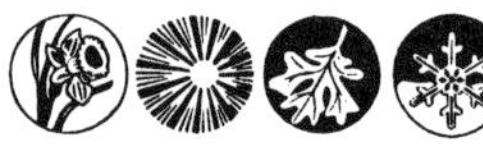

K, KV, KP
Serves 2

1/2 head of red cabbage
1 medium onion
1/2 tsp sunflower oil
1 tbs natural sauerkraut

Shred cabbage and onion and sauté in oil in a cast-iron skillet over medium heat for a few minutes. Add sauerkraut; cover and cook for 15 minutes over medium-low heat. Serve hot.

## Creamed Corn

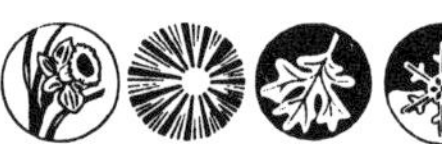

ALL TYPES, OCCASIONALLY
Serves 4

9 ears corn, husked
1/2 c soy flour
1/2 tsp umeboshi paste
1/4 tsp rock salt
1/4 c water

Using a hand grater, grate kernels from each ear of corn. Preheat oven to 350 degrees F. Toast soy flour in a cast-iron skillet until golden. Combine corn kernels, flour, umeboshi paste, salt, and water. Pour corn mixture into a baking dish and bake uncovered for 20 minutes. Serve hot.

## Steamed Artichokes

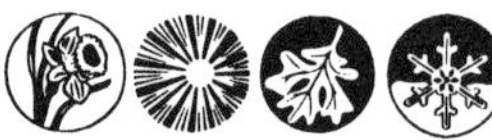

ALL TYPES
Serves 4

4 artichokes
1 tbs sunflower oil
1 tsp cumin seeds

Steam artichokes in a large saucepan for about 25 minutes or until individual leaves can be easily plucked from artichoke. Heat oil in small skillet and sauté cumin seeds until golden brown. Pour seeds over artichokes and serve hot.

## Brussels Sprouts in Lemon Sauce

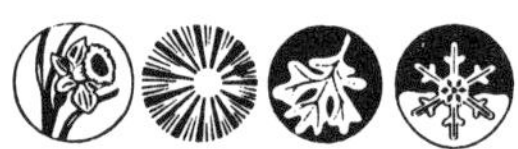

P, PK, K, KP
Serves 2

2 c Brussels sprouts
4 c water
1 tbs lemon juice
1/2 tsp lemon rind
1 tbs mirin
1/2 tsp coriander powder
1/4 tsp turmeric
1/4 tsp salt
1 tsp agar-agar

Boil Brussels sprouts in water over medium heat for 8 minutes. Reserve 1/2 cup of cooking water; drain sprouts and allow to cool. To reserve cooking water, add lemon juice and rind, mirin, coriander, turmeric, and salt. Add agar-agar to spiced water and stir until it thickens. Remove mixture from heat and pour over sprouts.

## SPICED VEGETABLES AND CURRIES

### Aviyal

*From Kerala in South India, Aviyal is a thick stew of yogurt and vegetables.*

P, PV, V, VP
Serves 2

3 carrots
1 green plantain
1 lb green beans
1 tsp cumin seeds
1/4 c freshly grated coconut
1 tsp olive oil
1/2 tsp turmeric
1/4 tsp sea salt
1/8 c water
2 tbs water
1/2 c fresh plain yogurt

*Garnish:*
1 tbs minced fresh cilantro

Wash vegetables. Cut carrots into matchsticks; peel plantain and slice into 2" rounds; cut green beans into 2" pieces. In a small cast-iron skillet, dry-roast cumin and coconut until golden.

In large skillet, heat oil. Add vegetables, turmeric, and salt and sauté over medium-low heat. Add 1/8 cup of water and simmer, covered, for 25 minutes. Using a hand grinder, grind roasted coconut and cumin with 2 tablespoons water into a paste; add to cooked vegetables. Stir in yogurt. Pour aviyal into an attractive serving bowl and garnish with fresh cilantro.

### Spiced Broccoli

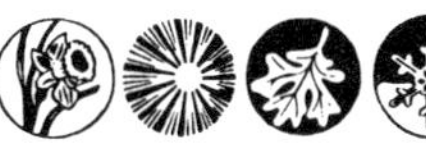

V, VK, K, KV
Serves 2

1/4 c yellow split peas
1/4 c split urad dhal, without skins
2 dried red chili peppers
1/4 c sunflower oil
1/2 tsp black mustard seeds
Pinch of asafoetida
2 stalks broccoli with florets
1/2 c water

*K types: use only 1 teaspoon oil.*

Wash dhals until the water runs clear. In a small, cast-iron skillet dry-roast peas, urad, and chili peppers until medium brown. Remove from skillet and heat 1 teaspoon of oil; roast mustard seeds, and when they pop, add asafoetida. Using a small hand grinder, grind entire mixture to a paste. Warm the remaining oil and add to spice mixture.

Cut broccoli into thin, long spears; steam for 5 minutes. Add 1/2 cup water to the spicy paste and use as a sauce over broccoli.

## Cassava Masala

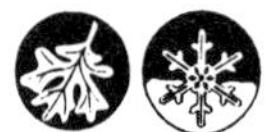

ALL TYPES, OCCASIONALLY
Serves 2

1 lb cassavas
2 c water
2 tsp sunflower oil
1/4 tsp black mustard seeds
1/4 c diced onion
2 tbs minced fresh cilantro
1/2 tbs lemon juice
1/4 tsp turmeric
1/4 tsp sea salt

*V types: serve with appropriate dhal, to lend moisture.*

Peel cassavas and split into halves lengthwise. Cut into 2" half-rounds. Boil in water for 20 minutes until tender; drain.

In a large skillet, heat oil and roast mustard seeds until they pop. Add onion and sauté until translucent. Mix in cilantro, lemon juice, turmeric, and salt; sauté for an additional 2 minutes. Add boiled cassavas and brown for 5 minutes over low heat.

## Asparagus with Besan

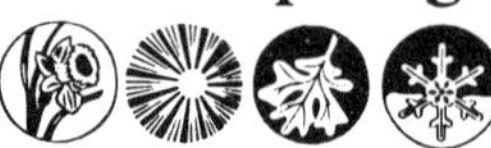

ALL TYPES
Serves 2

1/8 c soy milk
1/4 c chickpea flour (besan)
1 tsp rasam masala (see page 304)
1/4 tsp turmeric
1/8 c water
1 tsp split urad dhal, without skins
1 tsp coriander seeds
12 spears fresh asparagus, trimmed

*V types: substitute fresh, plain yogurt for soy milk.*

Combine soy milk, chickpea flour, rasam powder, turmeric, and water into a batter. In a medium cast-iron skillet, dry-roast urad and coriander seeds until medium brown. Add batter and toast over low heat for about 10 minutes, until the batter is baked and flaky. Steam asparagus for about 5 minutes until al dente. Crumble toasted batter over asparagus and serve.

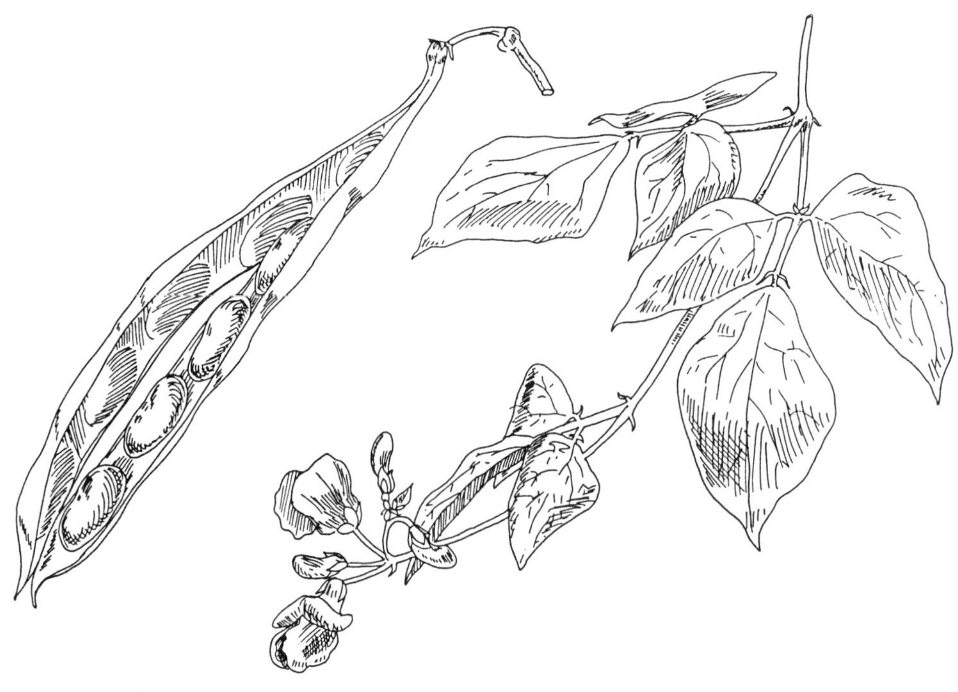

**Scarlet Runner Bean and Flower**

## Vegetable Pullau

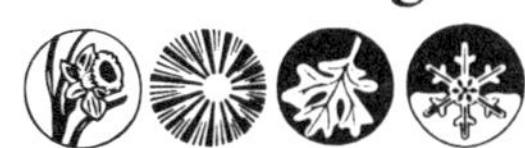

ALL TYPES
Serves 6

1 tsp sunflower oil
1 tbs yellow split peas
1 tsp coriander seeds
1 tsp cumin seeds
$^1/_2$ tsp whole peppercorns
3 dried crushed curry leaves
6 whole cloves
2" cinnamon stick, broken into small pieces
4 large cardamom pods
1$^1/_2$ tsp sunflower oil
$^1/_2$ c diced white onions
$^1/_2$ c diced carrots
$^1/_2$ c diced celery
$^1/_2$ c string beans, cut into 1" pieces
$^1/_2$ c fresh peas
$^1/_4$ tsp turmeric
$^1/_4$ tsp sea salt
2 c brown basmati rice
4$^1/_2$ c boiling water
$^1/_8$ c raisins

*V types: omit fresh peas.*
*K types: substitute millet for rice.*

In a medium skillet, heat 1 tablespoon oil. Brown split peas, coriander and cumin seeds, peppercorns, and curry leaves. Using a hand grinder, grind to a fine powder.

In a small skillet, dry-roast cloves, cinnamon, and cardamom. Remove seeds from cardamom pod and using a small hand grinder, grind all dry-roasted spices into a coarse mixture.

Heat 1$^1/_2$ teaspoons oil in the medium skillet and sauté onions for 3 minutes. Add vegetables, turmeric, and salt; sauté for 5 minutes.

Place vegetables in a medium pot along with spice mixtures from the two skillets. Wash rice and place over vegetables. Add boiling water and raisins; cover and simmer over low heat for 35 to 40 minutes until grain is cooked and fluffy.

## Cauliflower with Mustard Seeds

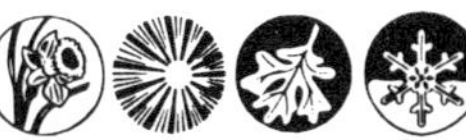

K, KP, PK
Serves 2

$^1/_2$ tsp sunflower oil
1 tsp black mustard seeds
2 c cauliflower
$^1/_4$ c water

Heat oil in skillet and roast mustard seeds until they pop. Cut the cauliflower florets and stems into small pieces and add to skillet; brown lightly. Add water, cover, and simmer for a few minutes, until cauliflower is tender. Serve warm.

## Sweet Potato Curry

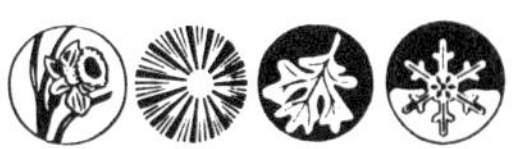

V, VP, VK, P, PV, PK
Serves 2

3 sweet potatoes
1 tsp sunflower oil
$^1/_2$ c diced onion
1 tbs curry powder
$^1/_2$ tsp garam masala
1 tsp cumin seeds
$^3/_4$ c water
Pinch of sea salt

*K types: substitute 3 white potatoes for sweet, add 2 green chili peppers, and reduce oil to $^1/_2$ teaspoon.*

Scrub potatoes well and cut into 1" cubes. In a large skillet, heat oil and sauté onion and spices for a few minutes. Add potatoes and sauté over low heat for 3 minutes. Add water and salt. Stir, cover, and simmer for 45 minutes over low heat until curry is fairly thick. Serve with appropriate grain.

## Spiced Vegetables

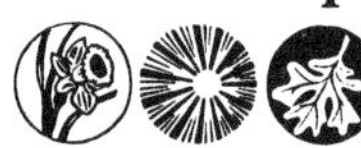

K, KV, KP
Serves 2

1/4 tsp sunflower oil
1 tsp black mustard seeds
1 tsp split urad dhal, without skins
1/4 tsp fenugreek powder
1/2 tsp cayenne pepper
1/4 tsp turmeric
Pinch of asafoetida
Pinch of salt
1/4 c diced red bell peppers
1/4 c finely cut collard stems
1/2 c finely cut cauliflower pieces
1/2 c finely cut broccoli florets and peeled stems
1/2 c water
1/2 c shredded collard greens

*KP types: omit cayenne and fenugreek.*

In a medium skillet, heat oil. Brown mustard seeds until they pop; add urad dhal and fenugreek. Add cayenne, turmeric, asafoetida, and salt. Stir in bell peppers, collard stems, and cauliflower and broccoli pieces. Add water, cover, and simmer over low heat for 10 minutes. Add shredded collard greens and simmer for another 3 minutes. Serve hot.

## Karelas with Yogurt Sauce

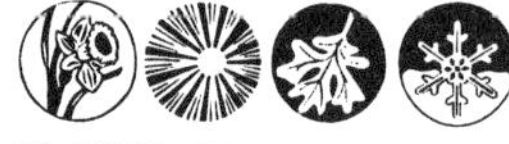

V, VK, K, KV
Serves 2

1/2 c fresh plain yogurt
2 tbs chickpea flour (besan)
1 c water
1/2 tsp sunflower oil
1/2 tsp minced ginger
1/2 tsp minced green chili peppers
3 dried crushed curry leaves
1/4 tsp cumin powder
Pinch of turmeric
4 karelas
1 1/2 tsp sunflower oil
Pinch of sea salt

*K types: use 1/4 cup yogurt and only 1 teaspoon oil.*

Blend yogurt, chickpea flour, and water to a smooth consistency. In a medium skillet, simmer over low heat, stirring constantly to prevent curdling. In another skillet, heat 1/2 teaspoon of the oil and sauté ginger, chili peppers, curry leaves, cumin, and turmeric for 3 minutes over low heat. Stir into yogurt mixture (dadhi) and remove mixture from heat.

Cut karelas in half lengthwise; core and rinse. Slice into 1/4" half-rounds. Reheat skillet and add remaining oil. Sauté karelas over medium heat for 5 minutes. Add salt, cover, and simmer over low heat for 25 minutes. Uncover and simmer an additional 15 minutes, until karela pieces are crisp. Pour yogurt sauce over karela and serve.

## Roasted Peppers

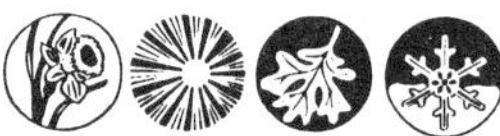

ALL TYPES
Serves 2

2 large green bell peppers

Wash both peppers and, holding with tongs, place each one directly over a medium open flame. Turn as needed to roast evenly. When completely blackened, place in a bowl of cold water. Remove the blackened skin by hand and cut open pepper to remove stem and seeds. Be careful not to burn your hands. Slice peppers and serve with a salad or dressing. They can also be used as a garnish.

# UNIVERSAL BEAN DISHES AND DHALS

## Baked Beans

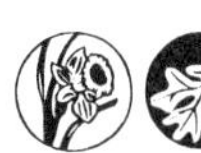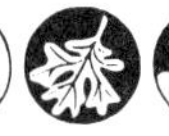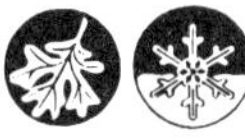

P, PV, PK, K, KV, KP
Serves 2

1 c navy beans
3" piece kombu seaweed
3 1/2 c water
1/8 tsp black mustard seeds
1/2 tsp grated ginger
1 tbs sunflower butter
1/4 tsp rock salt

Preheat oven to 300 degrees F. Wash beans and soak in 3 cups of water for 2 hours. To wash kombu, place in a small bowl of water and rub gently to remove salt. Combine beans and kombu in a pot with water and bring to a boil. Cover and simmer over medium heat for 1 hour. Dry-roast the mustard seeds and add to beans, along with the ginger, butter, and salt. Bake for 45 minutes.

## Soybeans

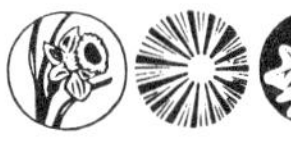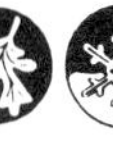

P, PV, PK
Serves 2

1 c soybeans
1 ear corn, husked
4 c boiling water
1 very finely chopped carrot
1/2 c minced onion
1/4 tsp sea salt
1/2 tsp cinnamon powder
1/4 tsp whole cloves
Pinch of turmeric
1/2 tsp orange peel

Wash soybeans and soak in 3 cups cold water overnight. Strip kernels from corn ear. Drain soybeans and add to boiling water along with carrot, onion, corn kernels, stripped corn cob, salt, and spices. Cover and simmer over medium heat for 1 1/2 hours. Remove from heat. Remove and discard the stripped cob and add orange peel. Allow dish to sit for 15 minutes. Serve warm.

## Mung Humus

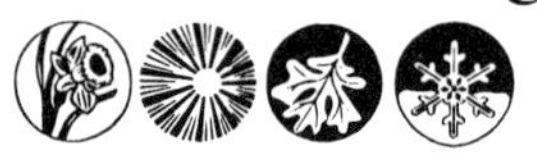

ALL TYPES
Serves 2

$^{1}/_{2}$ c split mung dhal
1 c boiling water
Pinch of sea salt
$^{1}/_{2}$ tsp fine black pepper
$^{1}/_{4}$ c minced onion
2 tsp olive oil
2 tbs minced parsley
1 tsp lemon juice
1 tbs sunflower butter

*V types: use tahini instead of sunflower butter.*
*V and K types: add 1 minced clove garlic.*
*P and K types: substitute chickpeas for mung.*
*K types: use $^{1}/_{4}$ teaspoon sunflower oil instead of the butter.*

Wash mung dhal until water runs clear. Add to boiling water and cook over medium heat for 8 minutes. Remove mung from water when cooked but still firm. Using a potato masher, mash mung in a bowl and add salt and pepper.

Sauté onion in olive oil for 3 minutes. Add minced parsley and sauté for an additional 3 minutes. Combine mung, onions/parsley mixture, and lemon juice in a suribachi and grind to a fine paste. Add the sunflower butter and blend into the paste. For K and P types, serve on appropriate toast or crackers. For V types, serve on moist, freshly baked bread.

## Chickpeas and Onions (PC)

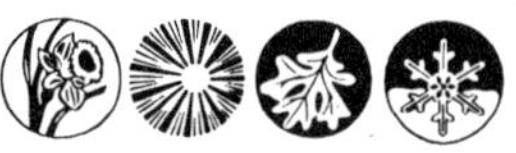

P, PV, PK, K, KV, KP
Serves 2

$^{1}/_{2}$ c chickpeas
2 c water
1 tsp coconut oil
$^{1}/_{4}$ c minced onion
1 tbs minced fresh cilantro
Pinch of sea salt

*K types: add $^{1}/_{2}$ teaspoon cayenne and substitute $^{1}/_{2}$ teaspoon of sunflower oil for the coconut oil.*

Soak chickpeas in 3 cups of water overnight. Drain and add, along with 2 cups water, to pressure cooker. Cover without locking and bring to a boil. Lock cover and bring to pressure. Cook over medium heat for 25 minutes. Remove from heat and allow pressure to fall naturally; drain. (For conventional cooking, bring chickpeas to a boil in 4 cups of water. Cover and cook over medium heat for 45 to 50 minutes.)

In a large skillet, sauté onion in oil for 3 minutes. Add cilantro and sauté for an additional 2 minutes. Add drained chickpeas and salt. Allow to sit over low heat for 3 minutes. Remove and serve warm.

## Plain Dhal

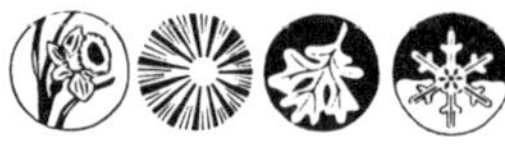

ALL TYPES
Serves 2

$^{1}/_{2}$ c split mung dhal
2 c boiling water
Pinch of sea salt
$^{1}/_{4}$ tsp turmeric
$^{1}/_{2}$ tsp sunflower oil
1 tsp cumin seeds

*P and K types: add $^{1}/_{2}$ cup yellow split peas, if desired.*

Wash split mung dhal until the water runs clear. Add to boiling water with salt and turmeric. Cover and simmer over medium-low heat for 20 minutes.

In a small skillet or large tablespoon heat oil and brown cumin seeds. Add to dhal. Remove from heat. Cover and allow to sit for 5 minutes. Serve with appropriate grain.

## Whole Mung Dhal

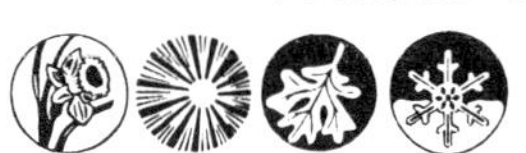

V, VP, VK, K, KV, KP
Serves 2

1 c whole mung dhal
2 1/4 c water
1/4 tsp turmeric
Pinch of sea salt
1 tbs ghee
1 minced green chili pepper
1/2 tsp grated ginger
1/2 tsp cumin seeds
1 tsp coriander powder
Pinch of asafoetida
1 tsp fresh lemon juice

Wash mung dhal until water runs clear. Soak in 3 cups of cold water overnight. Drain. Boil 2 cups of the water and add dhal, turmeric, and salt. Cover and simmer over medium heat for 50 minutes.

In a small skillet, heat ghee and brown chili pepper, ginger, and cumin seeds for a few minutes. Add the powdered spices toward end of the browning. Add to dhal with lemon juice and remaining water. Cover and continue to simmer for an additional 30 minutes over low heat.

## Chana Dhal

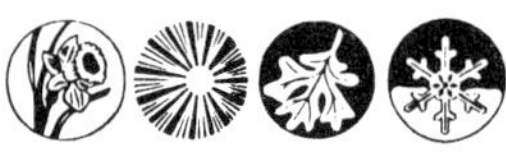

P, PV, PK, K, KV, KP
Serves 2

1/4 c chana dhal (or yellow split peas)
4 c water
Pinch of rock salt
1/2 tsp sunflower oil
1/2 tsp cumin seeds

*P types: use 1/2 teaspoon ghee instead of oil.*

Wash chana dhal until water runs clear. Soak dhal in 2 cups of cold water for 2 hours; rinse and drain. Boil dhal in remaining 2 cups of water for 20 minutes. Add salt. In a small skillet or large tablespoon, heat oil and roast cumin seeds until light brown. Add seeds and oil to dhal. Cover and allow to sit for 3 minutes. Serve warm with cooked grain or chapati.

## Split Pea Dhal

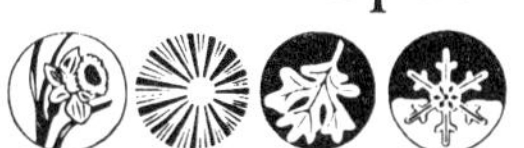

P, PV, PK, K, KV, KP
Serves 2

1 c yellow split peas
3 c boiling water
1/2 tsp turmeric
Pinch of sea salt
1 tsp sunflower oil
1 tbs minced fresh cilantro
1 tsp garam masala (see page 302)

Wash yellow split peas until water runs clear. Soak in 3 cups water for 30 minutes. Drain and add to boiling water with turmeric and salt. Cover and simmer over low heat for 1 hour.

In a small skillet, heat the oil and sauté cilantro for 2 minutes; add garam masala and sauté for 1 minute. Pour into cooked dhal. Cover and allow to sit for 3 minutes. Serve warm.

## Aduki and Shallot Dhal (PC)

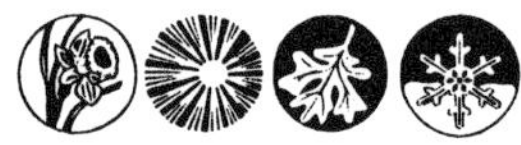

ALL TYPES
Serves 2

1/2 c aduki beans
3 c water
1/2 c thinly sliced shallots
1/2 tsp minced ginger
1 tsp sunflower oil
1/2 tsp lemon juice
1/2 tsp turmeric
1/2 tsp black mustard seeds

*Garnish:*
Minced fresh parsley

Soak beans in 3 cups of cold water for 5 hours. Drain and rinse. Add beans and water to pressure cooker. Cover without locking and bring to a boil. Lock cover and bring to pressure. Cook over medium heat for 10 minutes. Remove from heat and allow pressure to fall naturally. (For conventional cooking, bring aduki beans to a boil in 3 1/2 cups of water. Cover and simmer over medium heat for 1 hour.)

Sauté shallots and ginger in oil for 3 minutes; add to beans with lemon juice and turmeric. Cover and simmer for 40 minutes over medium-low heat.

Dry-roast mustard seeds until they pop; add to dhal. Remove dhal from heat. Allow to sit for 5 minutes. Garnish with minced parsley.

## Soybeans and Red Cabbage Dhal (PC)

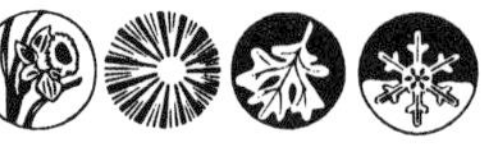

P, PK
Serves 2

1/2 c soybeans
3 c water
1 c shredded red cabbage
1 tbs minced fresh parsley
1 tsp coriander powder
Pinch of sea salt
1/2 tsp coarse black pepper
1 tsp avocado oil
1 tsp cumin seeds

*Garnish:*
Minced fresh arugula

Soak beans in 3 cups of cold water for 5 hours. Drain and rinse. Add beans and 3 cups water to pressure cooker. Cover without locking and bring to boil. Lock cover and bring to pressure. Cook over medium heat for 10 minutes. Remove from heat and allow pressure to fall naturally. (For conventional cooking, bring soybeans to boil in 3 1/2 cups of water. Cover and cook over medium heat for 2 hours.) Add cabbage, parsley, coriander, salt, and black pepper. Cover and simmer over medium heat for 45 minutes.

In a small skillet or large tablespoon, heat oil and brown cumin seeds; add to dhal. Remove from heat and allow to sit for 15 minutes before serving. Garnish with fresh arugula.

## RASAM AND SAMBAR

Originating in South India, rasam is a thin, clear broth made of dhals and spices. It has a slightly sour base that stimulates the digestive enzymes. Sambar, also sour, is a stew of spicy vegetables and dhal. Both are excellent for V types and may be taken occasionally by K types. They are basically too sour for the high powered digestive enzymes of P types. However, these recipes may be modified to suit P types, if used only occasionally.

### Toor Rasam

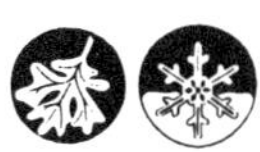

V, VP, VK, K, KV

2 tbs toor dhal
4 crushed curry leaves, preferably fresh
1 tsp black mustard seeds
3 c boiling water
2 tsp tamarind paste
1/8 c rasam liquid
1/4 tsp turmeric
1 tsp rasam masala (see page 304)
2 sprigs minced fresh cilantro

*VP: use sparingly.*

Dry-roast toor dhal until dark golden. Remove from pan and dry-roast curry leaves and mustard seeds. Add to boiling water along with toor dhal. Dilute tamarind paste in 1/8 cup rasam liquid and add along with turmeric and rasam powder, to rasam. Simmer for 5 minutes over medium heat. Remove from heat and add fresh cilantro. Cover and steep for 3 minutes. Strain broth and serve warm.

### Coconut Sambar

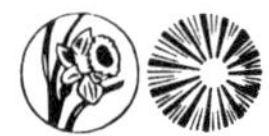

V, VP, VK, K, KV, KP
Serves 2

1 c masoor dhal
2 1/2 c boiling water
1/4 c freshly grated coconut
3 fresh curry leaves
1/8 tsp dried fenugreek leaves
Pinch of sea salt
1/4 tsp coriander powder
Pinch of asafoetida
1/2 tsp tamarind paste
1/8 c sambar liquid
2 cubed (1/2") parsnips

*VP types: use sparingly*
*K types: use 2 tablespoons coconut, and substitute 2 turnips for parsnips.*

Wash masoor dhal until water runs clear. Soak in 3 cups of cold water for half and hour. Add dhal to boiling water. In a small skillet, dry-roast coconut, curry leaves, and fenugreek.

In a separate small skillet, dry-roast salt and powdered spices. Add both batches of roasted ingredients to sambar. Dilute tamarind paste in 1/8 cup of sambar liquid and add, along with parsnips, to sambar. Cover and simmer over medium heat for 40 minutes, until dhal and vegetables are completely cooked. Serve as a soup–gravy with grain, or with idli (see pages 205–206).

## Mixed Vegetable Sambar (PC)

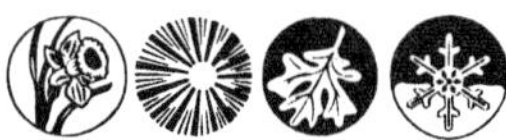

ALL TYPES
Serves 2

1 c toor dhal
3 c water
6 fresh asparagus stalks
1 small broccoli stalk with florets
1/4 tsp tamarind paste
1/4 c warm water
1/4 c chopped onion
1 small diced carrot
1 tsp sunflower oil
1 tsp split urad dhal, without skins
1 tsp black mustard seeds

Wash toor dhal until the water runs clear. Place in a pressure cooker with 2 cups of the water. Cover without locking and bring to a boil. Lock cover and bring to pressure. Cook over medium heat for 10 minutes. Remove from heat and allow pressure to fall naturally. (For conventional cooking, bring toor dhal to boil in 3 cups water. Cover and cook over medium heat for 25 to 30 minutes.) Purée with a wooden spoon and set aside.

Wash and cut asparagus and broccoli into 1" pieces (using peeled stems as well). Dilute tamarind paste in 1/4 cup of warm water. Put diluted tamarind in a large pan and add asparagus and broccoli, along with onion and carrot pieces. Cover and simmer over low heat for 5 minutes. Add remaining water as needed to maintain moisture.

In a small skillet, heat oil and roast urad dhal until golden brown. Add mustard seeds during last few minutes and roast until they pop. Stir mixture into sautéed vegetables and add puréed toor dhal and sambar powder. Cover and simmer together over low heat for 20 minutes. Serve warm.

## Tridosha Sambar (PC)

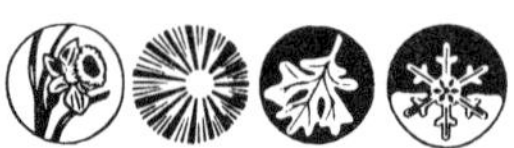

ALL TYPES
Serves 2

1 c whole mung dhal
1/2 c cubed (1/2") sweet potatoes
1/4 tsp turmeric
3 c water
1/2 lb green beans
1/4 tsp tamarind paste
1/4 c warm water
1/2 c cubed (1/2") daikon
1/4 tsp grated ginger
1/4 tsp chili powder
1/2 tsp coarse black pepper
1/2 c minced cilantro, plus extra for garnish
1 tsp coriander seeds
1/2 tsp cumin seeds
1/2 tsp black mustard seeds
1 tsp sunflower oil

*P types: omit chili powder.*
*K types: use white potato.*

Wash whole mung dhal until water runs clear. Drain and put mung, potatoes, and turmeric, along with 2 1/2 cups of the water, in a pressure cooker. Cover without locking and bring to a boil. Lock cover and bring to pressure. Cook over medium heat for 12 minutes. Remove from heat and allow pressure to fall naturally. (For conventional cooking, bring mung dhal and potatoes to boil in 4 cups of water. Cover and cook over medium heat for 25 minutes.)

Cut green beans into 1" pieces. Dilute tamarind paste in 1/4 cup of warm water. Put diluted tamarind in a small pan and add green beans and daikon. Cover and simmer over low heat for 5 minutes, before adding to the sambar.

Coarsely mash cooked mung and potatoes with a wooden spoon or potato masher. Add green bean/daikon mixture. Add ginger, chili powder, black pepper, cilantro, coriander seeds, and vegetables. Add remaining 1/2 cup water; cover and simmer for 15 minutes.

In a preheated skillet, heat cumin seeds and mustard seeds in oil until mustard seeds pop; add to sambar. Simmer for an additional 5 minutes. Serve hot. Garnish with fresh cilantro.

## Orange Rasam

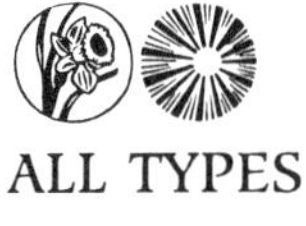

ALL TYPES
Serves 2

**1/8 c toor dhal**
**3 c boiling water**
**1/8 tsp turmeric**
**1 tbs rasam masala (see page 304)**
**2 curry leaves, preferably fresh**
**1 tsp black mustard seeds**
**2 tbs orange juice**
**1/2 tsp orange rind**

Wash toor dhal until water runs clear. Add dhal to 2 cups of the boiling water, along with turmeric and rasam powder. Cover and cook over medium heat for 35 minutes; using a potato masher, mash dhal until it has consistency of a thin purée. In a skillet, dry-roast curry leaves and mustard seeds; add to rasam, along with remaining water, orange juice, and orange rind. Cover and simmer for 10 minutes.

## Spinach Sambar (PC)

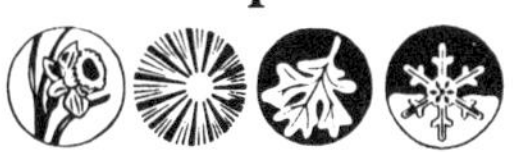

ALL TYPES
Serves 2

**1/2 c toor dhal**
**2 c water**
**1/2 bunch spinach**
**1/2 tsp tamarind paste**
**4 tbs warm water**
**4 fresh curry leaves**
**1/4 tsp turmeric**
**2 tsp sambar powder (see page 304)**
**1 tsp black mustard seeds**
**1 tsp sunflower oil**

*P types: use only 1/4 teaspoon of tamarind paste.*
*V types: use only 2 curry leaves.*
*Okra may be used instead of spinach by all types.*

Wash toor dhal until water runs clear. Soak dhal in 2 cups of cold water for 30 minutes. Place dhal and soaking water in pressure cooker. Cover without locking and bring to a boil. Lock cover and bring to pressure. Cook over medium heat for 10 minutes. Remove from heat and allow pressure to fall naturally. (For conventional cooking, bring toor dhal to boil in 3 cups of water. Cover and cook over medium heat for 25 to 30 minutes.)

Wash spinach thoroughly and cut into small pieces. Dilute tamarind paste in 4 tablespoons of warm water.

Purée dhal with a potato masher; add tamarind water, curry leaves, turmeric, and sambar powder. Cover and simmer for 30 minutes. Pop mustard seeds in hot oil; add to sambar and serve.

## KUTTU

Kuttu is a South Indian dish that is served traditionally during holiday festivities and wedding ceremonies. This delightful combination of dhal, vegetables, and spices is cooked into a fairly thick mixture. It is sometimes served as the second course, instead of sambar, in the traditional Tamil dinner. The vegetables most often used in India when preparing this dish are bitter gourd, snake gourd, ash gourd, eggplant, and plantain. Using a basic combination of vegetables, dhal, and spices, the Kuttu can be balanced to suit each individual body type.

### Mung and Spinach Kuttu

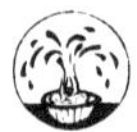

ALL TYPES
Serves 2

**1 c whole mung dhal**
**5 c boiling water**
**1/4 c dried coconut**
**2 tsp cumin seeds**
**1/4 tsp black mustard seeds**
**2 tbs split urad dhal, without skins**
**1/4 tsp coarse black pepper**
**1 bunch spinach**

Wash mung dhal until water runs clear. Soak in 4 cups of cold water for 2 hours. Drain and add to boiling water. Simmer, covered, over medium heat for 15 minutes.

In a cast-iron skillet, dry-roast the coconut, cumin, mustard seeds, urad dhal, and black pepper until coconut is golden. Add to mung dhal. Clean spinach thoroughly and tear into small pieces. Add to the dhal. Cover and continue to cook for 35 minutes over medium heat until the mung is tender. Add water if necessary. Kuttu should be fairly thick.

### Toor Dhal and Cabbage Kuttu

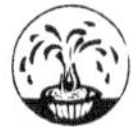

V, VP, VK, K, KV, KP
Serves 2

**1 c toor dhal**
**3 c boiling water**
**1/4 tsp sea salt**
**1/4 tsp turmeric**
**3 crushed curry leaves, preferably fresh**
**2 tsp cumin seeds**
**1/2 tsp black mustard seeds**
**1/2 tsp tamarind paste**
**1/4 c dhal cooking water**
**1/4 head shredded cabbage**

*V types: add the same herbs as K types (see above); substitute asparagus for cabbage.*
*P types: replace tamarind with 1 teaspoon minced fresh cilantro.*
*K types: add 1 chopped green chili pepper and 1/4 teaspoon minced ginger. Lightly dry-roast the chili and ginger; add to dhal before the roasted spices.*

Wash toor dhal until water runs clear. Drain and add to boiling water with salt and turmeric. Cover and simmer over medium heat for 7 minutes.

In a cast-iron skillet, dry-roast curry leaves, cumin, and mustard seeds for a few minutes. Dilute tamarind in 1/4 cup warm dhal water. Add to dhal, along with roasted spices and cabbage. Cover and simmer over medium-low heat for an additional 25 minutes.

## Toor Dhal and Eggplant Kuttu

**K, KV, KP**
**Serves 2**

**1/2 c toor dhal**
**2 c boiling water**
**Pinch of sea salt**
**Pinch of asafoetida**
**1/4 tsp turmeric**
**1 c cubed (1/2") eggplant**
**1/2 tsp sunflower oil**
**1/4 tsp tamarind paste**
**1/4 c warm water**
**4 dried red chili peppers**
**1/2 tsp coarse black pepper**
**1/2 tsp black mustard seeds**
**1/8 c split urad dhal, without skins**

***V types: substitute green papaya for eggplant and increase the oil to 2 teaspoons.***

Wash toor dhal until water runs clear. Drain and add to boiling water with salt, asafoetida, turmeric, and eggplant. Cover and simmer over medium heat for 15 minutes.

In a small cast-iron skillet, heat the oil. Dilute tamarind paste in 1/4 cup warm water. Add red chili peppers, black pepper, diluted tamarind, and mustard seeds; roast evenly for a few minutes. When mustard seeds begin to pop, remove spices from heat and add to toor dhal.

Roast urad dhal in another small skillet until dark golden. Add to toor dhal; cover and simmer for another 30 minutes. Add water, if necessary; final mixture should be fairly thick.

## Plantain Kuttu

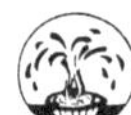

**ALL TYPES**
**Serves 2**

**1/2 c split mung dhal**
**2 c boiling water**
**Pinch of sea salt**
**1/4 tsp coarse black pepper**
**1/4 tsp turmeric**
**1 c peeled and cubed (1/2") green plantain**
**1/8 c split urad dhal, without skins**
**1/4 tsp tamarind paste**
**1/4 c warm water**
**1 tsp sunflower oil**
**1/2 tsp black mustard seeds**

***V and K types: add 1/8 teaspoon of asafoetida.***
***K types: reduce oil.***

Wash mung dhal until water runs clear. Add to boiling water with salt, black pepper, turmeric, and plantain cubes. Cover and simmer over medium heat for 10 minutes.

In a cast-iron skillet, dry-roast urad dhal until dark golden. Add to mung dhal along with tamarind diluted in warm water. Add oil to skillet and, when hot, roast mustard seeds until they pop; pour into the kuttu. Cover and simmer for 15 minutes over medium heat until plantain is tender and the kuttu is fairly thick.

# GRAIN AND BEAN COMBINATIONS

## Black Bean Chili (PC)

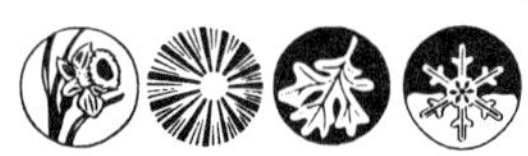

V, VP, VK, P, PV, PK
Serves 4

2 c black beans
1 c wheat berries
7 c water
1/2 tsp rock salt
1/2 tsp cumin seeds
1/2 tsp dried thyme
1 tsp coriander powder
1/2 tsp dried oregano
1 tbs sunflower oil
1/2 c minced onion
1/2 c grated carrots
1/2 tsp minced fresh basil
1 tsp fresh spearmint

Wash black beans and wheat berries separately until water runs clear. Soak separately overnight in enough cold water to cover by 2"; drain and rinse each. Place water, beans, wheat berries, and salt in a pressure cooker. Cover without locking and bring to a boil. Lock cover and bring to pressure. Cook over medium heat for 35 minutes. Remove from heat and allow pressure to fall naturally.

Preheat oven to 425 degrees F. In a small saucepan, sauté cumin seeds and dried herbs in oil for a few minutes. Add beans and wheat berries. Stir in fresh herbs and vegetables, mixing thoroughly. Lightly grease crock pot (ceramic bean pot) and fill with chili mixture. Bake for 15 minutes. Remove and allow to cook an additional 15 minutes before serving. Serve topped with mashed potatoes, if desired.

## Rice and Aduki Beans (PC)

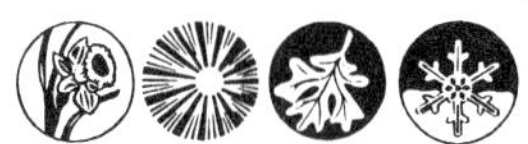

V, VP, VK
P, PV, PK OCCASIONALLY
Serves 2

1 c short-grain brown rice
1/2 c aduki beans
1/4 c fresh chestnut halves
4 c water
Pinch of salt

Wash rice and aduki beans until water runs clear. Soak rice, beans, and chestnuts in 4 cups of cold water for 1 hour. Drain; peel chestnuts and place all in pressure cooker with water. Cover without locking and bring to a boil. Add salt. Lock cover and bring to pressure. Cook over medium-low heat for 45 minutes. Remove from heat and allow pressure to fall naturally for 15 minutes. Serve hot.

## Basmati and Split Mung Beans

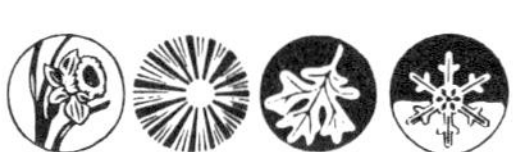

ALL TYPES
Serves 2

1 c brown basmati rice
1/2 c split mung dhal
3 c water
1 tsp roasted black cumin seeds
4 curry leaves, preferably fresh
Pinch of turmeric
Pinch of salt

Wash rice and mung until water runs clear. Place in water and bring to a boil. Add roasted cumin seeds, curry leaves, turmeric, and salt. Cover and simmer over medium-low heat for 30 minutes. Serve hot.

## Rice and Whole Mung Beans (PC)

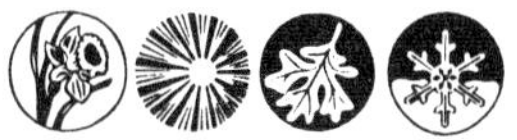

V, VP, VK, P, PV, PK
Serves 2

1 c medium-grain brown rice
1/2 c whole mung dhal
3 1/2 c water
1 tsp roasted cumin seeds
4 curry leaves, preferably fresh
Pinch of salt

Wash rice and mung dhal until water runs clear. Soak rice and mung together in 4 cups of cold water for 30 minutes; rinse and drain. Place in pressure cooker and add water. Cover without locking and bring to a boil. Add cumin seeds, curry leaves, and salt. Lock cover and bring to pressure. Simmer over medium-low heat for 35 minutes. Remove from heat and allow pressure to fall naturally. (For conventional cooking, add rice and mung dhal to 4 1/2 cups boiling water. Cover and cook over medium heat for 1 hour.) Serve hot.

## Red Lentils and Basmati Rice

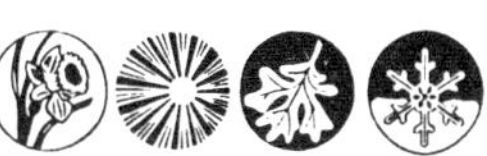

ALL TYPES (K TYPES, SPARINGLY)
Serves 4

2 c white basmati rice
1/2 c red lentils
3 1/2 c boiling water
3 curry leaves, preferably fresh
Pinch of sea salt
1 tsp ghee

Wash rice and lentils until water runs clear; drain. Add both to boiling water, along with curry leaves and salt. Cover and simmer over medium-low heat for 15 to 20 minutes until rice and lentils fluff. Remove from heat; mix in ghee. Serve hot.

## Sweet Rice and Aduki Beans (PC)

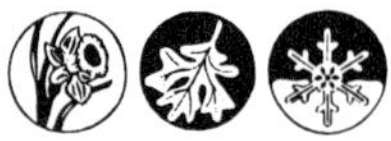

V, VP, VK, P, PV, PK
Serves 4

2 c sweet rice
1 c aduki beans
3 1/2 c water
Pinch of sea salt
Gomasio

Wash rice and aduki beans until water runs clear. Soak rice and beans together in 5 cups of cold water for 2 hours; rinse and drain. Add rice, beans, water, and salt to pressure cooker. Cover without locking and bring to a boil. Lock cover and bring to pressure. Cook over medium-low heat for 40 minutes. Remove from heat and allow pressure to fall naturally. (For conventional cooking, add rice and aduki beans to 4 cups boiling water. Cover and cook over medium heat for 1 hour.) Serve with gomasio.

## Barley and Whole Mung Beans

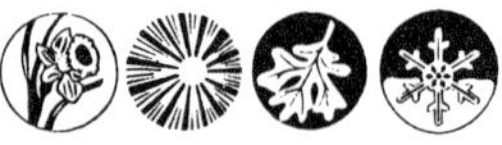

P, PV, PK, K, KV, KP
Serves 4

1/2 c whole mung dhal
2 c pearled barley
3 1/2 c boiling water
3 curry leaves, preferably fresh
6 whole cardamom pods
Pinch of sea salt

Wash mung dhal until water runs clear. Soak in 2 cups of cold water for 8 hours or overnight; rinse and drain. Wash barley and add to boiling water, along with dhal, curry leaves, cardamom, and salt. Cover and simmer over medium heat for 45 minutes. Serve warm.

## Tofu Fried Rice

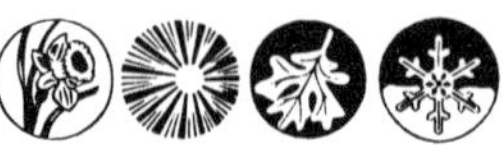

V, VP, VK
Serves 6

1 lb firm tofu
1/4 c barley flour
1/4 tsp sea salt
1 tbs sunflower oil
1/4 c bamboo shoots
1/2 c diced daikon
1/2 c diced onion
1/2 c fresh corn kernels
3 c medium-grain brown rice, cooked

*V types: substitute 1 pound cooked seitan for tofu.*
*P, PV, and PK: substitute 3 cups of either cooked barley or cooked wheat for brown rice.*
*K, KV, and KP: substitute 3 cups cooked millet for brown rice; reduce oil and salt.*

Cut tofu into 1" cubes. Pour flour, salt, and tofu pieces into a paper bag and shake. Heat a medium frying pan with 1/2 tablespoon of the oil and brown tofu pieces on each side. Set aside.

In a large skillet, add remaining oil and sauté all vegetables. Cover and simmer for 7 minutes over medium heat, adding a little water as needed. Add fried tofu pieces to vegetables. Place cooked rice on top of vegetables. Mix together and simmer over low heat for 5 minutes. Serve warm.

## KICHADI

*Kichadi* means the mixture of a grain and a bean. The White Basmati Kichadi is particularly nourishing and easy to digest. A mono-diet of this kichadi is recommended for anyone receiving panchakarma, Ayurvedic cleansing therapy, since it facilitates the cleansing process.

### Barley and Mung Kichadi

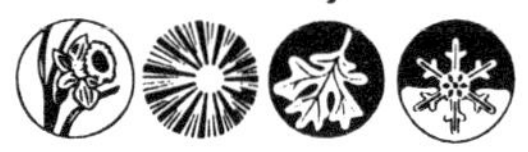

P, PV, PK, K, KV, KP
Serves 2

1 c hulled barley
1/2 c whole mung dhal
1 tbs ghee
1/8 tsp turmeric
4 curry leaves, preferably fresh
1/2 tsp black cardamom
1/4 tsp coarse black pepper
1/2 tsp coriander powder
1/4 tsp sea salt
3 c boiling water

*K types: use only 1 teaspoon ghee.*

Wash barley and mung until water runs clear. Soak mung in 2 cups cold water for 2 hours; drain. In a very large pot, heat ghee and sauté the spices and salt over low heat for 2 minutes. Add the barley and mung. Sauté for 4 minutes. Add boiling water, stir, and cover. Cook over medium-low heat for 1 1/2 hours, stirring occasionally. Serve warm.

### Brown Rice Kichadi

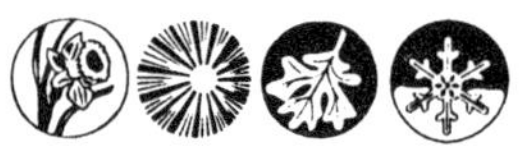

V, VP, VK, P, PV, PK
Serves 2

1 c brown basmati or short-grain brown rice
1/2 c whole mung dhal
1 tbs ghee
1 tsp black peppercorns
2 tsp cumin seeds
1/2 tsp minced ginger
8 c boiling water
Pinch of turmeric
Pinch of sea salt

*P types: omit ginger.*

Wash rice and beans until water runs clear. Soak mung in 2 cups water for 2 hours; drain. In a large pot, heat the ghee and sauté the peppercorns, cumin seeds, and ginger for a few minutes. Add rice and beans. Sauté over low heat for 3 minutes. Add boiling water (reduce water for a thicker kichadi), turmeric, and salt. Cover and simmer gently for 1 hour over low heat, stirring occasionally. Serve warm.

## Millet and Mung Kichadi

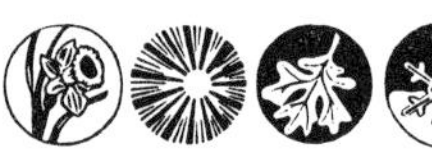

K, KV, KP
Serves 2

1 c millet
1/2 c split mung dhal
1 tsp of ghee
2 tsp cumin seeds
4 curry leaves, preferably fresh
1/8 tsp turmeric
Pinch of asafoetida
Pinch of sea salt
6 c boiling water

Wash millet and mung until water runs clear. In a large pot, heat the ghee and sauté the cumin seeds and curry leaves for 2 minutes. Add the millet, mung, turmeric, asafoetida, and salt. Sauté for a few minutes over medium heat. Add boiling water and stir. (Reduce water for a thicker kichadi.) Cover and simmer for 35 minutes.

## White Basmati Kichadi

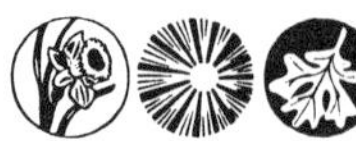

ALL TYPES—USE FOR CLEANSING
Serves 2

1 c white basmati rice
1/2 c split mung dhal
1 tbs ghee
Pinch of turmeric
Pinch of asafoetida
6 c boiling water

Wash rice and beans until water runs clear. In a large pot, heat the ghee and sauté the turmeric and asafoetida for a few minutes. Add rice and mung. Sauté over low heat for 3 minutes. Add boiling water. (Reduce water for a thicker kichadi.) Stir, cover, and simmer gently over low heat for 35 minutes. Serve warm.

# UNIVERSAL PASTA AND SAUCES

Most health food stores carry a wide variety of whole grain pastas. There are also many eggless pastas available today—whenever possible, buy fresh pasta.

Pastas are an acceptable food for all types, used occasionally. Pasta is easy to digest but it also promotes weight gain. K types, therefore, should use it sparingly. The best pasta for K types is made from rye or buckwheat.

## Sautéed Broccoli Pasta

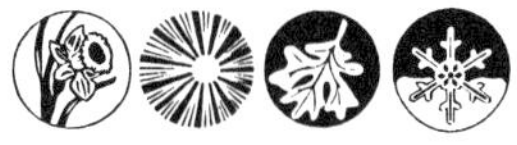

ALL TYPES
Serves 4

4 stalks broccoli with florets
1 tsp coarse black pepper
1 minced garlic clove
1 tbs olive oil
1 lb whole wheat linguini, cooked
 (see following recipe on page 258)

*V types: garnish with grated Romano cheese, if desired.*
*P types: omit garlic.*
*K, KV, and KP: substitute 1/2 tablespoon sunflower oil for the olive oil.*

Trim 1/2" from broccoli stalks and slice into long spears. Boil until soft but firm and remove from water. In a large skillet, sauté black pepper and garlic in oil for a few minutes; add broccoli. Cover and simmer for a few more minutes. Toss linguini and broccoli together.

## Linguini

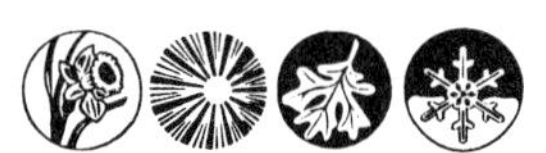

V, VP, VK, P, PV, PK
Serves 4

1 lb whole wheat linguini

Add whole wheat linguini to an ample amount of boiling water to which a touch of oil has been added. Stir occasionally. Cook until al dente (cooked, but firm); never overcook pasta. Drain and serve with broccoli or sauce.

## Tofu Lasagna

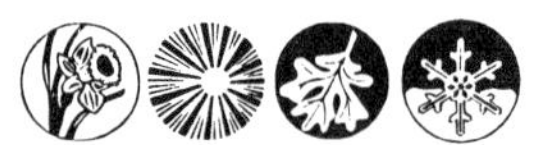

V, VK, VP, K, KV, KP
Serves 4

*Pasta:*
9 strips of whole wheat pasta, 2" wide
6 c boiling water
1/4 tsp olive oil

*K types: use rye or buckwheat lasagna, if available.*

*Filling:*
2 large leeks
1/4 tsp thyme
1/4 tsp oregano
1/4 tsp basil
2 tbs sunflower oil
2 lbs soft tofu
1 tbs sunflower seed butter
1/2 c warm water
Pinch of salt
1/2 tsp chili powder

*Carrot Sauce:*
4 sliced carrots
1/4 c minced onion
1 tbs sunflower oil
1/4 c minced fresh parsley
1/2 tsp fine black pepper
1/4 tsp salt

Place pasta in boiling water and add oil. Boil over medium heat, separating strips occasionally, until pasta is al dente. Drain and set aside until filling and sauce have been prepared.

Finely chop white part of leeks. In a large skillet, sauté leeks with thyme, oregano, and basil in oil for 5 minutes. Crumble tofu and add to leeks. Dilute sunflower butter in 1/2 cup water and pour over tofu-leek mixture. Add salt and chili powder. Stir, cover, and simmer over low heat for 15 minutes.

Preheat oven to 350 degrees F. To make Carrot Sauce, boil carrots; using a hand grinder, purée with onions. Add oil, parsley, pepper, and salt. Lightly oil a large baking dish. Place three pieces of pasta on bottom of dish, slightly overlapping edges. Spread 1/3 of the filling on the pasta. Place another layer of pasta on top, and then the rest of the filling, followed by the rest of the pasta. Pour the carrot sauce over the lasagna. Bake for 40 minutes. Let lasagna set for 20 to 30 minutes so that cut pieces will retain their form.

### PASTA SAUCES

Choose the appropriate pasta for your type and serve with the following sauces.

## Pesto for V Types

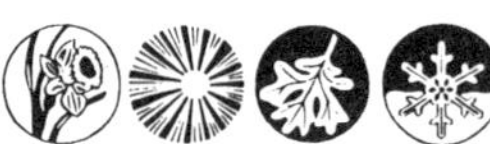

V, VK, VP
Serves 2

1/2 c Italian parsley
1/2 c fresh basil leaves
2 tbs pine nuts
1 clove garlic
1/8 c olive oil
Pinch of sea salt
2 tbs water
Grated Parmesan cheese (optional)

Using a hand grinder, purée the parsley, basil, pine nuts, garlic, and olive oil. Add salt and water. Serve over 1 pound cooked whole wheat linguini. Garnish with grated Parmesan cheese, if desired.

## Pesto for K Types

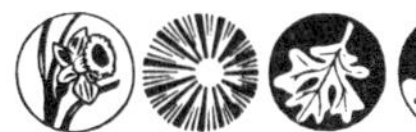

K, KV, KP
Serves 2

$^1/_2$ c Italian parsley
$^1/_2$ c fresh basil leaves
1 garlic clove
2 tsp sunflower oil
$^1/_4$ c plus 2 tbs water
Pinch of salt

*Garnish:*
Roasted sunflower seeds

Using a hand grinder, purée parsley, basil, garlic, oil, and water. Add salt. Serve over 1 pound cooked soba noodles. Garnish with roasted sunflower seeds.

***Note:** Most ingredients in a pesto are too pungent for P types, so no recipe is provided.*

## Sesame and Onion Sauce

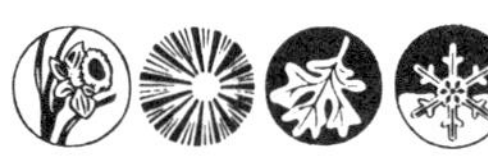

V, VP
VK OCCASIONALLY
Serves 2

1 c thinly sliced onion
$^1/_2$ tbs sesame oil
$^1/_4$ tsp turmeric
2 tbs tahini
$^1/_8$ c warm water
1 tbs tamari

*Garnish:*
2 tbs roasted sesame seeds

In a medium pan, sauté onion in hot oil until translucent; add turmeric. Dilute tahini in warm water and add to onion. Cover and simmer over low heat for 10 minutes. Stir in tamari and serve over hot udon noodles topped with roasted sesame seeds.

## Tofu and Ricotta Cheese Sauce

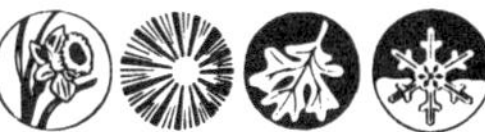

V, VP, VK, K, KV, KP
Serves 4

1 lb soft tofu
$^1/_2$ lb ricotta cheese
1 c grated carrots
$^1/_2$ c minced onion
1 minced garlic clove
3 tbs minced fresh parsley
1 tsp dried basil
1 tsp dried oregano
1 tbs olive oil
1 tsp chili powder
6 dried organic tomatoes, sliced
$^1/_4$ tsp sea salt
1 c water

***K types:** omit cheese and substitute 1 teaspoon sunflower oil for 1 tablespoon olive oil.*

Crumble tofu and combine with ricotta. In a large skillet, sauté carrots, onion, garlic, parsley, basil, and oregano in oil for a few minutes until onions are translucent. Add tofu mixture, chili powder, dried tomatoes, salt, and water; sauté an additional 4 minutes. Stir, cover, and simmer over low heat for 35 minutes. Serve over appropriate pasta shells or spirals.

## Beet Sauce

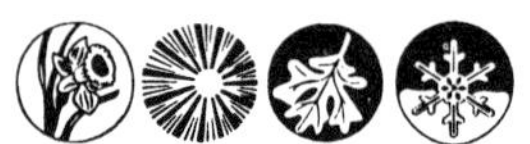

V, VP, VK, K, KV, KP
Serves 4

2 c peeled and cubed (1/2") beets
1/2 c minced onion
2 minced garlic cloves
1 tbs dried oregano
1 tbs minced fresh basil
2 tbs minced fresh parsley
1/2 tbs minced fresh marjoram
2 tbs olive oil
4 c water
1 bay leaf
1/4 tsp sea salt
1 tbs lemon juice

*K types: substitute 1 tablespoon sunflower oil for 2 tablespoons olive oil.*

Cook beets until tender. In a large pot, sauté onion, garlic, oregano, basil, parsley, and marjoram in oil for a few minutes. Using a potato masher, coarsely purée beets; add sautéed onions, water, bay leaf, and salt. Cover and simmer over medium heat for 30 minutes. Add lemon juice. Serve over appropriate pasta.

## Burdock and Mushroom Sauce

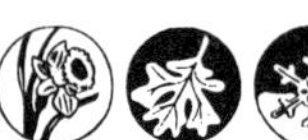

P, PV, PK, K, KV, KP
Serves 2

2 burdock roots
1 c thinly sliced mushrooms
1/4 c thinly sliced onion
1/2 tbs sunflower oil
1 tbs brown bean sauce
1/2 c warm water
2 tbs toasted corn flour
1/4 tsp coriander powder
3 sprigs fresh cilantro
1/2 c water

Scrub burdock and cut into matchsticks. Prepare mushrooms and onion. In a medium pan, heat oil and add vegetables. Cover and simmer over low heat for a few minutes. Dilute brown bean sauce in 1/2 cup of warm water and add to vegetables, along with corn flour and spices. Add 1/2 cup water and cook, covered, over low heat for 40 minutes. Serve over appropriate pasta.

***Note: Brown bean sauce, which is lima beans fermented in malt, is available at Oriental food stores.***

## Sunflower Sauce

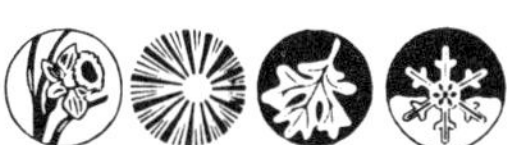

ALL TYPES
Serves 2

1/4 c sunflower seed butter
1 tsp natural mustard
1/2 c warm water
1/4 c diced white onion
Pinch of sea salt
1/4 tsp coriander powder
1 tbs sunflower oil
8 asparagus spears, cut into 1" pieces
1/2 c water

*Garnish:*
Minced fresh dill

*V, P types: serve over udon noodles.*
*P types: omit mustard and add 1/4 teaspoon cardamom and pinch of turmeric.*
*K types: serve over soba noodles.*

Dilute sunflower seed butter and mustard in 1/2 cup warm water. In a medium pan, sauté onion, salt, and coriander in oil for 5 minutes; add sunflower butter and mustard mixture, along with asparagus and 1/2 cup water. Cover and simmer over medium heat for 8 minutes. Serve over appropriate pasta and garnish with fresh dill.

# TOFU DISHES

The soybean plant was first cultivated in Korea and China more than two thousand years ago. The Chinese consider it to be one of the five sacred grains. Tofu making has been and continues to be a sadhana for Japanese tofu masters; they demonstrate great form and prowess when preparing this wholesome food. The making of tofu, considered to be an art, represents the traditional attitude toward work and sustenance common to the Japanese culture.

Tofu was first prepared in China. The curdling methods were adapted from the great milk nation to the south, India, and from the Mongols to the north. The Ming Dynasty is said to have considered tofu a delicacy, and many auspicious tofu dishes were served during that period. *Doufu* is the original Chinese name for tofu.

To prepare tofu, soybeans are first boiled in huge caldrons, and the whey of the beans is drained off. The remaining soy milk is curdled with the natural coagulant *nigari.* Once the curds and whey are separated, the soy curds are pressed in barrels, to yield bricks of tofu.

Tofu arrived in Japan early in the 1500s. The first book about tofu, *Tofu Hyaku Chin,* was written in 1782. The vegetarian Buddhist monks were the originators of the first tofu shops in Japan. These were actually set up inside the temples. Today there are approximately forty thousand tofu shops in Japan. The first tofu shop in the United States was established in San Francisco in 1906 by Quong Hop and Company Recently, tofu has found its way into mainstream supermarkets. There are as many grades of tofu as there are cheeses. Avoid tofu packed with preservatives. Most health food stores carry prime quality tofu in bulk. Tofu is inexpensive and can provide nourishing meals that are fat-free, cholesterol-free, and high in protein and calcium.

## Ramps and Tofu Stew

*Ramps, also known as wild leeks, grow throughout the East Coast from North Carolina to Maine. A pungent member of the scallion family, they have a flavorful, seafood-like taste when cooked.*

K, KV, KP
Serves 2

1 tsp sesame oil
1/2 lb sliced mushrooms
1/8 c minced onion
1 lb firm tofu
1/4 tsp sea salt
1/4 tsp coarse black pepper
4 stalks of ramps, thinly sliced
  or 4 scallions, if ramps are unavailable

In a medium pan, heat oil and sauté mushrooms and onions for a few minutes, adding a small amount of water. Crumble tofu into mixture and add salt, pepper, and thinly sliced ramps. Cover and simmer over medium heat for 12 minutes. Serve over rye toast.

## Sloppy Joes

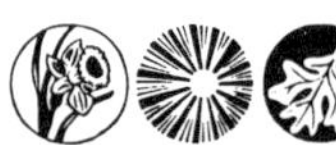

ALL TYPES
Serves 2

1 lb soft tofu
1/4 tsp turmeric
1 tbs sunflower oil
1/4 c minced onion
1/4 c grated daikon
1/4 c grated potato
1/4 tsp sea salt
1/2 tsp dried fenugreek leaves

*V types: substitute 1/4 cup grated carrots for potatoes, use 2 tablespoons sesame oil for the sunflower oil, and add 1/4 cup of buttermilk, if desired.*
*P types: omit fenugreek leaves and add fennel seeds.*

Crumble tofu into a large bowl; mix in turmeric. In a large skillet, heat oil and sauté vegetables. Add tofu, salt, and fenugreek. Cover and simmer over low heat for 20 minutes. Serve over a slice of freshly baked bread.

## Tofu and Broccoli

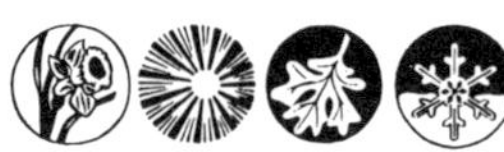

ALL TYPES
Serves 2

1/2 lb firm tofu
2 tbs barley flour
3 stalks broccoli with florettes
1 tsp olive oil
1/4 c thinly sliced onion
1 minced garlic clove
4 minced dried red chili peppers
1/4 tsp sea salt
1 tsp mirin
1/4 c water
1 tsp kudzu (or arrowroot)

*P types: omit red chili peppers and garlic.*

Slice tofu into 1" × 1/2" pieces. Put flour in a small paper bag; add tofu pieces and shake. Wash broccoli and cut into small pieces.

In a large skillet, heat oil and pan-fry tofu pieces for a few minutes. Add onions, garlic, chili peppers, and salt. Cover and simmer over low heat for 2 minutes. Add broccoli, mirin, and 2 tablespoons of the water. Cover and simmer for 10 minutes. Dilute kudzu in remaining water and add to mixture. Stir and simmer uncovered until kudzu becomes clear. Serve over appropriate grain.

## Lemon Broccoli Tofu

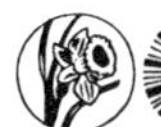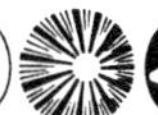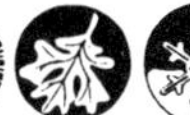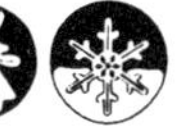

V, VP, VK, K, KV, KP
Serves 2

**3 stalks broccoli with florets**
**1 tbs sunflower oil**
**1/2 c thinly sliced firm tofu**
**1 minced garlic clove**
**1/2 tbs grated lemon peel**
**1/2 tbs rice vinegar**
**1/2 tbs rice syrup**
**3 tbs water**

Cut broccoli in florets; peel stems and cut into small pieces. Boil in water to cover for 3 minutes. In a large skillet, heat oil and sauté tofu with garlic. Add broccoli pieces to tofu. Combine lemon peel, vinegar, rice syrup, and water; toss into broccoli-tofu mixture.

## Pan-Fried Tofu

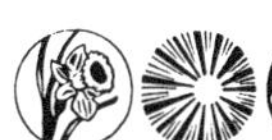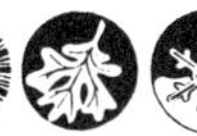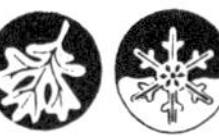

ALL TYPES (V TYPES, OCCASIONALLY)
Serves 2

**1/4 c corn flour**
**Pinch of salt**
**1/2 lb cubed (1") firm tofu**
**2 tbs sunflower oil**

Put flour and salt into a brown paper bag; add cubed tofu and shake. In a cast-iron skillet, heat oil until hot but not smoking. Reduce heat slightly; add tofu and brown on each side for a few minutes. Serve with Burdock Sauce (see following recipe) and appropriate grain.

## Burdock Sauce

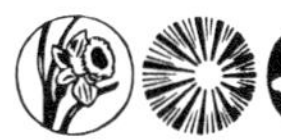

ALL TYPES
Serves 2

**1/2 tsp ginger juice (see page 194)**
**2 medium burdock roots**
**2 carrots**
**1/2 c minced onion**
**1/2 tsp sunflower oil**
**2 tbs water**
**Pinch of turmeric**
**Pinch of salt**
**1/4 c water**
**1 tbs kudzu (or arrowroot)**

***V, VP, and VK: substitute sesame oil for sunflower oil.***

Make the ginger juice and set aside. Scrub burdock roots and carrots; cut into matchsticks. In a medium pan, sauté roots and carrots with onions in oil. Add 2 tablespoons of water, cover, and simmer for 3 minutes. Add ginger juice, turmeric, and salt, and 1/8 cup of water. Continue simmering for 15 minutes. Dilute kudzu in remaining water and stir into hot vegetables.

Add pan-fried tofu cubes (see preceding recipe) and simmer over very low heat for 3 minutes. Serve over appropriate grain with steamed greens.

## Sweet and Sour Tofu

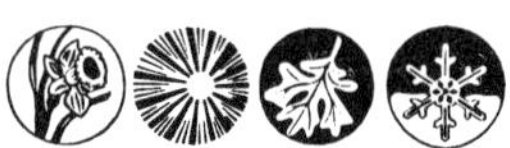

V, VP, VK
Serves 2

1 lb semi-firm tofu
1/2 c fresh cubed (1") pineapple
1 tsp walnut oil
1/2 tsp mirin
1/2 tsp rice vinegar
1/2 minced garlic clove (optional)
2 tbs water
Few strands of saffron
4 umeboshi plums, seeds removed
1/2 c pineapple juice
1 tbs kudzu (or arrowroot)
1/2 c warm water

Cut tofu into 1" cubes. In a large skillet, sauté with pineapple in oil until tofu begins to brown. Add mirin, vinegar, and garlic. Add 2 tablespoons of water and cover for 2 minutes. Add saffron, umeboshi plums, and pineapple juice. Simmer over low heat for 5 minutes. Dilute kudzu in 1/2 cup water and add to tofu mixture, stirring until it begins to thicken. Serve hot over appropriate grain.

## Tofu Tempura

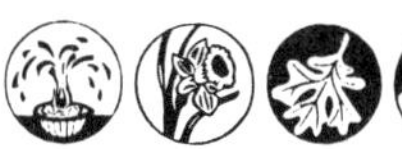

ALL TYPES
Serves 2

1 lb semi-firm tofu
1/4 c corn flour
Pinch of salt
1/4 c sunflower oil

Cut tofu into 1" cubes. Put flour, salt, and tofu in a paper bag and shake. Pour oil into a thin 6" stainless steel skillet. Heat until very hot but not smoking. Lower heat slightly and put 8 cubes of tofu in at a time. Use wooden chop sticks to turn cubes until golden brown on each side. Place on two pieces of cheesecloth in a colander in sink to soak up excess oil. Serve with Mild Sweet and Sour Sauce (see following recipe).

*Tempura Batter Variation:*
1 tsp agar-agar powder
1/4 c warm water
1/2 c whole wheat flour
Pinch of sea salt
1/2 c water

Dilute agar-agar in 1/4 cup warm water. Mix ingredients together and whip into a smooth batter. Add enough water to make batter thick, but fluid. Dip tofu pieces in batter and fry. Serve hot.

## Mild Sweet and Sour Sauce

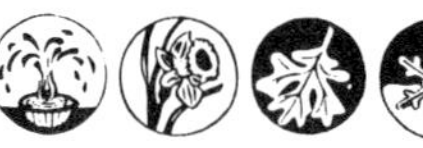

ALL TYPES
Serves 2

1 tbs ginger juice (see page 194)
1/4 c fresh orange juice
1/4 c fresh carrot juice
1/2 tsp coarse black pepper
Pinch of turmeric
1 tbs rice vinegar
1 tbs kudzu (or arrowroot)
1/4 c water
*Garnish:*
Grated daikon

Make the ginger juice. Add to orange and carrot juices. In a small pan, heat the three juices together for a few minutes. Add spices and vinegar. Dilute kudzu in water and add to juices. Stir and serve over Tofu Tempura or other tofu dishes. Garnish with freshly grated daikon.

## Natto-Stuffed Tofu

*Natto is cooked soybeans that have been mixed with specific enzymes and fermented.*

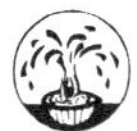

V, VK, K, KV
Serves 2

1/4 c natto
1/2 tsp umeboshi paste
1 lb firm tofu
1 sheet nori seaweed
1/2 tbs sunflower oil
*K types: use sparingly.*

Whip the natto and umeboshi paste together until frothy. Cut tofu in 4 large squares, 3/4" thick. Scoop 1 tablespoon tofu from the center of each square without piercing the bottom. Gently place 1 tablespoon natto-umeboshi mixture into each indentation.

If you have a gas stove, warm nori sheet briefly over an open flame; otherwise use sheet as is. Cut lengthwise into 4 pieces. Sandwich two pieces of natto-filled tofu together and wrap with a strip of nori, which will stick to the damp tofu. In a cast-iron skillet, heat oil and sauté for approximately 4 minutes until golden brown. Use a spatula to turn tofu squares so they brown evenly. Serve warm.

## Carrot and Raisin-Stuffed Tofu

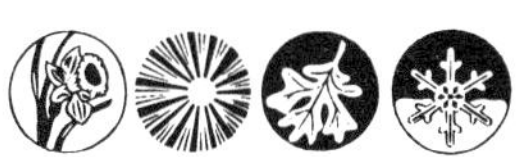

V, VP, VK, P, PV, PK
Serves 2

2 tbs raisins
1/2 c hot apple juice
1 tsp mirin
1/4 c grated carrots
1/2 tsp cinnamon powder
1/4 tsp fine black pepper
1 tbs walnut oil
1 sheet nori seaweed
1 lb firm tofu

Soak raisins in hot apple juice and mirin for 2 hours.

In a medium skillet, cook soaked raisins with liquid, carrots, and spices in oil over medium heat for 2 minutes. Follow the same procedures for cutting, scooping, filling, wrapping, and cooking as for Natto-Stuffed Tofu (above). Serve warm.

## Ricotta and Tofu Quiche

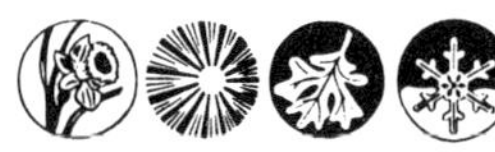

V, VP, P, PV
PK OCCASIONALLY
Serves 2

1 whole wheat pie crust dough (see page 311)
*Filling:*
1/2 c crumbled soft tofu
1/2 c ricotta cheese
1/2 c soy milk
Pinch of fine black pepper
Pinch of turmeric
1 tsp cumin powder
2 tbs sunflower oil
1/4 c water

Preheat oven to 375 degrees F. Mix all filling ingredients together in a large bowl. Lightly grease pie pan. Roll out pie crust dough and press dough into pan. Pour filling into pie crust, leveling the top. Bake for 35 minutes. Serve warm.

## Baked Spiced Tofu

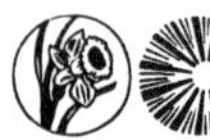 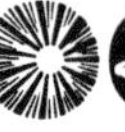 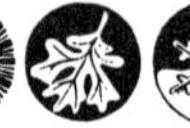 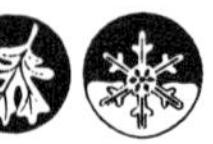

**V, VK, K, KV, KP**
**Serves 2**

**1 lb firm tofu**
**1/2 tsp curry powder**
**1/2 tsp tamari**
**1/2 tsp grated ginger**
**1/2 tsp minced garlic**
**1/2 c water**

Cut tofu into 1/2" slices. Mix spices with water and bring to boil. Remove from heat and marinate tofu in the mixture for 30 minutes. Preheat oven to 375 degrees F. Bake marinated tofu until dry (about 35 minutes). Allow to cool and store in refrigerator for use in sandwiches.

## Tofu-Stuffed Squash

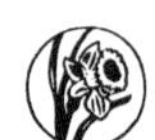 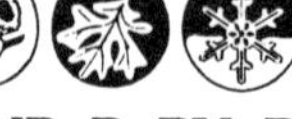 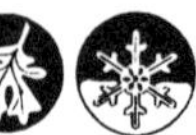

**V, VP, P, PV, PK**
**Serves 2**

**1/2 c crumbled soft tofu**
**1/2 c stale whole wheat bread, crumbled**
**1/2 c sliced fresh mushrooms (regular or shiitake)**
**1/4 c diced celery**
**1/4 c diced carrots**
**1/4 c diced onion**
**1/4 tsp rock salt**
**1/4 tsp turmeric**
**1 tsp coriander powder**
**2 tsp sunflower oil**
**2 c vegetable or grain water**
**1 buttercup squash**

***V types: omit celery and mushrooms.***

Preheat oven to 375 degrees F. Mix all ingredients except squash together in a large bowl. Lightly grease baking pan. Cut squash in half lengthwise, scoop out seeds, and fill the centers with tofu-vegetable stuffing. Bake for 45 minutes or until squash is tender. Serve hot.

# SEITAN DISHES

Seitan, a traditional food of Japan and China, is used mostly as a meat substitute. Made from the gluten of whole wheat flour, seitan is very high in nutrients. It is available prepackaged in health food stores. The following instructions tell you how to make your own at home.

## Seitan

Serves 4

**4 lbs whole wheat flour**
**9 cups water**

Place flour in large bowl; add enough water to knead into a bread-dough consistency; knead about 7 minutes. Cover with water and let sit for 1 hour. Knead in soaking water for a few minutes. Pour off the milky water and reserve.

To wash: Place dough in a large strainer and set in a large bowl of water. Knead dough in the strainer. Discard milky water. Repeat this washing process, alternating between cold and warm water in the bowl, until the bran and starch are worked out of the dough. The last rinse should be in cold water to contract the gluten.

Cut gluten ball into 4" pieces, place in 2 cups boiling water or stock, and boil for 40 minutes over medium heat. The milky rinse water may be used for thickening stews and gravies, or may be added to your bath water. Reserve seitan boiling water if you are making Stuffed Seitan or Seitan, Daikon, and Carrot Stew.

For Soft Seitan: Place gluten in a covered container in the oven with pilot light on, or in direct sun, for 4 hours. Dough will become light and pliable, making it ideal for stuffing. (See recipe on page 268.)

Quick Method: Place flour in a large bowl. Add enough water to form a batter of cookie-dough consistency. Knead for 5 minutes until flour is mixed thoroughly with water. Cover loaf with four cups of warm water and allow to sit for 10 minutes. Knead again in soaking water for 1 minute, then wash as above.

## Stuffed Seitan

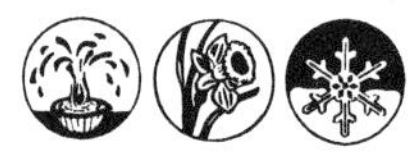

V, VP, VK, P, PV, PK
Serves 2

2 tbs unsweetened apricot jam
1/2 tsp rice vinegar
1/4 lb stale, unyeasted rye bread
2 tbs sesame oil
4 diced celery stalks
1/4 cup grated carrots
6 thinly sliced fresh shiitake mushrooms
4 diced crookneck squash
6 minced water chestnuts
6 dried apples, in pieces
1/4 c apple cider
2 4" pieces soft seitan
2 c reserve seitan water

Heat jam and vinegar together until thick and smooth. Set aside.

In a large bowl, shred 1/2 cup of coarse bread crumbs. In a large skillet, heat oil and add celery, carrots, mushrooms, squash, chestnuts, and apples. Mix all ingredients together except cider and seitan, and cook for 2 minutes over medium heat. Stir in cider; cover and simmer over low heat for 10 minutes.

Preheat over to 350 degrees F. With your hands, shape each seitan piece into approximately a 9" × 6" rectangle. Fill each center with stuffing. Wrap seitan around filling; tie together with cotton string and close the ends with toothpick. Using a baking dish with a cover, fill dish one-quarter full with reserve seitan boiling water. Add stuffed seitan and bake, covered, for 45 minutes. With a slotted spoon, remove seitan from liquid. Brush on apricot–vinegar mixture. Serve with freshly steamed collard greens.

## Stripped Tarragon Seitan

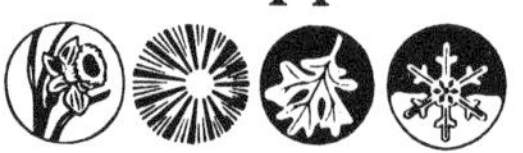

V, VP, VK, P, PV, PK
Serves 2

2 whole scallions, chopped
4 sprigs minced fresh tarragon
1/4 tsp coarse black pepper
1 tsp sesame oil
Few drops of lemon juice
2 4" pieces firm seitan, cut into 10 strips
Pinch of salt
1/4 c water

In a large skillet, sauté scallions, tarragon, and pepper in oil over medium heat for a few minutes. Add lemon juice, seitan, salt, and water. Cover and simmer for 5 minutes over medium heat.

## Chickpea and Seitan Stew

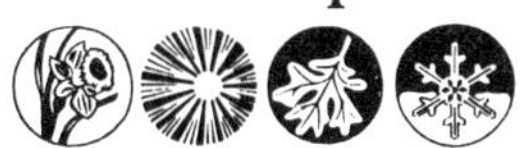

P, PK, PV, K
Serves 2

1 c chickpeas
4" piece of kombu seaweed
6 c water
1/4 tsp sea salt
2 tbs olive oil
1/2 c chopped shallots
1 c diced carrots
1/4 c diced burdock root
1/4 c chopped celery
1/2 tsp cumin powder
1/2 c seitan, cut into 1" pieces

*Garnish:*
1/4 c minced fresh fennel

Soak chickpeas overnight. Drain and rinse. Wash kombu by placing in a small bowl of water and rubbing gently to remove salt. Place kombu on the bottom of a large stew pot. Add water, salt, and chickpeas, and bring to a boil. In a large skillet, heat oil and sauté vegetables and spices for 5 minutes. Add the sautéed vegetables and seitan pieces to the chickpeas. Cover and simmer over medium heat for 35 minutes. Garnish with minced fresh fennel and serve hot.

## Seitan, Daikon, and Carrot Stew

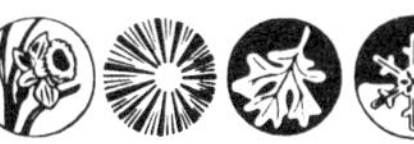

V, VP, P, PV
K, KV, KP, VK OCCASIONALLY
Serves 2

1/2 tbs sesame oil
1/2 c sliced onion
1/4 tsp grated ginger
1/4 tsp coriander powder
Pinch of salt
12 pieces firm seitan
4 carrots, cut in 1" chunks
2 daikon radish, cut in 1" chunks
1 burdock root, cut in 1" chunks
1/4 c reserve seitan water

In large skillet, heat oil. Sauté onion with ginger, coriander, and salt over medium heat for a few minutes. Add seitan, carrots, daikon, burdock, and reserve seitan water. Cover and simmer for 20 minutes over medium-low heat. Serve over appropriate grain.

# SALADS

## PRESSED SALADS

Pressed salads refer to sliced vegetables that have been combined with a pickling agent and pressed. These salads, which use a quick form of pickling, have been present in Japanese cuisine for centuries. Because of their sour and/or salty taste, small amounts are eaten to activate the digestion of the various body types. Use either a pickle press or a heavy rock. (Place salad in a bowl and put a shallower bowl, filled with a heavy rock, on top of salad.)

Pressed salads may sit for 30 minutes to 3 hours, depending on the strength desired. The longer it is pressed the more pickled, and thus more sour, the salad becomes. Unless otherwise specified, K and P types may use salads pressed for 30 minutes to 1 hour; V types may use salads pressed for 1 to 3 hours.

## Pressed Sprouted Mung and Cabbage Salad

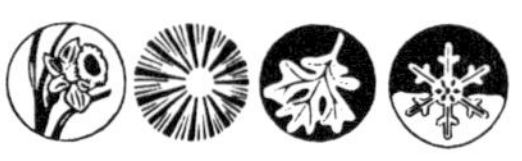

ALL TYPES
V TYPES: IN SMALL QUANTITIES
Serves 4

**1/2 c sprouted mung dhal**
**1 c thinly sliced red cabbage**
**2 tbs rice vinegar**
**2 tsp sea salt**

***V types: add 1 tablespoon warm walnut oil.***

Mix ingredients together. Press for 1 hour. Rinse off salt and serve.

## Pressed Endive and Cucumber Salad

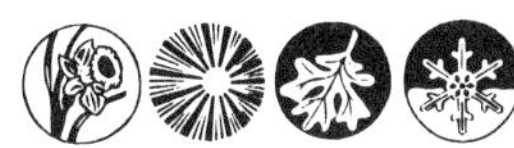

ALL TYPES
Serves 2

2 Belgian endives
1 thinly sliced cucumber
1 tsp salt
½ tsp umeboshi vinegar

*V types: add ½ tablespoon warm olive oil.*

Thinly slice endives diagonally and combine with cucumber slices. Toss with salt and vinegar. K and P types press for 30 minutes; V types press for 1 hour. Rinse off salt and vinegar. Serve cool.

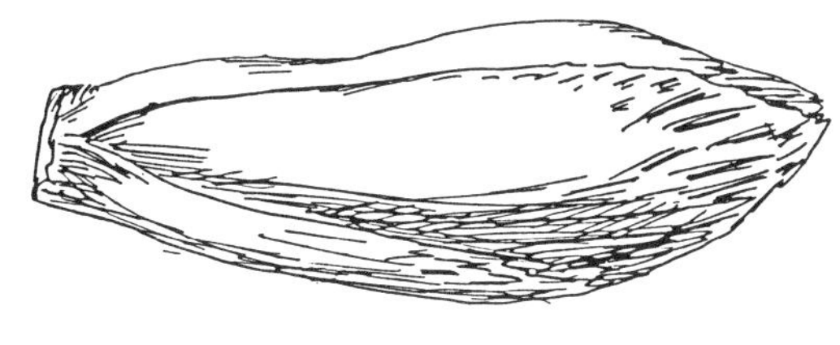

Belgian Endive

## Pressed Red Radish Salad

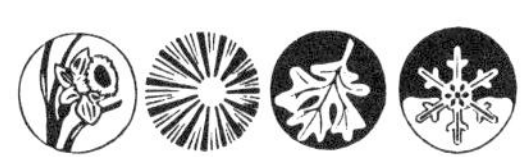

ALL TYPES
Serves 2

1 bunch red radishes, thinly sliced
1 tsp sea salt
2 tbs roasted sesame seeds

*V types: add ½ tablespoon warm sesame oil.*
*PK, K, KV, KP: use sesame seeds sparingly.*

Toss sliced radishes with salt and press for 1 hour. Rinse off salt and sprinkle with sesame seeds.

## Pressed Bibb Lettuce Salad

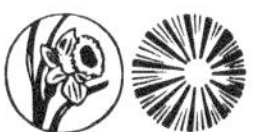

ALL TYPES
Serves 2

12 Bibb lettuce leaves
1 tsp sea salt

*V types: add 1 tablespoon warm sesame oil.*

Toss lettuce with salt and press for 30 minutes (1 hour for V types). Rinse off salt and serve.

*Note: Romaine or leaf lettuce may also be used.*

## Pressed Ginger Salad

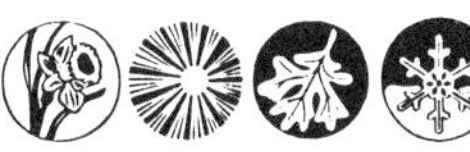

V, VK, K, KV
Serves 4

¼ c thinly sliced ginger root (peeled)
1 tbs umeboshi vinegar
1 tsp salt

Toss sliced ginger with vinegar and salt and press for 3 hours. Rinse and serve as a condiment.

## Pressed Onion Salad

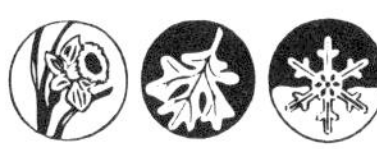

K, KV
Serves 4

¼ c thinly sliced onion
4 umeboshi plums, peeled
2 tsp sea salt

Slice onion thinly. Mix in plum and sea salt. Press for 2 hours. Rinse off salt and serve as a condiment.

## Pressed Watercress and Tamarind Salad

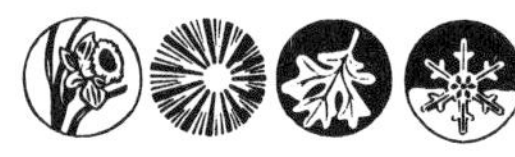

ALL TYPES
Serves 4

2 tbs tamarind paste
2 tbs warm water
1 tsp sunflower oil
1 tsp rice vinegar
1 tbs rock salt
1 bunch of watercress

Thin tamarind paste with warm water. Mix in oil, vinegar, and salt. Add watercress, toss, and press for 1 hour. Rinse off salt and diluted paste and serve. (Remaining diluted paste water may be used in sauces for V types.)

## Pressed Cabbage and Radish Salad

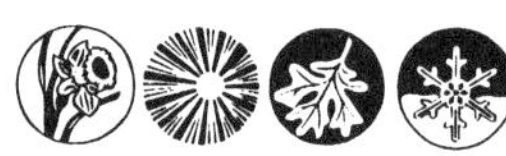

K, KV, KP
Serves 4

1/2 head of Chinese cabbage
4 red radishes
1 2" piece ginger root
1/2 tsp umeboshi vinegar
1/2 tsp sea salt

Shred cabbage, thinly slice radishes, and peel and thinly slice ginger root. Combine all ingredients and press for 1 1/2 hours. Rinse off salt thoroughly and use as a condiment.

## Pressed Cucumber and Dill Salad

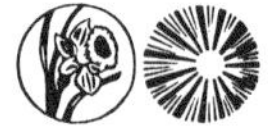

ALL TYPES
Serves 4

1 cucumber
3 sprigs fresh dill
2 tbs dill vinegar
1 tsp sea salt

Peel and thinly slice cucumber. Chop dill into large pieces. Mix all ingredients and press for 1 1/2 hours. Rinse thoroughly and serve as a condiment.

# FRESH SALADS

## Arugula Salad

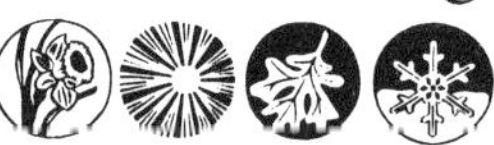

P, PK, K, KP
Serves 2

1 bell pepper
1 bunch arugula

Thinly slice pepper and blanch in boiling water for 3 minutes. Wash arugula. Arrange pepper slices on top of greens and serve with Fennel Dressing.

Fennel Dressing:
1/2 tbs olive oil
1 tsp rice vinegar
1/4 c apple cider
1 tbs minced fresh fennel
1/4 c water

Combine ingredients in a bottle and shake. Pour over arugula.

## Cauliflower and Endive Salad

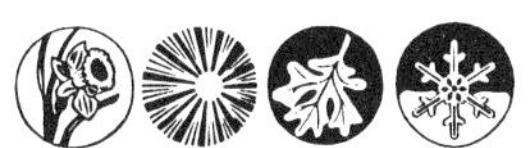

P, PK, K, KP
Serves 2

2 c cauliflower florets
2 Belgian endives

*Garnish:*
1/4 c roasted pumpkin seeds

Boil cauliflower pieces for 5 minutes. Remove from water and combine with whole endive leaves. Add Orange Dressing and garnish with roasted pumpkin seeds.

*Orange Dressing:*
1/4 c fresh orange juice
Few strands of saffron
1/2 tbs mild herbal vinegar
2 tsp sunflower oil

Heat orange juice; add saffron, vinegar, and oil. Pour over Cauliflower and Endive Salad.

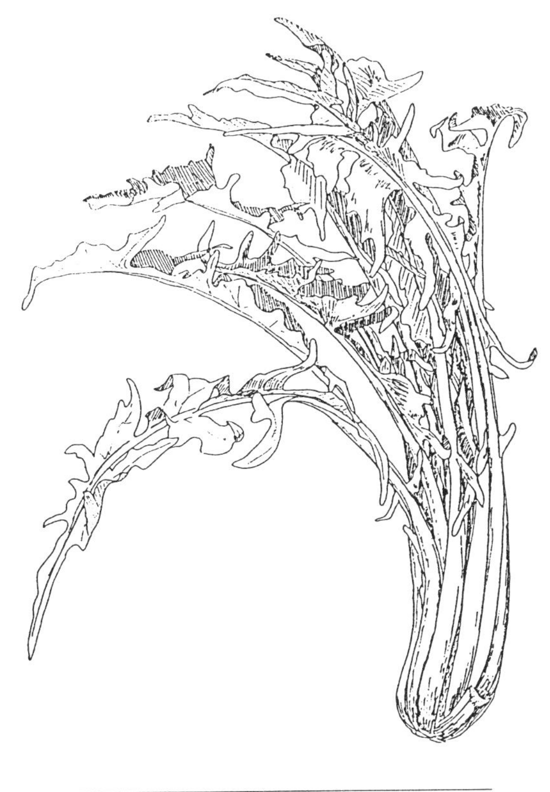

Catalonia Chicory

# GRAIN SALADS

## Buckwheat and Pea Salad

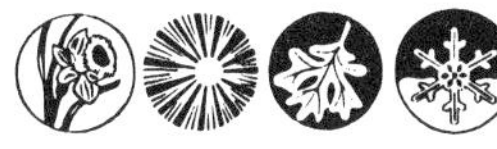

K
KV, KP OCCASIONALLY
Serves 4

2 c buckwheat groats
3 1/2 c boiling water
1/2 c fresh peas
2 c water
1/2 c fresh corn kernels
1 tbs minced fresh marjoram
1 tbs minced fresh basil
1/2 tsp lemon juice
Pinch sea salt

*Garnish:*
Whole sprigs of marjoram and 5 petalled red radishes

Wash buckwheat until water runs clear and add to boiling water. Cover and cook over medium heat for 30 minutes. Remove from heat and allow buckwheat to cool for 10 minutes. In a separate pan, boil peas in 2 cups water until just tender; add corn and boil for an additional 5 minutes. Remove vegetables and reserve water.

Combine marjoram, basil, lemon juice, and salt. Toss grain, vegetables, and herbs with 1/2 cup reserved water. Garnish with whole sprigs of marjoram and petalled red radishes.

## Millet and Quinoa Salad

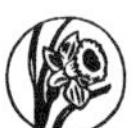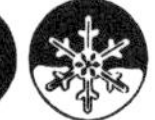

K, KV, KP
Serves 2

1/2 c millet
1/2 c quinoa
2 1/2 c boiling water
1 bay leaf
4 stalks celery
1 c water
1 red bell pepper
1/4 c celery water
1 tsp sunflower oil
1 tsp lime juice
1/2 tbs minced fresh rosemary

Wash grains and combine. Add to boiling water with bay leaf. Cover and simmer over low heat for 25 minutes. Remove from heat and allow to cool for 10 minutes. Cut celery into 1/2" pieces and boil in 1 cup of water for 3 minutes; reserve water. Thinly slice bell pepper and marinate in 1/4 cup celery water, oil, lime juice, and rosemary leaves for 30 minutes. In a large wooden bowl, toss grains, celery, and marinated pepper mixture. Serve warm.

## Almond and Carrot Rice Salad

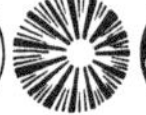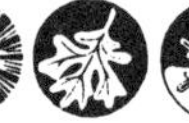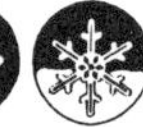

P, PV, PK
V, VP, VK OCCASIONALLY
Serves 4

2 c medium-grain brown rice
4 c boiling water
6 medium carrots, cut into matchsticks
2 c water
1/8 c almonds
1 tsp light sesame oil
4 tbs fresh orange juice
2 tbs minced fresh basil
2 tbs minced fresh oregano

Wash rice until water runs clear and add to boiling water. Cover and cook over medium heat for 45 minutes. Remove from heat and allow to cool for 10 minutes. In a separate pan, boil carrots in 2 cups water for 8 minutes; reserve water. Blanch almonds in hot carrot water for a few minutes; peel and sliver. Combine oil, orange juice, basil, oregano, and 2 tablespoons carrot water. Toss rice, carrots, almonds, and oil-herb mixture in a big wooden bowl. Serve warm.

## Barley, Onion, and Carrot Salad (PC)

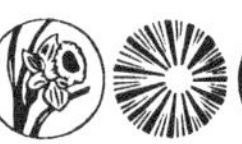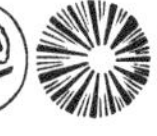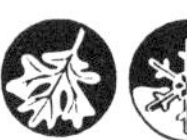

ALL TYPES
Serves 4

2 c pearl barley
1/4 tsp sea salt
3 c water
1 tsp sunflower oil
2 c diced onion
4 carrots, cut into matchsticks
3 tbs water
1 tbs orange juice
1 tsp umeboshi vinegar

*V types: use 1 teaspoon sesame oil instead of sunflower oil.*

Wash barley until water runs clear. Place barley, salt, and water in a pressure cooker. Cover without locking the lid and bring to a boil. Lock cover, and bring to pressure. Cook over medium heat for 45 minutes. Remove from heat and allow pressure to fall naturally. (For conventional cooking, bring barley to boil in 4 cups of water. Cover and cook over medium heat for 55 to 60 minutes.) In a skillet, heat oil and sauté onion and carrots. Add 3 tablespoons water; cover and simmer for 30 minutes. Combine vegetables and cooked barley. Mix juice and vinegar and stir into the grain salad. Serve warm.

## Barley and Pea Salad

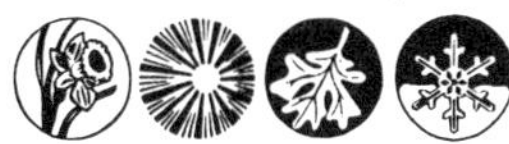

ALL TYPES
Serves 2

$^1/_2$ c hulled barley
$^1/_4$ c fresh peas
$^1/_4$ c cubed ($^1/_2$") carrots
$^1/_4$ c chopped collard stems
4 big collard leaves
1 tsp ghee
1 tsp orange rind
$^1/_4$ tsp rice vinegar

Wash barley until water runs clear. Place in 2 cups of water and bring to a boil. Lower and simmer, covered, over medium-low heat for 45 minutes.

Boil peas, carrots, and collard stems in $1^1/_2$ cups water until just soft. Reserve the vegetable water. In a separate pan, steam whole collard leaves for a few minutes. To make dressing, combine $^1/_4$ cup warm vegetable water, ghee, orange rind, and vinegar. Arrange collard leaves in bottom of a wide bowl. Toss vegetables and barley together and place on leaves. Add dressing and serve.

## Lime and Raisin Rice Salad

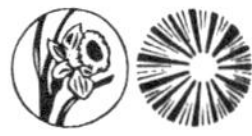

V, VP, VK
P, PV, PK OCCASIONALLY
Serves 4

$^1/_8$ c raisins
$^1/_4$ c warm water
2 c brown basmati rice
$^1/_2$ tsp sea salt
4 c boiling water
1 tsp walnut oil
1 tsp fresh lime juice
2 tbs minced fresh dill
1 tsp minced fresh marjoram

Soak raisins in warm water for 20 minutes. Wash rice until water runs clear and add, with salt, to boiling water. Cover and cook over medium heat for 40 minutes. Remove from heat and allow to cool for 10 minutes. Combine oil, lime juice, dill, marjoram, and soaked raisins; toss with rice. Serve warm.

## Millet and Snow Pea Salad

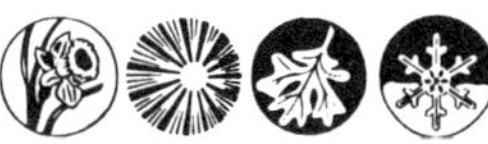

K, KV, KP
Serves 2

1 c hulled millet
2 c boiling water
Pinch of sea salt
$^1/_4$ lb snow peas
$^1/_2$ c diced shallots
$^1/_2$ c grated daikon
$^1/_2$ c grated carrots
2 tsp grated ginger
1 tsp light sesame oil

*Garnish:*
$^1/_4$ c minced fresh parsley and 2 tsp grated orange rind

Wash millet until water runs clear and toast in a skillet until dry and light brown. Pour into boiling water and add salt; cover and simmer over low heat for 20 minutes. In a separate pan, blanch snow peas for 5 seconds. In a frying pan, sauté shallots, daikon, carrots, and ginger in oil over medium heat for 2 minutes. Toss vegetables and millet together. Garnish with minced parsley and grated orange rind.

# SAUCES AND DRESSINGS

## Carrot and Oat Sauce

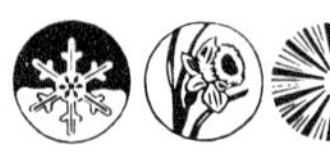

ALL TYPES
Serves 2

$^1/_4$ c rolled oats
$^1/_2$ c water
3 carrots, cut into chunks
2 tbs sunflower seed butter
1 tsp lemon juice
$^1/_4$ tsp salt

*K types: use rolled rye instead of oats.*

In a small saucepan with lid loosely in place, cook rolled oats in water over medium heat until sticky. Blanch carrot chunks and purée in a blender. Add sunflower butter, lemon juice, cooked oats, and salt. Add a touch of water and combine until smooth. Serve over vegetables.

## Tamari and Ginger Sauce

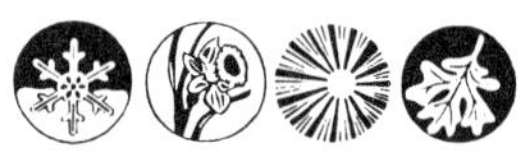

V, VP, VK
Serves 2

1 tbs mustard oil
1 tsp minced garlic
2 tbs chopped scallions
$^1/_4$ c plus 2 tbs tamari
$^1/_4$ c plus 2 tbs water
$^1/_2$ tsp ginger juice (see page 194)

In a frying pan, heat oil; add garlic and scallions and sauté over medium heat for a few minutes. Add tamari, water, and ginger juice. Reduce heat and simmer for 2 minutes. Serve over dumplings.

## Cilantro and Coconut Sauce

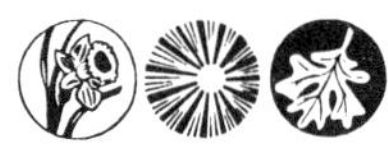

P, PV, PK
Serves 2

2 tbs pine nuts
2 sprigs cilantro
1 tbs avocado oil
2 tbs coconut milk (see page 194)
1 tbs minced fresh coconut
Pinch sea salt
1/4 c plus 2 tbs hot water

Dry-roast pine nuts over medium heat until golden brown. Place all ingredients, except water, in a small hand grinder and purée. Stir in water and serve.

## Basil and Parsley Sauce

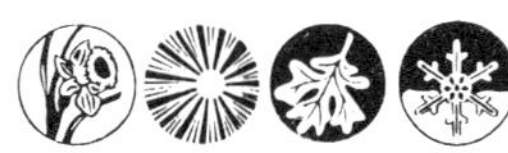

V, VK, K, KV
Serves 2

2 tbs split mung dhal
1 tsp black mustard seeds
8 leaves fresh basil
3 sprigs parsley
3 hot chili peppers (red or green)
1 tbs sunflower oil
Pinch sea salt
1/4 c plus 2 tbs hot water

In a cast-iron skillet, dry-roast the mung dhal and mustard seeds over medium heat for a few minutes. Place all ingredients, except water, in a small hand grinder and purée. Stir in water and serve.

## Burdock and Mushroom Sauce

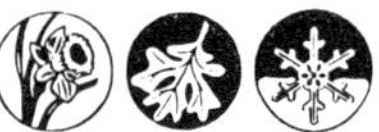

P, PV, PK, K, KV, KP
Serves 2

2 tbs corn flour
2 burdock roots
1 c fresh mushrooms
1 white onion
1/2 tbs sunflower oil
1/4 tsp coriander powder
3 fresh, finely chopped sprigs cilantro
1 tbs brown bean sauce
1 c warm water

In a cast-iron skillet, toast the corn flour over medium heat for a few minutes. Set aside. Scrub burdock roots and cut into matchsticks. Thinly slice mushrooms and onion.

In a medium skillet, heat oil; add vegetables, coriander powder, and cilantro; cover and simmer over low heat for a few minutes. Dilute brown bean sauce in warm water; add sauce, along with toasted corn flour, to vegetables. Add remaining water and cook, covered, over low heat for 40 minutes. Serve over noodles.

*Note: Brown bean sauce, which is lima beans fermented in malt, is available at Oriental food stores.*

## Burdock Gravy

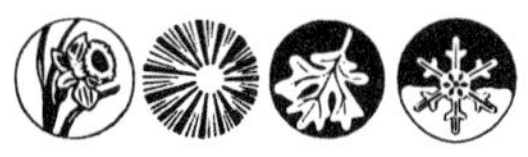

P, PV, PK
Serves 2

1 tsp soy oil
½ c burdock root, cut into matchsticks
½ tsp mirin
1½ c water
Pinch of rock salt
½ tsp tamari
1 tsp kudzu (or arrowroot)
3 tbs cold water

In cast-iron skillet, heat oil; sauté burdock root over medium heat for a few minutes. Add mirin and stir. Add water and salt. Cover and simmer 20 minutes over low heat. Remove the cooked burdock and serve separately. Add tamari to mixture. Dilute kudzu in cold water. Stir into sauce until it thickens; remove from heat. Serve warm over grains, vegetables, tofu, tempeh, or seitan.

## Mild Tamari Sauce

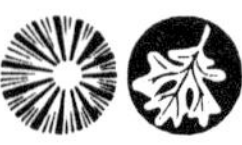

V, VP, VK
P, PV, PK, K, KP OCCASIONALLY
Serves 2

1 tbs tamari
⅛ c water
½ tsp coriander powder
¼ tsp turmeric
Pinch of dried ginger
1 tsp light sesame oil

In a small saucepan, combine tamari with water. Add spices, cover, and simmer for 3 minutes. Add sesame oil and serve over stir-fried dishes.

## Hollandaise Sauce

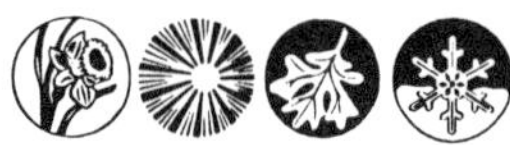

ALL TYPES
Serves 2

1 tbs soy flour
Pinch of salt
2 tbs corn oil
¼ c fresh plain yogurt
Pinch of turmeric
1 tsp honey
¼ c water

*P, PV, and PK types: use 2 tablespoons coconut oil instead of corn oil.*

Dry-roast flour and salt in a cast-iron skillet for 4 to 5 minutes until golden. Add oil, yogurt, and turmeric. Mix honey in warm water and stir into sauce. Serve warm.

## Brown Gravy

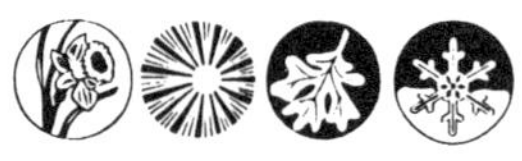

V, VP, P, PV, PK
Serves 2

½ c soy flour
2 c soy milk
1 tbs maple syrup
½ tsp mirin
1 c water
Pinch of rock salt
1 tsp cumin powder
Pinch of turmeric
¼ c puréed onion (optional)

Dry-roast soy flour over medium heat until golden brown. In a small saucepan, heat milk, maple syrup, mirin, and water; add roasted flour, salt, spices, and onion, if desired. Stir to a smooth consistency. Cover and allow to simmer over medium heat for 25 minutes. Stir occasionally to avoid sticking. Serve over grains or stuffed squash.

## Garlic and Ginger Sauce

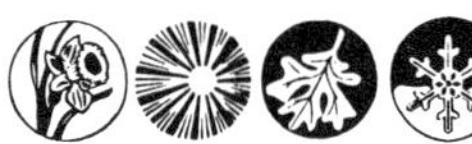

V, VK, K, KV
Serves 2

1/2 c vegetable water
1/2 tsp minced garlic
1/2 tsp minced ginger
1 tsp light sesame oil
1/4 tsp turmeric
2 tbs tamari

*K types: use only 1 tablespoon tamari and substitute 1 teaspoon sunflower oil for sesame oil.*

Bring water to boil and add garlic and ginger. Simmer over medium heat for 10 minutes. Add oil, turmeric, and tamari; remove from heat. Allow to sit for 5 minutes before serving with stir-fries, steamed vegetables, or nori rolls.

## Lemon Kudzu Sauce

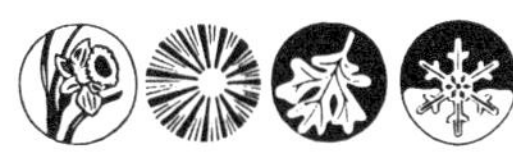

ALL TYPES
Serves 2

1 tbs kudzu (or arrowroot)
1/8 c cold water
1/4 c fresh lemon juice
1/2 tsp rice vinegar
1 tsp finely minced mint leaves
Pinch of salt

*P and K types: omit rice vinegar.*

Dilute kudzu in cold water; heat in a heavy saucepan over very low heat. Add lemon juice, vinegar, mint leaves, and salt. Remove from heat and serve over vegetables.

## Peppered Oil

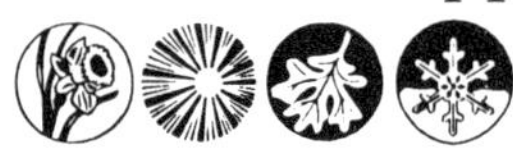

V, VK, PK, K, KV
Serves 2

1/2 tsp coarse black pepper or chopped garlic
1 tsp sunflower oil
1/4 tsp ghee

*V types: use 1 teaspoon sesame oil.*

Dry-roast pepper (or garlic) in a skillet for 3 minutes; remove from heat. Add oil and ghee. Drizzle over corn on the cob or toast.

## Cumin Dressing

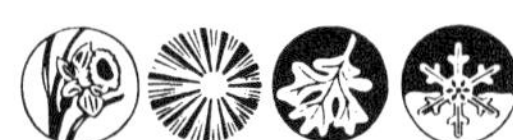

ALL TYPES
Serves 2

1 tbs roasted cumin seeds
1/4 c vegetable water
1 tsp olive oil
1 tsp lime juice
Pinch of coarse black pepper
Pinch of turmeric
1/2 tsp rock salt

Place all ingredients into a bottle, tightly cover, and shake. Pour over salad.

## Basil Dressing

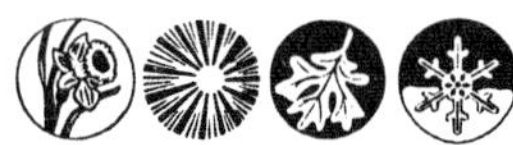

ALL TYPES
Serves 2

1 tsp olive oil
1/2 tsp umeboshi vinegar
1 tbs minced fresh basil
Pinch of turmeric

Place all ingredients into a bottle, cover tightly, and shake. Pour over salad.

## Thyme and Vinegar Dressing

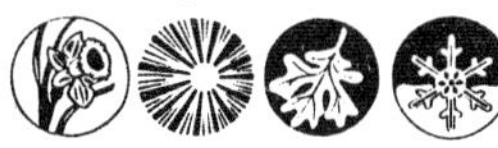

K, KV
Serves 2

1 tsp corn oil
1/2 tsp rice vinegar
3 tbs vegetable water
Pinch each of turmeric, black pepper, cayenne, and thyme

Place all ingredients into a bottle, cover tightly, and shake. Pour over salad.

## Orange Fennel Dressing

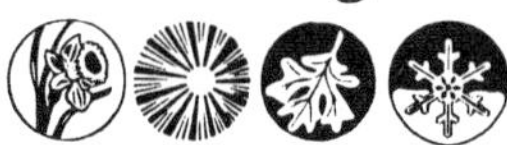

V, VP, P, PV, PK
Serves 2

1/4 c fennel seeds
1/4 c barley cooking water (or spring water)
1/2 tsp orange rind
Pinch of turmeric
Pinch of black pepper
1/4 tsp rice vinegar
1/2 tsp maple syrup
1 tsp light sesame oil

Steep fennel seeds in 1/4 cup boiling water for 15 minutes. Strain seeds and combine tea and all remaining ingredients in a saucepan. Cover and simmer over low heat for 5 minutes. Allow to cool and serve over barley salad.

# SOUPS

## Vegetable Stock

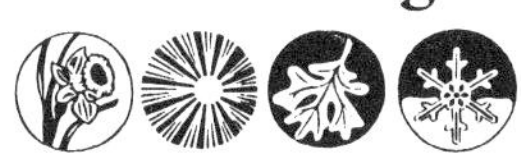

V, VP, VK

**8 c water**
**3 c leftover vegetable ends**
**1 c diced onion**
**1/4 c mugi (barley) miso**
**1/4 c cold water**

In a large soup pot, bring 8 cups of water to boil. Add vegetable ends and onions Dilute miso in cold water and add to broth. Cover and simmer over medium heat for 3 hours. Allow to cool. Put colander over large bowl or pan and drain. Reserve stock and discard vegetable leftovers.

*Note: Vegetable ends may be saved in a basket and kept in a dry place for up to one week.*

## Rye Croutons

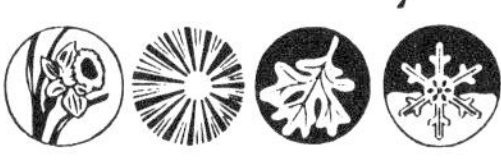

K, KP

**Unyeasted rye bread, several days old**

Dice bread into small pieces. Toast in a dry skillet over low heat for 15 minutes.

## Whole Wheat Croutons

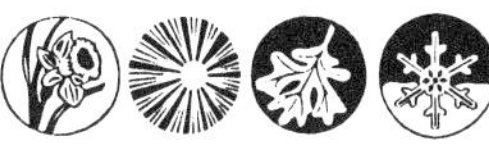

V, VK, P, PK

**Unyeasted whole wheat bread, several days old**

***V types: soak croutons in soup before eating.***

Cut bread into small cubes and toast in an oiled skillet over low heat for 15 minutes.

## Leek and Chickpea Soup

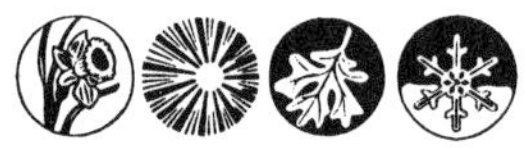

P, PK, K, KV, KP
Serves 2

1 c chickpeas
5 c soup stock (recipe follows)
2 c chopped leeks
1 whole garlic clove
Pinch of turmeric
Pinch of coarse black pepper
Pinch of salt
2 tbs canola oil
1/2 c eggless pasta shells, cooked

*P and PK: use whole wheat pasta shells.*
*K and KP: use rye or buckwheat shells.*

Soak chickpeas for 2 hours. Make soup stock (see below). Drain chickpeas and add to soup stock. Sauté leeks, garlic, turmeric, black pepper, and salt in oil for 5 minutes. Add to soup stock, along with cooked pasta shells and cooked kombu that remains from soup stock. Simmer over medium heat for 25 minutes. Remove kombu and, using a wooden spoon, mash until soup has consistency of a coarse purée. Serve hot.

*Soup Stock:*
3" piece of kombu seaweed
1/2 c minced onion
1/2 c hulled barley
6 c water

To wash kombu, place in a small bowl of water and rub gently to remove salt. Boil kombu, onion, and barley in water over low heat for two hours. Strain and use 5 cups of liquid for soup stock.

## Clear Ginger and Corn Soup

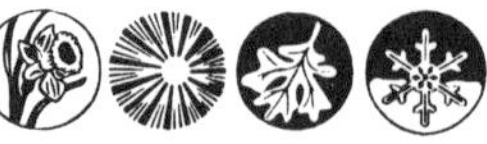

ALL TYPES, OCCASIONALLY
Serves 2

2 ears corn, husked
5 c water
2 sprigs fresh parsley, chopped
5 whole scallions
1 tbs grated ginger
1/2 c sliced onion
2 c fresh corn kernels
1/2 lb semi-firm cubed tofu
1/4 c chopped scallions
Pinch of asafoetida
1/4 tsp sea salt
2 tsp light sesame oil
3 tsp kudzu (or arrowroot)
1/4 c cold water

Strip kernels from corn ear. To make soup stock, in a large pot boil 5 cups of water with stripped corn cobs, parsley, scallions, ginger, and onion covered, over medium heat, for 20 minutes. Strain stock and add corn kernels, tofu, chopped scallions, asafoetida, salt, and oil. Simmer covered over low heat for 7 minutes. Dilute kudzu in cold water and add to soup. Stir and serve.

## Black Bean Soup (PC)

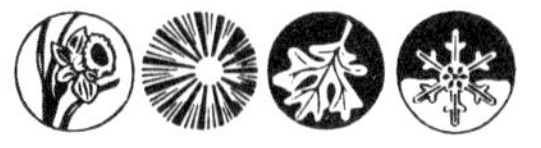

P, PV, PK, K, KV, KP
Serves 2

1 c black beans
2 ears corn, husked
3" piece of kombu seaweed
6 c water
1 c diced summer squash
1/2 c diced onion
1/4 tsp sea salt
1/4 c soy flour
1 tbs ghee
1 tsp coriander powder

*K types: garnish with cayenne pepper or red chili peppers.*

Soak beans in 4 cups water for 1 hour. Rinse and drain. Strip kernels from corn ears. To wash kombu, place in a small bowl and rub gently to remove salt. Place water, beans, stripped corn and cobs, kombu, squash, onion, and salt in a pressure cooker. Cover without locking and bring to a boil. Lock cover and bring to pressure. Cook over medium heat for 50 minutes. Remove from heat and allow pressure to fall naturally. (For conventional cooking, bring ingredients to a boil in 8 cups of water. Cover and cook over medium heat for 2 hours.)

In a cast-iron skillet, toast soy flour until golden. Remove from skillet. Add ghee to skillet and sauté corn kernels and coriander for 5 minutes. Pour into bean soup. Remove corn cobs and kombu. Stir in toasted flour and add water to desired thickness. Simmer for 10 minutes. Using a wooden spoon, mash until soup has consistency of a coarse purée. Serve hot.

## Millet and Corn Soup

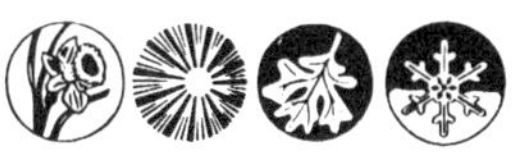

K, KV, KP
Serves 2

4 ears corn, husked
5 c water
1/2 c millet
1 c fresh corn kernels
1/2 c diced carrots
8 finely chopped fresh basil leaves
1/2 tsp coarse black pepper

*Garnish:*
2 scallions, trimmed and sliced

Strip kernels from corn ears. Boil stripped corn cobs in water for 10 minutes, then discard cobs. Wash millet and toast in skillet until dry. Add millet, corn kernels, carrots, basil, and black pepper to corn water. Cover and simmer over medium heat for 40 minutes. Garnish with fresh scallions.

## Millet and Squash Soup

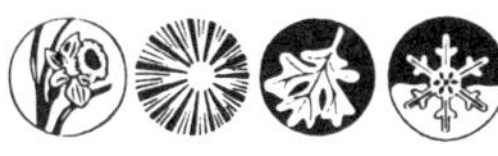

ALL TYPES
Serves 2

1 buttercup squash
1 c millet
6 c water
1/2 c diced onion
1/4 tsp sea salt
1/2 tsp coarse black pepper
1 tsp finely chopped fresh tarragon

Scrub squash; core and cut into 1" cubes. In a large pot, add millet and squash to water and bring to boil. Add onion, salt, pepper, and tarragon. Cover and cook over medium heat for 45 minutes. Serve hot.

## Barley and Squash Soup (variation 1)

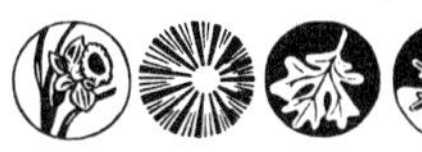

V, VK, K, KV
Serves 2

1/2 c pearl barley
1/2 c toor dhal
1 c diced crookneck squash
6 c water
2 chopped scallions
1 tsp cumin powder
1/4 tsp turmeric
1/4 tsp cayenne pepper
Pinch of asafoetida
Pinch of sea salt

In a large pot, bring barley, dhal, and squash to boil in water. Add scallions, spices, and salt. Cover and simmer over medium heat for 45 minutes. Using a wooden spoon, mash until soup has consistency of a coarse purée; serve hot.

## Barley and Squash Soup (variation 2)

V, VP, P, PV
Serves 2

1/2 c hulled barley
2 c water
1 small butternut squash
1/2 c diced onion
Pinch of salt
1 tsp ground coriander
4 curry leaves, preferably fresh
1/4 tsp turmeric
1 tsp ghee

*Garnish:*
2 sprigs finely minced cilantro

Soak barley for 1/2 hour in water. Scrub squash; core and cut into 1" cubes. Pour soaked barley (with water), squash, and onion into a large pot and bring to boil. Add salt, coriander, curry leaves, and turmeric. Cover and simmer over medium heat for 55 minutes. Using a wooden spoon, mash until soup has consistency of a coarse purée; add ghee. Garnish with cilantro and serve.

## Leek and Potato Soup

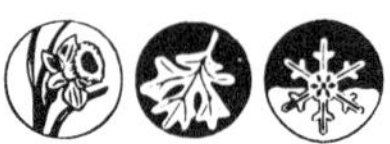

ALL TYPES
Serves 2

2 whole leeks
2 large white potatoes
5 c water
4 sprigs dill
1 tsp curry powder
1/4 c minced onion
1/4 tsp sea salt
1 tsp ghee
1/2 tsp coarse black pepper

*V types: substitute equal amount of parsnips or sweet potatoes for white potatoes.*

Wash leeks well and thinly slice; use both green and white parts. Scrub potatoes and cut into large pieces. Add, with water, to a large pan and bring to boil. Add chopped dill, curry powder, onion, leeks, and salt. Cover and boil over medium heat for 45 minutes. Using a wooden spoon, mash until soup has the consistency of a coarse purée. In a small pan, heat ghee and sauté black pepper until ghee begins to bubble; add to soup. Remove from heat and serve.

## Lima Bean Soup

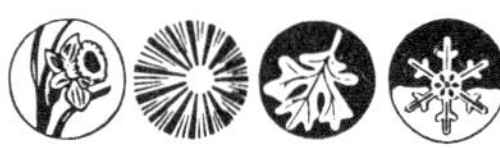

P, PK, K, KV, KP
Serves 2

1 c fresh lima beans
3" piece kombu seaweed
6 c water
1/2 c diced onion
3 sprigs freshly minced dill
1/4 tsp sea salt
1/2 tbs sunflower oil

*Garnish:*
Fresh minced dill

To wash kombu, place in a small bowl of water and rub gently to remove salt. In a large pot, soak lima beans and kombu in 2 cups of the water for 30 minutes. Add remaining water, onion, dill, salt, and oil; cover and cook over medium heat for 45 minutes. Garnish with fresh dill and serve hot.

## Clear Noodle Soup

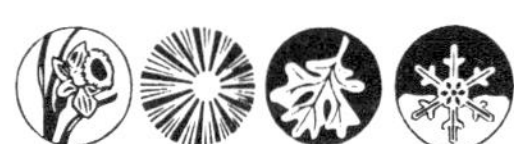

ALL TYPES, OCCASIONALLY
Serves 2

4 oz bijun noodles
1 oz small snow peas
5 c vegetable soup stock (see page 281)
4 c boiling water

Add noodles to boiling water and cook for a few minutes until tender. Drain, reserving noodle water. Boil noodle water and blanch snow peas; drain; discard water. Add noodles and snow peas to warmed soup stock. Cover and simmer for about 5 minutes and serve.

## Leek, Potato, and Barley Soup

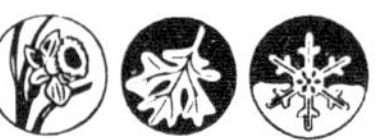

ALL TYPES
V, VP OCCASIONALLY
Serves 2

1 tsp olive oil
1 tsp coriander seeds
1/2 c minced onion
1/2 c pearl barley
6 c water
2 leeks, thinly sliced
3 large white potatoes, diced
3 sprigs finely chopped dill
4 curry leaves, preferably fresh
Pinch of salt

*V types: garnish with roasted black sesame seeds, gomasio, or whole wheat croutons.*
*P types: garnish with cottage cheese and whole wheat croutons.*
*K types: garnish with fresh green chili peppers and rye croutons.*

In a skillet, heat oil and sauté coriander seeds with onion until onion turns golden brown. Remove from skillet. In a large pot, cook barley in water over medium heat for 20 minutes; add leeks, potatoes, and onion/coriander mixture. In onion skillet, sauté dill with curry leaves for 3 minutes. Rinse spice skillet with soup liquid and add to soup, along with salt. Cover skillet and simmer over medium heat for 45 minutes.

## Squash and Seaweed Soup

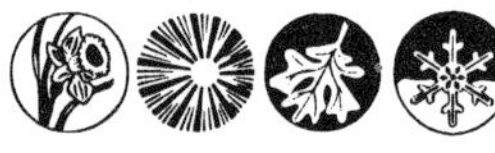

V, VP, VK, K, KV, KP
K TYPES: USE SPARINGLY
Serves 2

1 butternut squash
2 ears corn, husked
1 c diced onions
6 strands seaware seaweed
4 c water
1 tbs chickpea miso
1/4 c water

*Garnish:*
Minced fresh parsley

Scrub squash; core and cut into 1" cubes. Simmer corn ears, onions, and seaweed in water for 10 minutes. Add squash and cook over medium heat for 25 minutes. Dilute miso in 1/4 cup water and add to soup. Simmer for 3 minutes. Garnish with parsley. Serve hot.

## Carrot and Broccoli Soup

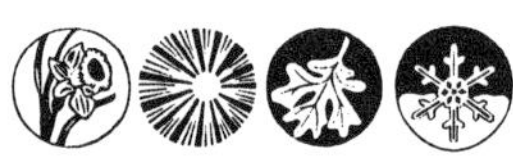

ALL TYPES
Serves 2

6 c water
2 c sliced carrots
1/2 c diced onion
2 c broccoli florets and peeled stem pieces
1/2 tsp grated ginger
1 tsp coriander powder
1/2 tsp sea salt
1 tbs grated orange peel

*Garnish:*
1/4 c minced fresh chives

Bring water to boil. Add carrots, onion, broccoli, ginger, coriander, and salt. Cover and boil over medium heat for 35 minutes. Remove from heat. Add orange peel; garnish with fresh chives.

## Buckwheat Soup

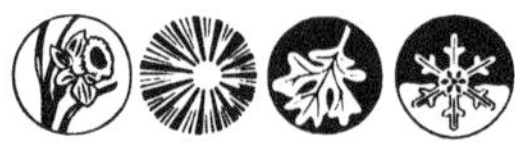

K
Serves 2

2 tsp corn oil
1/2 c diced onion
1/2 c shredded cabbage
1/2 c shredded daikon radish
1/4 c chopped celery
1/2 c buckwheat groats
1/4 tsp caraway seeds
1/4 tsp coarse black pepper
6 c water
Pinch of salt

*Garnish:*
Minced fresh fennel or parsley

In a large pot, heat oil and sauté the vegetables for 7 minutes. Dry-roast groats and caraway seeds in a cast-iron skillet over low heat, stirring constantly until golden. Add with pepper to vegetables. Stir in water and salt. Cover and simmer over low heat for 30 minutes. Serve hot. Garnish with fresh fennel or parsley.

## Vegetable Dumpling Soup

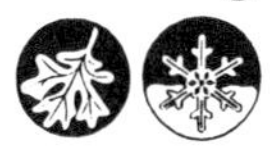

ALL TYPES, OCCASIONALLY
Serves 6

*Dumpling Dough:*
1 c whole wheat pastry flour
1 c unbleached white flour
Pinch of salt
Pinch of natural baking powder
3/4 c ice cold water

Combine dry ingredients; slowly mix in the water.

Knead dough for 10 minutes until tender but firm. Wrap in cotton cloth and chill for 1 1/2 hours. Tear with your fingers into 18 pieces. Roll each piece between your palms into a ball, 3" in diameter. Place a teaspoon of filling in center of each, fold over and fork-press edges together.

*Filling:*
2 tsp light sesame oil
1/2 c shredded carrots
1/4 c minced fresh shiitake mushrooms
1/4 c mung sprouts
1/4 c minced firm tofu
1/2 tsp sea salt
1/2 tsp ginger powder
1/4 tsp coarse black pepper
3 tsp water

In a large skillet, heat oil and add carrots, mushrooms, sprouts, tofu, salt, ginger, and black pepper. Stir in water, cover, and sauté for 5 minutes. Fill dumplings as indicated above. Add, along with vegetables of your choice, to vegetable soup stock (see page 281).

## Sweet Potato and Artichoke Soup

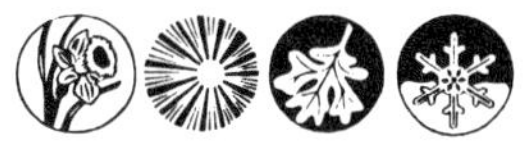

V, VP, VK, P, PV, PK
Serves 2

1 whole globe artichoke
2 sweet potatoes
1 tbs ghee
1 tsp whole black peppercorns
1 minced garlic clove
1 tsp salt
5 c boiling water
1/4 c fresh plain yogurt

*P types: omit garlic.*

Steam artichoke until tender and set aside. Scrub potatoes and dice. Heat ghee in small pan and sauté the peppercorns and garlic until garlic turns golden brown.

Add potatoes to boiling water in a large soup pot. Cover and cook over medium heat for 35 minutes. Using a wooden spoon, mash potatoes until soup has the consistency of a coarse purée. Add sautéed spices and salt. Rinse spice pan with soup water and pour back in to soup. Cover and simmer over low heat for 10 minutes. Peel the artichoke leaves and thinly chip the artichoke heart. Sprinkle the chips into soup and allow to cook for 30 minutes. Pour soup into 2 serving bowls and arrange as many leaves as you can on top to form a mandala. Place a dollup of yogurt in the middle and serve.

## Mung and Buckwheat Soup

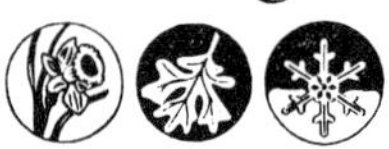

K, KV, KP
Serves 2

1/4 c buckwheat groats
1/2 c whole mung dhal
5 c water
1/2 c diced celery
1/2 c diced onion
1 clove garlic
1/4 tsp turmeric
1/4 tsp cumin
1/2 tsp ground coriander
1/2 tsp chili powder
Pinch of salt
1 tbs mustard oil
1 1/2 tsp mustard seeds

Soak buckwheat groats for 30 minutes, then drain. In a large pot, bring mung and buckwheat to boil in five cups of water. Add celery, onion, garlic, turmeric, cumin, coriander, chili powder, and salt. Cover and simmer over medium heat for 45 minutes. Remove from heat. In a small skillet, heat oil and sauté mustard seeds until they pop; add to soup. Serve hot.

## Mung and Wheat Berry Soup

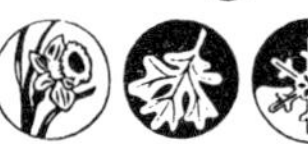

V, VP, P, PV
Serves 2

1/4 c wheat berries
1/2 c whole mung dhal
5 c water
1/2 c diced carrots
1/2 c diced onion
1/4 tsp turmeric
1/4 tsp cumin powder
1/2 tsp coriander powder
1/4 tsp cardamom powder
Pinch of salt
1 tbs avocado oil
1 1/2 tsp dill seeds

Soak wheat berries in 2 cups water for 2 hours. Drain. In a large pot, bring wheat berries and mung dhal to boil in five cups of water. Add carrots, onion, turmeric, cumin, coriander, cardamom, and salt. Cover and simmer for 1 hour. Remove from heat. Heat oil and sauté dill seeds for 3 minutes until dark brown; add to soup. Serve hot.

## Potato and Broccoli Soup

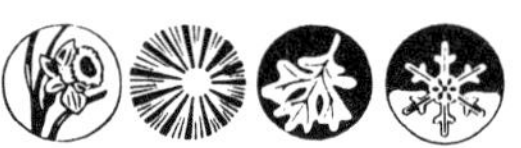

ALL TYPES
Serves 2

4 broccoli stalks with florets
2 large white potatoes
6 c water
1 tbs dried dill
1/2 tsp dried parsley
1/2 tsp sea salt
3 finely chopped scallions
1 tbs canola oil
1 tsp cumin seeds

*V types: garnish with grated natural cheddar cheese.*
*P types: garnish with whole wheat croutons.*
*K types: garnish with rye croutons.*

Cut broccoli florets and peeled stems into small pieces. Scrub potatoes and cut into 1" cubes. Place potatoes and broccoli in water and bring to boil. Add dill, parsley, and salt. Cover and simmer over medium heat for 45 minutes. Add scallions and cook for an additional 10 minutes; remove from heat. In a frying pan, heat oil and sauté cumin seeds for 3 minutes; add to soup.

## Karhi (Yogurt Soup)

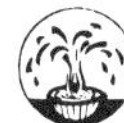

V, VP, VK, P, PV, PK
Serves 2

1 tbs chickpea flour (besan)
1 c fresh plain yogurt
1 c water
1/4 tsp coriander seeds
1 tsp maple syrup
3" stick of cinnamon
1/4 tsp orange rind
1 tsp walnut oil
3 dried curry leaves
1/2 tsp black cumin seeds
Pinch of grated ginger
2 whole cloves

*Garnish:*
Minced fresh parsley

*V, VP, and VK: add 2 dried red chili peppers and 1/8 teaspoon asafoetida.*

Toast chickpea flour in a skillet until golden; set aside. Beat yogurt with an eggbeater until smooth and creamy, and slowly add water. Blend in flour until mixture is smooth and fluid.

Dry-roast coriander seeds in a cast-iron skillet for a few minutes and grind to a very coarse powder. Add to yogurt-flour mixture. Transfer to a saucepan and bring to a boil. With lid ajar, simmer over low heat for 5 minutes. Add maple syrup, cinnamon, and orange rind. Cover and simmer an additional 4 minutes.

In a small skillet, heat oil and roast curry leaves, cumin seeds, and ginger until curry leaves crackle. Pour into soup, add cloves, and cover. Remove from heat and allow to sit for 7 minutes before serving. Garnish with fresh parsley.

## Lima and Cauliflower Soup (PC)

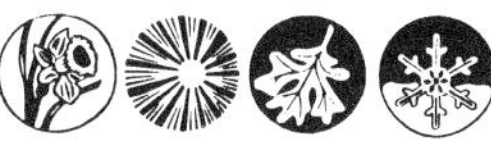

P, PK, K, KV, KP
Serves 4

1/2 c fresh lima beans
6 c water
1 c cauliflower, florets and stems
2 tsp dill powder
1/2 tsp coarse black pepper
Pinch of salt
1/2 tsp ghee

*P types: garnish with fresh cilantro or minced fresh dill.*

*K types: garnish with cayenne pepper and parsley.*

Combine beans and water in a pressure cooker. Cover without locking and bring to a boil. Lock cover and bring to pressure. Simmer over medium heat for 15 minutes. Remove from heat and allow pressure to fall naturally. (For conventional cooking, bring beans to a boil in 8 cups of water. Cover and cook over medium heat for 1 1/2 hours.) Add cauliflower, spices, and ghee. Cover without locking lid and simmer for 25 minutes. Garnish with fresh dill.

# SUMMER ASPICS

## Corn and Red Pepper Aspic

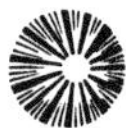

ALL TYPES
Serves 2

4 ears corn, husked
3 c water
Pinch of sea salt
1/4 c agar-agar
1/4 tsp fine black pepper
1 finely diced red bell pepper

Strip kernels from corn ears. In a medium pot, add water, stripped cobs, salt, and agar-agar and boil, covered, for 15 minutes. Add corn kernels, pepper, and diced bell pepper during the last 3 minutes. Pour into mold and refrigerate until mixture sets. Serve with steamed greens.

## Carrot and Cucumber Aspic

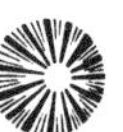

ALL TYPES
Serves 2

3 medium carrots
2 cucumbers
3 c water
1/4 c agar-agar
1/4 tsp ground cardamom
1/4 tsp fine black pepper
1/4 tsp sea salt

Scrub and dice carrots. Peel cucumbers and cut in half lengthwise; remove seeds with a spoon and dice. In a medium pan, add water and boil carrots for 10 minutes. Add agar-agar, spices, and salt. Continue boiling for an additional 5 minutes; remove from heat and add cucumber. Pour into mold and refrigerate until mixture sets. Remove and serve with appropriate grain salad.

## Squash and Onion Aspic

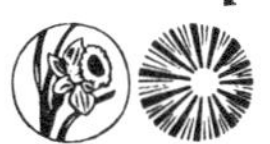

ALL TYPES
Serves 2

1 butternut squash
3 c water
1 large white onion
1/4 tsp fresh ginger juice (see page 194)
1 tbs freshly minced mint
1/2 tsp cardamom powder
1/2 tsp coriander powder
1/2 tsp coarse black pepper
1/2 tbs coconut oil
1/4 c agar-agar
*K types: use occasionally.*

Wash, core, and cut squash into large pieces. In a medium pot, add water and boil over medium heat for 15 minutes. Reserve squash water and remove skins from squash. Cut the onion in lengthwise slices and combine with squash, ginger juice, herbs, spices, and oil. Purée mixture, adding in the warm squash water. Return to pot with agar-agar and heat for 10 minutes. Pour into mold and refrigerate until mixture sets. Serve with sautéed watercress.

## Red Cabbage and Pepper Aspic

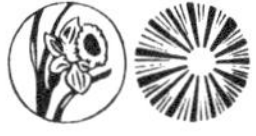

K, KV, KP
Serves 4

1/2 medium red cabbage
1 green bell pepper
1 white onion
1 small daikon
1/4 tsp chili powder
1/4 tsp curry powder
Pinch of salt
3 c water
1/4 c agar-agar

Shred cabbage, pepper, onion, and daikon. Add spices and salt and sauté with 8 tablespoons of water for 3 minutes. Add remaining water and agar-agar; simmer over low heat for 10 minutes. Pour into mold and refrigerate until mixture sets. Serve with a warm millet salad.

## Cherry, Lettuce, and Cucumber Aspic

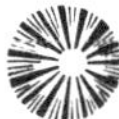

V, VP, P, PV
Serves 2

1 c fresh ripe cherries
1/2 head lettuce
1 cucumber
1 c cherry juice
1 tsp mirin
1/4 tsp ground clove
Pinch of salt
2 c water
1/4 c agar-agar

Remove seeds from cherries, leaving them whole. Shred lettuce. Peel cucumber and shred. In a large saucepan, add cherry juice, mirin, ground clove, and salt and boil for a few minutes. Add agar-agar and water; cover and simmer over medium heat for 10 minutes. Add lettuce, cucumber, and cherries. Remove from heat and allow to sit for 5 minutes. Pour into mold. Refrigerate until mixture sets. Serve with sautéed asparagus.

# SEAWEED DISHES

Seaweeds have been a part of the diet in China and Japan as far back as the sixth century. Mention of nori, wakame, miru, and koru moha (agar-agar) can be found in eighth century Japanese literature. Japan uses more seaweeds than most other countries combined.

The Chinese character ZAO refers to all plants growing in the sea. Translated, it means "that which is in water under the sound of the chirping birds." Seaweeds are man's primal connection to the waters of the earth. They contain photosynthetic pigments and are richly packed with nutritious minerals. Seaweeds contain complex carbohydrates, called polysaccharides, that selectively absorb the inorganic substances from the sea water. These polysaccharides cannot be digested by the enzyme a-amylase, which means seaweeds are also calorie-free in the human system. Minerals account for 10 to 38 percent of their dry weight. They are fortified with calcium, sodium, magnesium, potassium, phosphorus, iodine, iron, zinc, and trace elements. The calcium ratio of seaweeds is second only to that of milk. Seaweeds contain ten times the iron of spinach and egg yolks, as well as chlorophyll and carotenoid. The amino acid composition of seaweeds is similar to that of beans. They contain more Vitamin A, B, $B_2$, $B_6$, $B_{12}$, C, pantothenic acid, folic acid, and niacin than fresh fruits and vegetables.

Within their own environment seaweeds are odorless. Their strong fishy scent is due to the volatile element that decomposes when the weeds are out of their element. Because of their unappealing dark green color (which appears black), their strong smell, and our lack of familiarity with them, seaweeds are often regarded as a strange and unimportant source of food. They are, however, destined to become one of our most important replenishing food sources of the future, as our earth continues to disintegrate from carelessness and abuse.

While much research remains to be done into the curative potential of seaweeds, it has already been established that they are a great natural antibiotic, blood anticoagulant, and tumor preventive. Irish moss is used for respiratory disorders; green algae is used for stomach disease and hemorrhoids; undaria is used for cleansing the blood of a new mother; lamanaria is used in the bath reducing hypertension.

Once our mental obstacles are removed and we learn how to prepare seaweeds, we will find them to be a delicious addition to wholesome meals. Because seaweeds are high in sodium, Kapha and Pitta types will want to thoroughly soak and wash them before cooking. They should be used only occasionally, not daily, by these types. Vata types benefit the most from these nurturing underwater foods.

## Wakame and Bamboo Shoot Soup

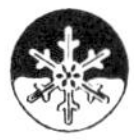

ALL TYPES, OCCASIONALLY
Serves 6

**8 oz wakame seaweed, soaked**
**4 oz bamboo shoots**
**8 c vegetable soup stock (see page 281)**
**5 sansho leaves**
**1 tsp tamari**
**1/2 tsp sea salt**

*P and K types: omit salt.*

Thoroughly wash and soak the wakame and bamboo shoots in water to cover for 10 minutes. In a large pot, boil the vegetable stock. Add seaweed to boiling stock water. Cover and simmer for 30 minutes. Add sansho leaves, tamari, and sea salt. Simmer for 5 minutes. Serve over thin rice noodles or clear noodles.

## Wakame Salad

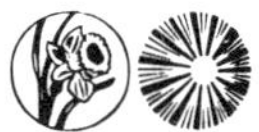

ALL TYPES, OCCASIONALLY
Serves 2

**2 oz wakame seaweed**
**4 red radishes**
**1 small Belgian endive**
**2 medium cucumbers**

Soak wakame in 3 cups cold water for 30 minutes; slice thinly. Slice radishes, endive, and cucumbers thinly. Toss together in a big wooden bowl and serve with the following dressing.

**Orange Rind Dressing:**
**1 tsp olive oil**
**1/4 tsp orange rind**
**1/2 c orange juice**
**1/2 tsp mirin**
**1 tsp rice vinegar**
**1/4 tsp coarse black pepper**

Shake all ingredients together in a bottle and pour over Wakame Salad.

## Rice and Wakame

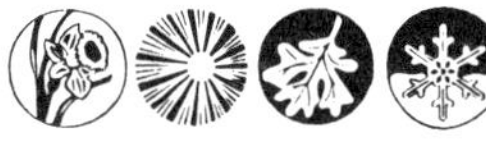

V, VP, VK, PV
Serves 6

**2 c medium-grain brown rice**
**3 1/2 c water**
**1 tbs sake**
**1/2 c diced carrots**
**1/2 tsp sea salt**
**1 oz wakame seaweed**

Rinse rice until water runs clear. In a heavy pan, add rice to water and boil for 15 minutes. Add sake, carrots, and salt. Cover and simmer for an additional 15 minutes. Toast dried wakame in a cast-iron skillet and crumble over cooked rice.

## Oden

*A traditional Japanese stew of vegetable roots, pan-fried tofu, and kombu cooked in a* mabe, *a Japanese-style clay pot.*

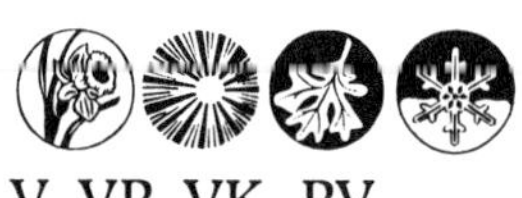

V, VP, VK, PV
Serves 2

2 strips kombu seaweed
1 c water
6 slices semi-firm tofu, 1/2" thick
1 tbs sesame oil
4 fresh shiitake mushrooms
1 tsp tamari
*Garnish:*
Fresh grated daikon

Soak kombu in a small bowl of water for 20 minutes. Rub gently to remove salt. Cut kombu lengthwise into 1/2" strips and tie into bows. Bring water to boil in a large pot. Lightly pan-fry tofu slices. Place kombu bows, tofu, oil, and mushrooms in separate areas of boiling water in the pot. Cover and simmer over medium heat for 15 minutes. Add tamari. Remove from heat and allow to sit for 5 minutes. Garnish with daikon radish. This dish is best cooked in a clay pot.

### TEMPURA

Tempura are deep-fried batter-dipped vegetables. A variety of vegetables may be used, such as broccoli, winter squash, and cauliflower. Once vegetables are cut into small, bite-sized pieces, dip them in the batter (recipe below) and deep-fry as follows. Pour a 1/4 cup of corn oil into a thin, 6" stainless-steel pan. Heat oil until hot but not smoking. Lower heat slightly as you begin to add vegetables. Fry a few pieces at a time for 3 minutes or until crisp and golden. When done, place in colander, lined with two pieces of cheesecloth, over the sink.

## Tempura Batter

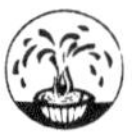

V, VP, VK, P
K, KP, KV RARELY
Serves 4

1/8 c soy flour
1/8 c unbleached white flour
Pinch of salt
Pinch of turmeric
2 tbs aloe vera gel
1/4 c water

Mix flours together with salt, turmeric, and gel. Add enough of the water to make a thin paste.

## Arame and Carrot "Tempura"

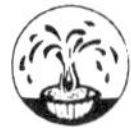

ALL TYPES
Serves 4

1 c arame seaweed
1 c carrots, cut into matchsticks
1 tbs sunflower oil
Garnish: fresh grated daikon

Wash arame by passing under cold water and combine with carrots. Mix into tempura batter (see recipe above). In cast-iron skillet, heat oil until it is hot but not smoking. Add spoonfuls of batter/vegetable mixture to the oil and, using a flat wooden ladle, press down on each patty. Brown on both sides. Remove with a slotted spoon and drain in a cheesecloth-lined colander. Garnish with fresh grated daikon and serve.

*Other combinations:*
P, PK, K, KP: arame/shredded cabbage
All types: arame/zucchini (cut into matchsticks); arame/sprouts/sliced onions

# VEDIC HERBS, SPICES, AND ACCENTS

### *Ajwan seed*

Bishop's weed. A relative of the caraway and cumin seed, ajwan resembles the minute celery seeds, and has the flavor of thyme. It is to be used mostly by Vata and Kapha types.

### *Amchoor*

A powder made from sun-dried slices of unripe mango. It has a pungent flavor and is often used like pomegranate seeds or lime juice in North Indian cuisine. It is to be used mostly by Vata types.

### *Ancho chili pepper*

This pod of the poblano chili is sun-dried to dark brown and used in the fried spice seasonings of curries and dhals. All chilis are good for Kapha types and occasionally for Vata types.

### *Asafoetida*

Also known as *hing* or *hingu*, asafoetida is a highly pungent dried gum resin obtained from the *ferula* plant. It is used in Ayurvedic medicine as well as in South Indian cuisine. Ayurvedic pharmacologists give it to breast-feeding mothers to cleanse and increase milk. This resin is used sparingly in foods for Vata and Kapha types.

### *Bala*

The Sanskrit name for an Ayurvedic herb that is cooling and sweet in nature. It is used mainly as a rejuvenating tonic for nervous conditions by both Vata and Pitta types. Available from Ayurvedic Resources and Supplies (see page 336).

### *Basil*

*Tulsi.* Two varieties of basil, one with purple-brownish leaves and the other with green leaves, are used for worshipping of Lord Krishna and Rama throughout India. The flowers and leaves of both varieties of this divine herb are used extensively in religious ceremonies. The camphor basil, known as *karpoor,* is the only basil used for Indian cooking. This herb is to be used mostly by Vata and Kapha types.

### Bay leaves

Sweet Laurel. This leaf resembles the cassia leaf, which is used in the cuisine of Bengal and the eastern regions of India. Bay leaves are highly aromatic and pungent, and should be used sparingly. This leaf is for Vata and Kapha use.

### Bhringaraja

The Sanskrit name for an Ayurvedic herb that is bitter, astringent, sweet, and cooling in nature. It is used as a rejuvenating tonic by all body types. Available from Ayurvedic Resources and Supplies (see page 336).

### Bibhitaki

The Sanskrit name for an Ayurvedic herb that is astringent, sweet, and heating in nature. It is used as a mild laxative and rejuvenating tonic for Kapha and Pitta types. Available from Ayurvedic Resources and Supplies (see page 336).

### Black cumin

*Shahi jeera* or royal cumin. Often called *kala jeera.* Black cumin grows abundantly as a wild annual of the Himalayas. The seed is black, slender, and is closely related to the common cumin seed. This cumin is used mostly in the Kashmir, Punjab, and Uttar Pradesh regions. This glorious seed may be used by all three doshas.

### Black salt

*Kala namak.* This is a dark crimson–grey salt that has a strong and pungent flavor. It is high in trace minerals and iron and is found almost exclusively in India. This salt is to be used mostly by Vata types and occasionally by Kapha types.

### Camphor

*Kacha karpoor.* This edible crystalline compound is obtained by distillation of the fragrant leaves of the Indian and Chinese evergreen. Very tiny pieces of this raw and natural camphor are used to flavor milk beverages, puddings, and sweets in the eastern regions of India. This crystal is also used in Ayurvedic medicine in Kapha remedies.

### Caraway

This aromatic seed grows on the wild *carum carvi* plant in the foothills of the Himalayas. In India, it is used predominantly in the Kashmir region. While best for Vata and Kapha use, it may be used occasionally by Pitta.

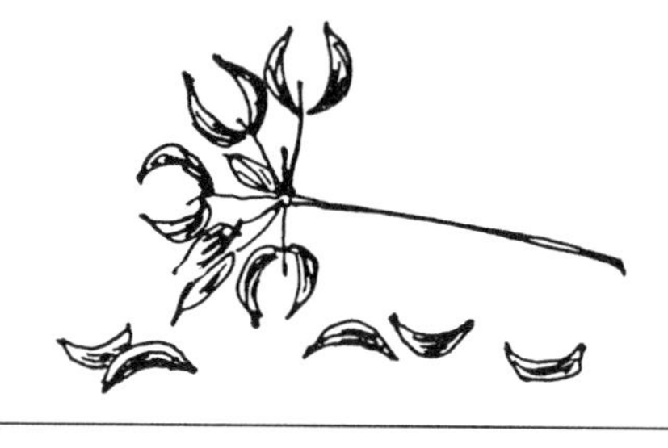

**Caraway**

### Cardamom

*Ela.* The cardamom plant is native to South India. The black seeds are encased in either small green pods or large black pods. The green pods are high in volatile oils, with a taste that resembles eucalyptus. The seeds of the green pods are mostly used in beverages, sweets, and pilafs. Cardamom has been used for centuries in Ayurvedic medicine. This seed is best for Vata and Kapha, but may be used occasionally by Pitta due to its aromatic flavor.

### Cassia leaves

*Tejpatta.* Native to Sri Lanka and South India, these 7"-long sun-dried leaves are olive green color. They are pungent in nature and are used as a fried herb seasoning in India's eastern regional cooking. They may be used by Vata and Kapha types.

### Cayenne peppers

*Puissi lal mirch.* These are red hot chilis sun-dried and ground into a highly potent powder. India exports great quantities of cayenne. It is used in Ayurvedic medicine to reduce phlegm and inflammation in the Kapha dosha.

## Charoli seed

*Chironji.* These large seeds, which have an almond flavor, are toasted and frequently substituted for almonds in many Indian desserts. These are best for Vata and, on occasion, for Kapha types.

## Chili Peppers

There are hundreds of varieties of red and green chili peppers from various capsicum plants. The heat and intense taste are mostly held in the seeds. The smaller the chili, the hotter it is; the large bell-shaped peppers are not very pungent. Chilis have been used even before the Vedic period in India. They are a mainstay of the Vedic kitchen. India has a large number of Kapha- and Vata-type people, which explains in part the use of so many heating and stimulating spices by this culture.

## Cilantro

See Coriander Leaves.

## Cinnamon

*Twak* or *dalchini.* Cinnamon, the dried bark of the *cinnamomum cassia* tree, is native to South India. Both the bark and the cassia leaves are used extensively in South Indian cooking. The cassia cinnamon is more pungent with a thicker stick than the thinner bark found in the West. Cinnamon is another essential ingredient in Ayurvedic remedy. It is good for Kapha and Vata because of its heating energy. Pitta may use it occasionally.

## Cloves

*Lasuna* or *laung.* Cloves are the small pointed dried buds of the evergreen tree. They contain the antiseptic volatile clove oil and are used in small amount as a ground spice in masala. Cloves are used extensively in Ayurvedic pharmacology. They are good for Vata and Kapha types.

## Colocasia leaf

Elephant ears, *arbi patta.* These plant leaves are blanched and used to wrap various kinds of stuffing. They are excellent for all three doshas.

## Coriander leaves

Cilantro, *har dhania.* This fragrant and cooling herb is grown profusely in South America, India, and most tropical climates. It is used predominantly in the Gujarat, Punjab, Rajasthan, and Maharastra regions of India. The cooling energy of cilantro is used to reduce high Pitta conditions, and the cilantro juice is used to neutralize the poisons of snake bites and insect stings. These leaves are good for all three doshas.

## Coriander seeds

*Dhania.* These round, light seeds are used extensively in Ayurvedic pharmacology and Vedic cooking. They are slowly roasted and powdered or crushed into a variety of masalas. Sweet and cooling in nature, they are the primary spice for Pitta types. Coriander seeds are good for all three doshas.

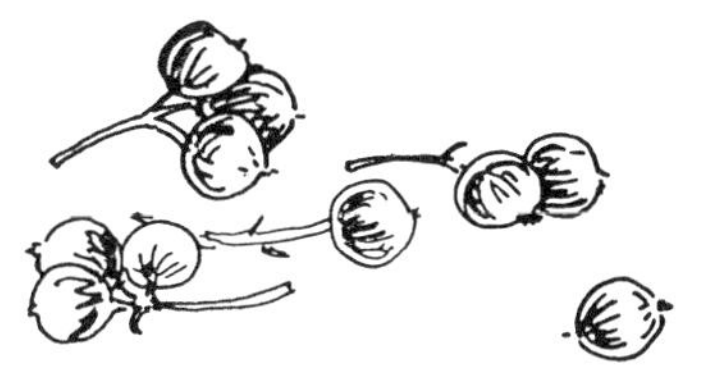

**Coriander**

## Cumin

*Jeera* or *safed jeera.* This ancient spice is a relative of caraway. Its golden aromatic seeds are used in cooking throughout India. They are dry-roasted and either ground into powder or coarsely crushed for vegetable dishes and dhals. They are also used as an accent in kichadi, a dish that forms part of a cleansing diet in Ayurveda. Like coriander seeds, the energy of cumin is suitable to all three doshas.

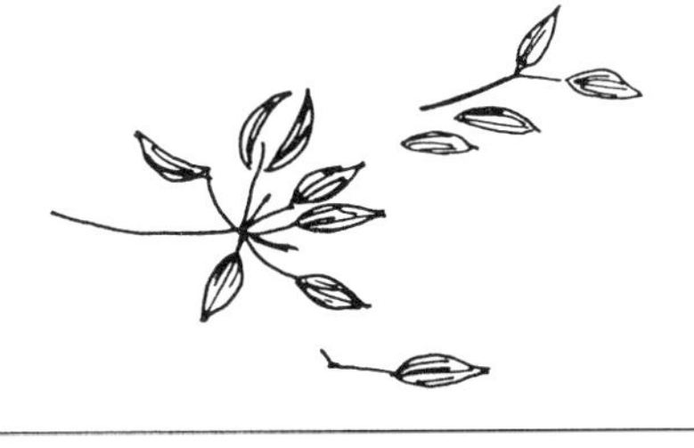

**Cumin**

## *Curry leaves*

*Neem, meetha neem,* or *kadhi patta.* Curry leaves have a highly fragrant scent with a slight touch of citrus. They look like a tiny version of the lemon leaf. Curry leaves have been used since Vedic times and are grown profusely throughout India. Due to their extensive presence in the *kari* dishes of South India, most Indian sauces became known as curries. They are a main ingredient in curry powders, even though many are made without them. Fresh neem juice, which is extremely bitter, is administered to diabetics and to persons with high Pitta conditions. It is also used for weight reduction. The neem leaf has a multitude of uses. The twigs have been used as toothbrushes to prevent tooth and gum decay. They are also used in companion planting as a natural pesticide.

## *Curry powder*

Curry powder is a truly exotic blend of some of India's finest spices. It can be either mild or hair-raisingly hot. While the most well-known curry powder comes from Madras, the elders in Guyana once made the most superb curry masala I have ever tasted. Generally, a curry masala is made from fresh curry leaves (or dried), cumin seeds, mustard seeds, fenugreek seeds, black peppercorn, chili peppers, coriander, and turmeric. This powder is best for Kapha types; Vata types may use occasionally, and Pitta types rarely.

## *Fennel seed*

*Saunf.* The fennel plant is similar to the dill plant; both the leaves and the seeds are used in cooking. Fennel is delicate and fragrant. The bulb and the stalks are valued for their post-digestive qualities. The seeds are similar in appearance to cumin and close in taste to the anise seed. The roasted seeds are ground in masalas or used as a breath refresher after meals, and as a digesting aid. Fennel seeds are excellent for the Pitta constitution and have been used in Ayurvedic pharmacology for thousands of years. It is an excellent seed for all three doshas.

## *Fenugreek leaf*

*Methi sak.* This leaf has a strong and unusual scent, and a densely bitter and pungent taste. Its energy, when added to vegetables, dhals, and other dishes, is very pervasive. It is a good stimulant for Kapha types, but too pungent for Pitta and too bitter for Vata. These leaves are used either fresh or sun-dried.

## *Fenugreek seed*

*Methi.* This seed is more like a small bean than a seed. It has a golden yellow color and has an odd shape. Generally methi is dried and moderately roasted before use. Like the leaves, the fenugreek seeds are also bitter; they are used mainly in pickles, dhals, and masalas.

The fenugreek seed is also used in Ayurvedic pharmacology to promote hair growth. For this purpose, the seeds are soaked overnight and mashed by hand into a paste. This paste is massaged into the scalp and kept on the hair for 30 to 45 minutes before rinsing. The hair is left gleaming with subtle oils. Fenugreek seed is good for Kapha types, although Vata may use occasionally. All types may use externally.

## *Ginger root*

*Sunthi.* This rhizome has been used in both Ayurvedic and Chinese medicine for over five thousand years. Native to Asia, ginger is widely used throughout Indian cuisine. Ginger has heating, cleansing, toning, and stimulating properties. It is used for a multitude of health purposes, such as digestive problems, muscular pains, and constipation. Hundreds of varieties, from the small green type to the delicate shell-pink ginger, are available in the spring in India. Many fresh chutneys and condiments are made with ginger. It is also used in various curries, dhals, and vegetable dishes. It is best for Vata and Kapha types, although Pitta may use occasionally. All types may use it externally.

## *Green mango*

*Kacha aam.* The young green mango is peeled and grated and used in many dhals, chutneys, and veg-

etable dishes in India. It is an excellent mango for pickling. It may be used in moderation for all three doshas.

### Horseradish root

This root is used moderately in areas such as Bengal and Orissa for its cooling qualities. It is best for Kapha types and may be used occasionally by Vata types.

### Lotus seeds

*Makhana.* Several varieties of lotus and water lilies exist in India. In summer the lotus stems, leaves, and pods are harvested along with water chestnuts and the fruits of the water bamboo. The lotus seeds are removed from the pods, peeled, dried, and then roasted in hot beach sand until they pop and become light and fluffy. This is a great delicacy in India. The dried seeds are pressured cooked with rice in Japan and are also used in soups. These seeds are good for Vata and Pitta types and for occasional use by Kapha types.

### Lotus roots

*Bhain, kamal.* These roots are native to the Kashmir region of India and also to China and Japan. The lotus flower, the most auspicious flower in the Hindu culture, symbolizes purity in yoga. The flowers are white, blue, and pink, and the stamens are used for tea by the yogis. The roots resemble the heart. When cross-cut, their open chambers resemble a chakra. They are used as a vegetable in North Indian cuisine. The dried roots are an important medicine in Ayurvedic pharmacology. They are used for Pitta and Vata conditions.

### Mace

*Javitri.* This fibrous covering of the nutmeg fruit can be dried, roasted, and ground into a masala with other spices, or used to flavor sauces. Since the fibers of mace do not dissolve, they are removed before the sauce is served. Mace is good for Vata and Kapha types, and for occasional use by Pitta types (infused in milk).

### Mint leaves

*Pudina.* Mint leaves are widely used in India. There are several varieties grown worldwide. While excellent in rice, dhals, and vegetable dishes, they are superb in mint chutneys. Most mints can be used by all three doshas.

### Mugwort

Pungent, bitter, and heating in nature, this herb is grown domestically and used to promote the removal of bodily wastes such as sweat and menstrual fluid. It is recommended for Vata and Kapha types.

### Nigella seeds

*Kalonji.* This tear-shaped black seed is incorrectly called a black onion seed. Aromatic and peppery, it is used in masalas and pickles in India. Kalonji is good for Vata and Kapha types and for occasional use by Pitta types.

### Nutmeg

*Jatiphala, jaiphal.* This sleep-inducing nut is found in the center of the fruit of the evergreen tree. The nut should be grated fresh. It is used in many milk beverages and in masala in Indian cuisine.

Nutmeg is excellent to induce sleep and relaxation for Vata types. It may also be used by Kapha types.

### Paprika

*Deghi mirch.* These mild chilis are grown in the Kashmir region of India. They are used for their mild pungency and red and orange colors in food. They are good for Vata and Kapha types, and may be used occasionally by Pitta.

### Peppercorn

*Marica, kali mirch.* Grown in profusion along the world's oldest spice shores, the Malabar Coast, and throughout the southwest regions of India. There are notably three colors: black, white *(safed mirch)*, and green. Peppercorns, used in a great variety of foods, are the dried berries of a vine. Harvested unripe and sun-dried, they are ground, crushed, or used whole. Great for digestive stimulation, peppercorns are one of the three heating spices used in the ancient Ayurvedic formula called *trikatu.* The other two ingredients are ginger and pippali. This pepper is excellent for Vata and Kapha types, and may be used occasionally by Pitta types.

## Poppy seeds

*Khas khas, pusta.* These tiny, off-white seeds of the poppy plant are used ground, wet-ground, or whole in many vegetable dishes. They have a high oil content like most seeds and lend a nutty flavor to foods. Both the cream and blue poppy seeds are available in the United States. Poppy seeds may be used by all three doshas.

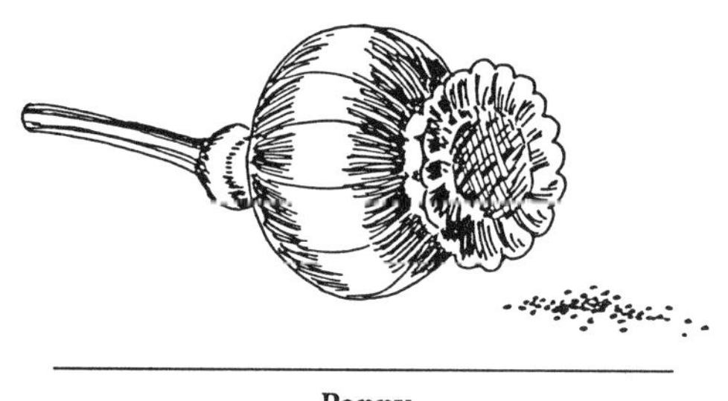

**Poppy**

## Rock salt

*Sendha namak.* A salt mined in its crystalline form from the underground dry sea beds. Recommended by Ayurveda for use with cooking foods, rock salt has the highest mineral content of any salt. Cooling in energy, it has an unusual oxidizing property not present in sea salt. Even when salt is prohibited in a diet, a certain quantity of rock salt is permitted by Ayurveda. Rock salt is good for all types; it is best for Vata, and for occasional use by Pitta and Kapha types.

## Saffron

*Kesar.* These stigmas of the saffron crocus have been cultivated in Asia Minor, India, China, and the Mediterranean. The deep carmine strands are very expensive and provide a sattvic accent to food. Saffron is used in many milky desserts to add a perfumed sweetness, and in Indian basmati rice dishes. The best saffron strands are available from Kashmir and Spain. It is excellent for Pitta, but may be used by all types.

## Sarsaparilla

This bitter, sweet, and cooling herb is grown domestically and is used as a mild diuretic and blood purifier by both Pitta and Kapha types.

## Sassafras

This pungent and heating herb is grown domestically and used as a mild blood cleanser and stimulant. It is good for both Kapha and Vata types.

## Sesame seeds

*Til.* These tiny, tear-shaped seeds come in black and ivory. Found in the pods of the sesame plant, these seeds are fragrant and rich in oil and protein. Once washed and roasted, they are ground or used whole in dhal, rice, and milk. Sesame seeds are very often used in religious ceremonies. The black seeds are generally used in ceremonies for the deceased and are not often used for cooking in India. Sesame oil is used extensively in the Ayurvedic massage therapies. These seeds are good for Vata types.

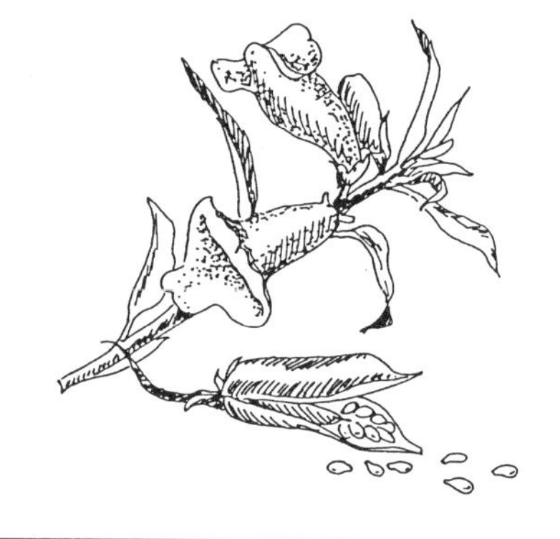

**Sesame**

## Tamarind

*Imli.* The tamarind tree is native to India. Its pulpy, podded fruit is used for its sour and fruity taste, and for its somewhat cooling effect in the hot weather. Found throughout India in dhals, vegetables, and rice, tamarind is also used to make confectionery. It is excellent for Vata types and may be taken occasionally by Pitta types.

### Turmeric

*Haldi.* Native to Southeast Asia and South India, this rhizome, like ginger, may be used dried or fresh. The roots are boiled, sun-dried for several weeks, and then ground. Turmeric is used in many masalas, curries, dhals, rice, vegetable dishes, and desserts in India. Although bitter, it is considered by Ayurveda to be good for all three doshas.

### Varak

Varak refers to the exquisite soft filigree foil sheets of gold and silver used in India since ancient time. These sheets are slivered and used to adorn various foods. This custom was derived from the Ayurvedic tradition of using precious metals and pieces of pearl and conch shell in *bhasma* (medicinal ash). The sheets are made by molding pure metal dust between parchment sheets, then hammering them until the dust sets into a foil. Gold varak may be used by Vata and Kapha types and silver by Pitta types.

### Wild pomegranate seeds

*Daru, anardana.* Grown in the foothills of the Himalayas, the daru fruit is not edible; only the seeds are used. Dried, roasted, and ground or used whole, the seed lends a sour taste to vegetables, soups, and dhals. This is an especially suitable spice for Vata types. Wild pomegranate seeds have been used in Ayurvedic medicine as far back as the Vedic period.

## VEDIC ESSENCES

Essences, called *ruh* in India, are concentrated flavorings extracted from herbs, spices, fruits, flowers, root, bark, wood, and tree leaves. They are used in foods to induce the body's natural aroma, in the form of remembering the cosmic nature of our beings. Fragrant scents and delightful tastes are both important forms of therapy in Ayurveda. Aromatic oils and essences invoke our sattvic nature.

Essences were in use even before the Vedic period. They are made by a water distillation process and extracted without the use of chemicals or alcohols. The most popular essences in Vedic cooking are from rose petals, vetiveri's roots, screw pine flowers, and sandalwood. Essences are used in the sweet brews, beverages, puddings, and desserts of India. Essences and essential oils are added to foods after the foods have been removed from the fire.

### Khus essence

*Khas khas.* Khus essence is extracted from the roots of vetiver grass, grown in tropical climates throughout the world. The roots are used for making hand fans. The essence of khus grass is sweet and cooling. Khus oil has a strong, deep aroma like that of a forest. This essence is good for all three doshas.

### Sandalwood essence

*Ruh chandan.* The wood is known as *chandan* and the oil as *chandan tel.* Sandalwood is native to India and grows in Tamil Nadu and Mysore. This most exquisite wood has been used to carve deities and build temples. The chandan paste is used in Hindu ceremonies and worn on the forehead as a constant reminder of our true nature. A cooling paste, powder, oil, or essence, sandalwood is used in Ayurvedic pharmacology and aromatherapy. It is also used in small amounts in Vedic cooking. The oil is mixed in a syrup and administered as a revitalizer.

Sandalwood paste can be made by taking a piece of sandalwood and rubbing it on a flat stone. Add a few drops of water to allow a paste to form. This essence is excellent for all three doshas.

### Screw pine essence

*Ruh kewra.* This essence comes from the screw pine trees, which grow mostly in South India. The screw pine bears beautiful perfumed flowers and sweet fruits. *Ruh kewra* is good for Vata and Kapha and for occasional use by Pitta.

### *Rose essence*

*Ruh gulab.* Rose essence is extracted from the petals of the rose; rose water, or *kewra,* is extracted through a process of infusion and distillation. The rose oil, essence, and water are used throughout India to accent sweet beverages. The rose essence and oil are used in Ayurveda's aromatherapy. Rose essence is excellent for both Vata and Pitta types.

## MASALAS AND CONDIMENTS

A masala is a combination of spices that have been ground and melded together. The spices are frequently dry-roasted before grinding. Spices begin to yield their potency and healing characteristics as soon as they are ground; after a certain time, only the shell of the spice remains—the body of flavor and energy evaporate with exposure to the elements. Practice grinding your masalas once a week for the following week's cooking needs and store in well-sealed jars in a cool place. Unique to all cultures, condiments are pungent, salty, sour, or sweet food items, taken in small quantities, that invigorate the taste buds and give excitement to a meal. Masalas and condiments are to be made fresh every fortnight.

## Garam Masala

***Every state in India has its own variation of garam masala. Peppercorn, nutmeg, ginger, sesame seeds, mace, cassia leaves, mustard seeds, and grated coconut may also be used in a variety of these masalas.***

ALL TYPES

*North Indian Style:*
1/4 c coriander seeds
1/2 c cumin seeds
1/8 c whole cloves
2 to 4 cinnamon sticks, 2" long
1/4 c green cardamom pods

***V and K types: use any combination of the above mentioned spices.***
***P types: substitute cumin, coriander, fennel, roasted coconut, saffron, and neem leaves for the cardamon; reduce cinnamon to one 2" stick.***

In a heavy cast-iron skillet, dry-roast the seeds, cloves, and cinnamon over medium-low heat for 10 minutes. Tap the cardamom pods to release the seeds (discard the pods). Using a grinding stone as a mallet, pound the cardamom seeds and roasted cinnamon sticks into small bits on a grinding stone. Combine the sticks and cardamom seeds and, using a hand spice grinder or a suribachi, grind into a fine powder. Store the masala in an airtight jar in a cool place.

*South Indian Style:*
1 c cumin seeds
1/4 c coriander seeds
1/2 tsp ajwan seeds
4 black cardamom pods
1 dried whole red chili pepper

*P types: substitute 1 teaspoon fennel seeds for the ajwan seeds and chili pepper.*

In a heavy cast-iron skillet, dry-roast the seeds and whole chili pepper over medium-low heat for 10 minutes. Using a hand mallet and grinding stone, pound the cardamom pods; discard the shells. Grind all the seeds and chili pepper together with a small hand grinder into a fine powder. Store the masala in an airtight jar in a cool place.

## Mild Garam Masala

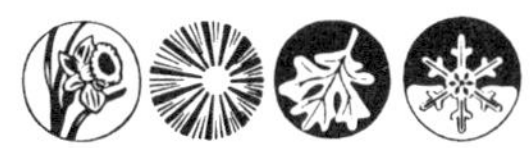

ALL TYPES

2 tsp coriander seeds
1 tsp cumin seeds
1/2 tsp fennel seeds (optional)
1/2 tsp whole black peppercorns
1/4 tsp whole cloves

Using a mortar and pestle, grind all the seeds and spices into a fine powder. Store in an airtight jar.

## Chat Masala

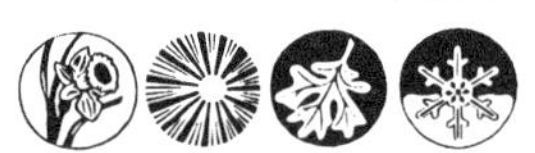

V, VP, VK

1 tbs cumin seeds
1/4 tbs fennel seeds
1/2 tbs mango powder
1/2 tbs garam masala (see page 302)
1/4 tbs black salt (or rock salt)
1/2 tsp cayenne powder
2 pinches asafoetida
1/8 tsp ginger powder

*P types: omit mango powder, cayenne, and asafoetida.*

In a heavy skillet, dry-roast the cumin and fennel seeds until golden brown. Remove and grind in a mortar and pestle. Combine with remaining ingredients, return to skillet, and dry-roast for a few more minutes. Store in a tightly covered jar in a cool place.

## Panch Puran: Bengali Masala

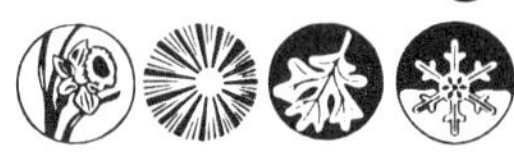

V, VP, VK, K, KV, KP

1/2 c cumin seeds
1/3 c nigella seeds
1/4 c fennel seeds
1/4 c black mustard seeds
1/8 c fenugreek seeds

In a heavy skillet, dry-roast all the seeds for 10 minutes over low heat. Stir gently. Using a suribachi, grind into a fine powder. Store in an airtight jar in a cool place.

## Madras Curry Powder

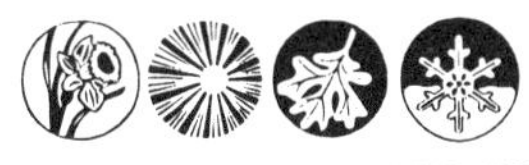

V, VP, VK, K, KV, KP

1 tbs cumin seeds
1 tbs black mustard seeds
1/4 tbs fenugreek seeds
1/4 tbs split urad dhal, without skins
4 fresh whole dried red chili peppers
1/2 tsp whole black peppercorns
12 fresh curry leaves
1 tbs turmeric powder
1/8 c coriander powder

In a heavy skillet, dry-roast cumin, mustard, and fenugreek seeds along with the dhal, chili peppers, peppercorns, and curry leaves over low heat for 8 minutes, stirring gently. Using a small hand grinder or a suribachi, grind spices until they are powdered. Lightly roast the turmeric and coriander powder, and combine with other spices. Place curry powder in an airtight jar and store in a cool place.

## Rasam Masala

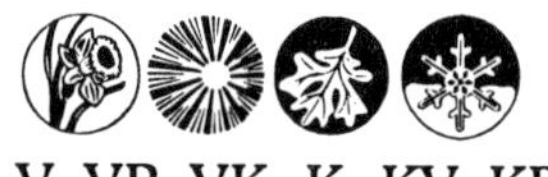

V, VP, VK, K, KV, KP

1 c coriander seeds
1/2 c dried red chili peppers
1/2 c whole black peppercorns
1/2 c plus 2 tbs cumin seeds
1/2 c black mustard seeds

In a large cast-iron skillet, dry-roast all the ingredients, stirring constantly. Maintain low, even heat until the seeds begin to pop and crackle. Using a wooden spoon, grind together. When cool, store in an airtight jar.

## Pudina (Mint) Masala

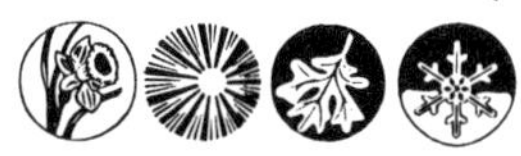

ALL TYPES

1 tbs sunflower oil
1/4 c split urad dhal, without skins
1 c dried mint leaves
1/8 c whole black peppercorns
2 tbs coriander seeds
1 tsp green cardamom seeds

In a large cast-iron skillet, heat the oil. Lower heat and slowly roast dhal until light brown. Add mint and roast for a few minutes. Using a small hand grinder, grind both to a fine powder. In a separate skillet, dry-roast peppercorns, coriander, and cardamom. Stir seeds constantly to ensure even roasting. Grind, then combine with dhal-mint mixture. When cool, store in an airtight jar.

## Sambar Powder

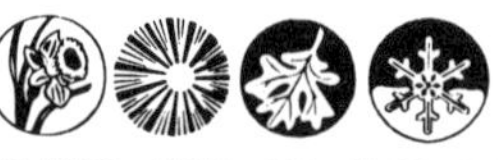

V, VP, VK, K, KV, KP

3/4 c coriander seeds
3/4 c cumin seeds
1/8 c chana dhal
2 tbs fenugreek seeds
1/2 c black mustard seeds
1/2 c dried red chili peppers
1/2 tsp sea salt
1/2 tsp asafoetida

*KP and VP: use sparingly.*

In a large cast-iron skillet, dry-roast coriander and cumin seeds and dhal. Add fenugreek, mustard seeds, and chili peppers after the dhal begins to turn light brown. Continue roasting over very low heat for an additional 5 minutes. Add salt and asafoetida at end of roasting. Using a small hand grinder, grind the ingredients together into a fine powder. When cool, store in an airtight jar.

## Cumin and Black Pepper Rasam

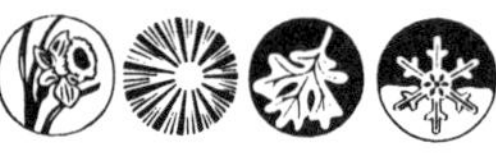

ALL TYPES

1/2 c whole black peppercorns
1/2 c plus 2 tbs cumin seeds
1/4 c coriander seeds

In a cast-iron skillet, dry-roast ingredients evenly over very low heat until cumin seeds turn light brown. Using a small hand grinder, grind to a fine powder. When cool, store in an airtight jar.

## Gun Powder

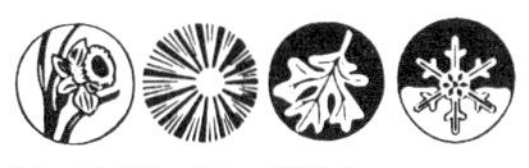

V, VK, K, KV

$^1/_2$ c split urad dhal,wihout skins
$^1/_2$ c yellow split peas
10 dried red chili peppers
$^1/_2$ tsp sea salt
$^1/_4$ tsp asafoetida
*K types: use $^1/_4$ teaspoon salt*

In a large cast-iron skillet, dry-roast urad dhal, split peas, and chili peppers evenly until dhal turns light brown. Remove from pan and add salt and asafoetida; toast for a few minutes. Grind ingredients together in a suribachi into a very fine powder. When cool, store in an airtight jar.

## Gomasio

*This Japanese condiment, made of salt and sesame seeds, is excellent for Vata types.*

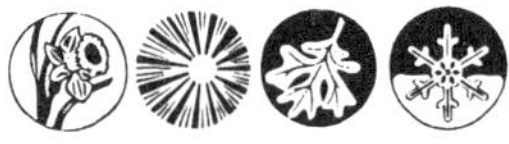

ALL TYPES, OCCASIONALLY

1 tbs sea salt
1 c sesame seeds, washed
*P types: use sparingly*

Place sea salt in a stainless-steel pan over medium heat. Dry-roast for two minutes until salt becomes dry. Using a mortar and pestle, grind salt to a fine powder. Place the washed sesame seeds in the pan over a medium heat and dry-roast for several minutes. Stir constantly with a wooden spoon to avoid burning; shake the pan frequently to brown the seeds evenly. When the seeds turn golden, place them in the mortar and pestle with the ground sea salt. Slowly but firmly grind into a coarse powder. Allow to cool completely before placing in an airtight glass or ceramic container.

## PICKLES

Pickles have been used for centuries by every culture to stimulate the digestive process, and to add the necessary sour taste to a meal. Nomadic tribes used pickles to accent foods; pickles needed little care and matured as they traveled. In the villages of India, travelers still often carry some dried dhal, pickles, fresh ground flour, and ghee. They park by the roadside and find small pieces of firewood and some dried cow dung to make a fire. After cooking the dhal, they bake the flour dough directly on the kindling embers. The bread and dhal will be served as a full meal, along with the pickles, which are called *achar*.

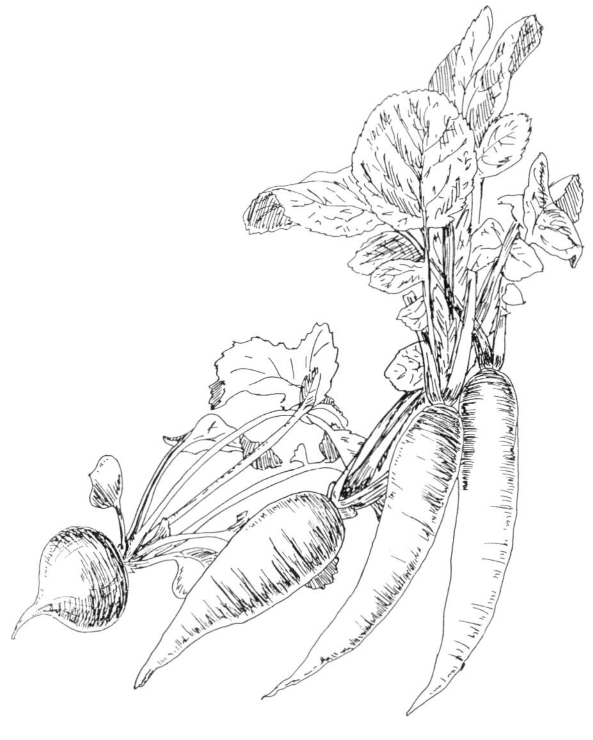

**Radish, Daikon, Turnip, Wild Radish**

The most common pickles in India are the lime and the green mango. Today, there are scores of different pickles, such as hot chili, fresh ginger, daikon, and gooseberry. Most watery vegetables, such as cauliflower and cabbage, are good for pickling.

Vedic pickling is done without vinegar, garlic, or onions, since these foods became too tamasic in nature when used in pickling. Vedic pickles are made from mustard oil, rock salt, and lime or lemon juice. They are left in the sun, which is the best heat for pickling. Sunlight retards the fermentation process, which allows the pickle to cure. All pickles are taken inside at night. The energy of the moon slows the natural process and diminishes the energy of a good pickle. Most commercial pickles in India today are saturated with oils, asafoetida, and spices. Making a good pickle is a fine art and a worthwhile accomplishment.

In Japan, the pickles of daikon, umeboshi plum, ginger, and a variety of vegetables also provide a ritual support to meals. Rice balls wrapped in nori with a piece of pickled umeboshi plum in the center is the mainstay of a traveller's repast.

Pickles are best for the Vata types, although tiny pieces may occasionally be taken by Kapha and Pitta types.

## Nimbu Achar (Lime Pickle)

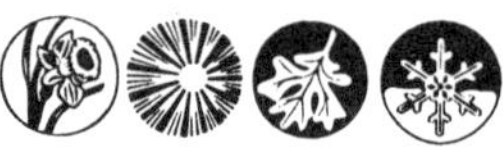

V, VP, VK

**6 thin-skinned limes**
**1/2 c mustard oil**
**3 tbs sea salt**

Wash the limes and sun-dry for 15 minutes. Cut lengthwise and squeeze juice. Reserve. Cut skin of each lime into eight sections. In a small stainless-steel pot, heat the mustard oil and add the lime juice. Remove from heat and stir in salt. Place, along with lime pieces, into a clean glass jar. Allow to cool and cover with a nonmetallic lid.

Set jar in the sun every day for 4 to 5 hours for four weeks. Bring jar in daily at dusk, and shake it occasionally. Store thereafter at room temperature.

## Mula Achar (Daikon Pickle)

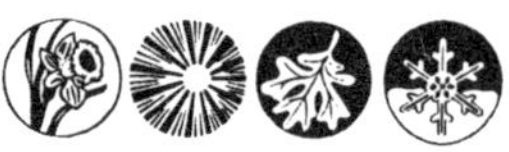

V, VP, VK

**2 1/2 c water**
**2 c thinly sliced daikon**
**1/2 c sesame oil**
**1 tbs black mustard seeds**
**4 whole cayenne peppers**
**2 tsp sea salt**

Boil water in a stainless-steel saucepan. Scrub the radishes and blanch for a minute. Drain and sun-dry for one hour. In a small stainless pan, heat the sesame oil. Mix the sun-dried radishes, black mustard seeds, cayenne pepper, and salt together and place in a clean glass jar. Add the warm oil. Allow to cool; cover with a nonmetallic lid.

Set the jar in sunlight every day for 4 to 5 hours for two weeks. Remember to bring jar in daily at dusk, and shake occasionally. Store in a cool place after opening.

## Nimbu Achar (Lemon Pickle)

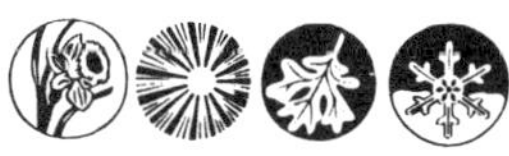

V, VK

**8 lemons**
**1 tbs black mustard seeds**
**1/4 c fine sea salt**
**1 tsp asafoetida**
**1/2 c cayenne**
**1/2 tsp turmeric**
**3 tbs sesame oil**

Cut each lemon into twenty-four pieces, leaving rinds intact. In a small cast-iron skillet, dry-roast mustard seeds until they pop. Turn off heat and slightly toast salt, asafoetida, cayenne, and turmeric.

In a separate pan, heat oil and pour onto lemon pieces. Allow to cool. Mix in spices thoroughly with clean hands. Place in a glass jar, cover with a muslin cloth, and allow to sit for one week in a warm place. Serve in small amounts as a condiment.

## Aam Achar (Green Mango Pickle)

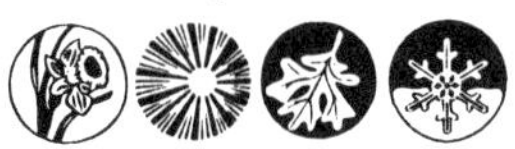

ALL TYPES, OCCASIONALLY
P TYPES: ONLY IN FALL AND WINTER

**3 medium unripe mangoes**
**2 tsp sea salt**
**1/3 c sunflower oil**
**2 tbs black mustard seeds**
**1/8 tsp cardamom powder**
**1/8 tsp ground mace**
**1/8 tsp ground cloves**
**1/4 c Sucanat or unrefined brown sugar**

Wash and peel mangoes. Remove pits and slice into thin slivers. Marinate slivers in sea salt for 1 hour. Heat oil in a stainless steel saucepan; add mustard seeds, cardamom, mace, and cloves and roast for a few minutes until the mustard seeds pop. Stir in sugar and remove from heat. Add marinated mangoes and place mixture in a clean glass jar; allow to cool.

Cover with a nonmetallic lid and place in the sun every day for 4 or 5 hours for two weeks. Remember to bring jar in daily before dusk, and shake it occasionally. Store in a cool place after opening.

## CHUTNEYS

Chutneys are an important accent to Vedic cuisine. They are made with a variety of ingredients, from dhals and nuts, to coconut and tamarind. A panoply of chutneys are made fresh for daily use and are cooked or marinated over a period of time to accompany ceremonial feasts and celebrations. Much like pickles, chutneys are a condiment that enliven any meal.

## Imli (Tamarind) Chutney

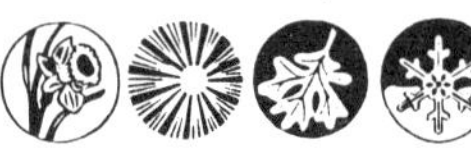

ALL TYPES

**1/4 c dried tamarind**
**1 c boiling water**
**1/2 tsp ajwan seeds**
**3 tbs dried shredded coconut**
**3 tbs finely chopped roasted peanuts**
**3 whole cayenne peppers**
**1 tsp sea salt**
**1 tbs minced fresh cilantro**
**1/2 tbs minced ginger**
***P types: use sparingly.***

In a glass bowl, combine dried tamarind and boiling water. Allow to sit for 30 minutes. With clean hands, mash and knead the tamarind into a smooth pulp. Strain the pulp through a sieve to remove tamarind fibers. Scrape the bottom of the sieve thoroughly to retrieve as much pulp as possible.

Heat a heavy cast-iron skillet and dry-roast the ajwan seeds, dried coconut, peanuts, cayenne, and salt over medium heat for 5 minutes. Combine roasted ingredients and tamarind pulp in a large glass bowl. Add the fresh cilantro and ginger. Serve fresh with rice or chapatis.

## Plum Chutney (Aloo Bukhara)

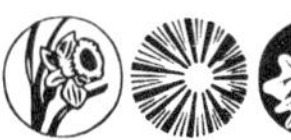

ALL TYPES

2 lbs ripe plums
2 tbs ghee
1/2 tsp minced ginger
1 tsp grated orange peel
1/4 tsp ground mace
1/4 tsp cinnamon powder
1/4 tsp coriander powder
1/8 tsp ground turmeric
1/8 tsp ground cloves
1/2 c grape juice
1/2 c Sucanat, unrefined brown sugar, or maple syrup
1/8 tsp sea salt

Wash plums; pit and cut into quarters. In a stainless steel saucepan, heat the ghee. Sauté ginger and orange peel for a few minutes. Add plums, spices, juice, sugar, and salt; bring to a boil. Lower heat and continue to cook, covered, for 30 minutes until the chutney becomes a thick jam. Allow to cool; place in a glass jar and store in a cool place. While this chutney is used mostly for festivities and celebrations, it may be used by all three doshas throughout the year as a condiment.

## Mango Chutney

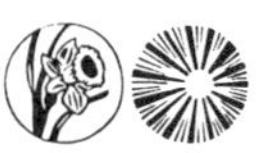

ALL TYPES

1 c peeled and finely chopped semi-ripe mango
1/2 c freshly grated coconut
1/2 c coconut milk (see page 194)
1/2 tsp sea salt
1/2 tsp black mustard seeds
1/2 tsp sunflower oil

Using a small hand grinder, grind mango pulp, coconut, coconut milk, and salt into a paste. Sauté mustard seeds in hot oil until they pop and mix into the paste.

## Mint Chutney

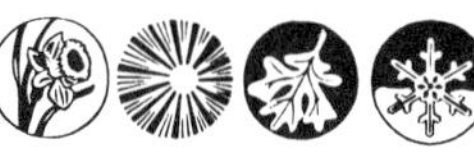

P, PV, PK, K, KV, KP

1/2 bunch fresh cilantro
1/2 bunch fresh mint leaves
1/2 tbs lemon juice
1/2 tsp roasted pomegranate seeds
1/4 tsp fine sea salt
2 tbs fresh plain yogurt

*P types: add 1 1/2 teaspoons maple syrup to yogurt, if desired.*

Grind all ingredients, except yogurt, together in a suribachi. Store in a glass jar and keep in a cool place. Mix in yogurt directly before serving.

## Dry Coconut Chutney

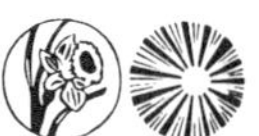

ALL TYPES

1 tbs sunflower oil
1/8 c split urad dhal, without skins
1/8 split chana dhal
1/4 tsp tamarind pulp
1 c freshly grated coconut
1/2 tsp black mustard seeds
1/4 tsp sea salt

*K types: use only 1 teaspoon oil and 1/8 cup grated coconut.*

Heat oil in a large cast-iron skillet. Lower heat and roast dhals evenly until light brown. Using a small hand grinder, grind into a dry paste. In a small skillet, dry-roast tamarind pulp and coconut (keeping them separated) over very low heat for 30 minutes until tamarind flakes. Remove tamarind and dry-roast mustard seeds until they pop. Remove coconut and allow to cool for thirty minutes. Grind coconut, tamarind, and mustard seeds into a powder. Combine with dhal powder and salt. When cool, store in an airtight jar.

## Orange and Cherry Chutney

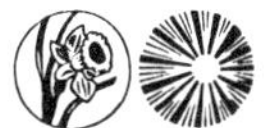

V, VP, P, PV

- 1/8 c fresh cherries, seeded
- 1/8 c orange pulp
- 1/8 c fresh orange juice
- 1/2 tsp cinnamon powder
- 1/4 tsp cardamom powder
- 2 tbs minced fresh mint leaves
- 1 tbs ghee
- Pinch of coarse black pepper
- Pinch of turmeric
- Pinch of sea salt
- 1 tbs mirin

Using a potato masher, mash cherries in a small saucepan until they have consistency of a coarse purée. Add orange pulp and juice, cinnamon, cardamom, and mint leaves; warm over very low heat for 15 minutes. In a separate pan, warm ghee and roast black pepper, turmeric, and salt for 2 minutes. Stir in mirin and add to orange/cherry mixture. Simmer for an additional 5 minutes. Allow to cool; place in a glass jar and store in a cool place. Serve with dosa or idli on festive occasions.

## Cilantro and Parsley Chutney

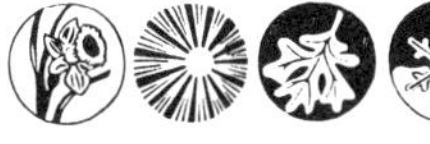

ALL TYPES

- 1/2 c minced fresh cilantro
- 1/4 c minced fresh parsley
- 2 tsp sunflower oil
- 1/8 c split urad dhal, without skins
- 1/2 tsp black mustard seeds
- 1/4 tsp dried tamarind
- 1/4 tsp salt

*K types: use 1 teaspoon oil.*

*V and K types: add 1/8 cup roasted red chili peppers and a pinch of asafoetida.*

Sun-dry minced cilantro and parsley for a few hours. Heat oil in a large skillet and roast urad dhal evenly over low heat until light brown. During the last few minutes, add mustard seeds and roast until they pop. Using a small hand grinder, grind mixture to a dry paste.

In a small skillet, dry-roast tamarind over very low heat for 30 minutes until it flakes. Add the sun-crisped cilantro and parsley and dry-roast for 5 minutes. Add salt during the last minute. Grind into a fine powder. Combine the dry paste and the powder. When cool, store in an airtight jar.

## Green Ginger and Coconut Chutney

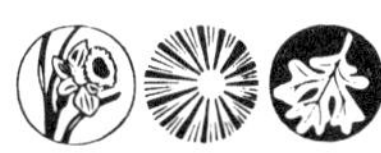

V, VP, VK, K, KV, KP

- 1/2 c freshly grated coconut
- 2 tbs minced green ginger
- 1 tbs minced fresh green chili peppers
- 2 tbs lemon juice
- 1/2 c water
- 1/4 tsp sea salt
- 1/2 tsp black peppercorns
- 1/2 tbs sunflower oil

*VK: use sparingly*

*K types: use 1/2 teaspoon oil and only 1/8 cup of coconut*

Grind coconut, ginger, and chili peppers together in a suribachi, adding lemon juice, water, and salt. Sauté peppercorns in oil and add to suribachi. Continue grinding and adding water until desired consistency is reached. Store in a glass jar.

## Hot Pepper Chutney

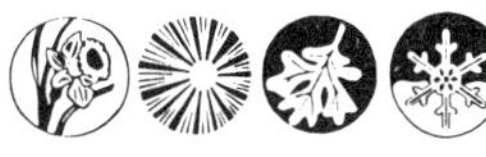

V, VK

- 1 tsp sea salt
- 1/4 c fresh red hot chili peppers
- 1/4 c rice vinegar

Lightly toast salt in a cast-iron skillet for 2 minutes. Finely mince chili peppers. In a small stainless steel pan, heat vinegar over low heat; mix in chili peppers and salt. Store in an airtight jar in a cool place.

## Zucchini Chutney

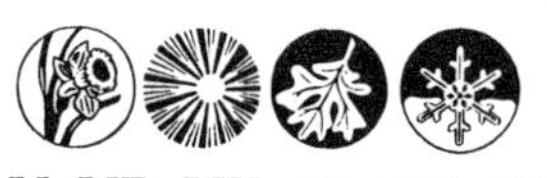

V, VP, VK, K, KV, KP

1 zucchini
1/2 tsp sunflower oil
2 tbs yellow split peas
1 tsp split urad dhal, without skins
4 green chili peppers
4 curry leaves, preferably fresh
Pinch of asafoetida
Pinch of sea salt
1/4 c water
1/2 tsp black mustard seeds

Cut zucchini into 1/2" slices. In a large skillet, heat oil and add split peas, urad dhal, chili peppers, curry leaves, asafoetida, and salt. Brown evenly over low heat for 5 minutes. Add zucchini and water. Cover and simmer for 5 minutes. Using a small hand grinder, grind zucchini mixture to pulp. In a separate pan, dry-roast mustard seeds over medium heat for 3 minutes and add to chutney. Serve as a condiment.

# RAITAS (YOGURT SALADS)

## Cucumber Raita

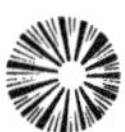

ALL TYPES (K TYPES, USE SPARINGLY)
Serves 4

1 cucumber
1 c plain yogurt
1/2 tsp cumin powder
1/4 tsp turmeric
1/4 tsp fine sea salt

*V and K types: add cayenne or chili powder.*

Peel cucumber and cut into thin slices. Combine yogurt, spices, and salt. Add cucumbers to yogurt and refrigerate for 10 minutes before serving. Use as a condiment.

## Lemon Raita

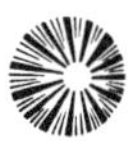

V, VP, VK
Serves 4

1 small lemon
1/2 c fresh plain yogurt
1/2 tbs honey
1/4 tsp cumin powder
1/4 tsp fine black pepper

Cut lemon into thin slices, discarding seeds but leaving rind intact. Combine yogurt, honey, and spices. Marinate lemon in yogurt mixture for 15 minutes and then refrigerate for 15 minutes. Serve as a condiment.

## Orange Raita

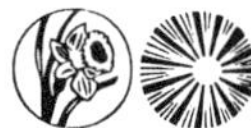

V, VP, VK, P, PV, PK
Serves 4

1 small peeled orange
1 tbs maple syrup
1 c fresh plain yogurt
1/4 tsp turmeric
1/4 tsp cardamom powder
1 tbs grated orange rind

Cut peeled orange into thin slices and discard seeds. Combine maple syrup with yogurt; add spices. Marinate orange slices in spiced yogurt for 20 minutes. Add the orange rind. Refrigerate for 30 minutes. Serve as a condiment.

# UNIVERSAL DESSERTS

Some of the recipes in this section call for certified raw milk. For those people who are lactose intolerant, the following substitutions are suggested: Soy milk for P and K types; almond or rice milk for V types.

## PIE DOUGH

### Whole Wheat Dough

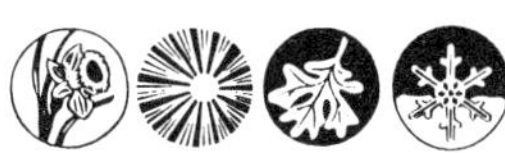

V, VP, P, PV
Makes double crust for three 9" pies

4 c whole wheat pastry flour
¼ tsp sea salt
¼ c light sesame oil, chilled
1 c cold water

Mix flour and salt together in a large mixing bowl. Add oil and mix well. Add water. Knead dough for 4 minutes; then allow to sit at room temperature for 15 minutes or chill for 30 minutes.

Divide dough in two pieces; roll one piece into a circle about 1½" larger than the bottom of your pie dish. Lightly oil the dish and press rolled dough into it, letting dough come up over edge of the dish a little. Fill with prepared filling.

Roll out second piece of dough to cover the top and edges of the dish. Place loosely over the filling; press edges of the upper and lower crusts together with your fingertips or the tines of a fork. Poke a few holes in the top of the pie with a fork to allow excess air to escape.

## Barley and Whole Wheat Dough

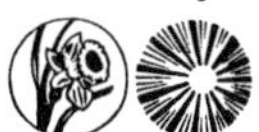

K, KV, KP

Makes double crust for two 9" pies

2 c barley pastry flour
1 c whole wheat pastry flour
1/4 tsp sea salt
1/8 c chilled corn oil
1 c cold water

Follow the same procedure for the Whole Wheat Pie Dough described on the preceding page.

# PIES

## Amasake and Cardamom Pie

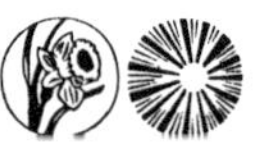

ALL TYPES

Fills two 9" pies

1 c amasake
1/4 tsp cardamom powder
1/4 tsp vanilla extract
1 c tangerine sections
1/4 tsp orange rind
2 tsp agar-agar
2 tbs warm water

*P and V types: add 2 tablespoons maple syrup, if desired.*

Preheat oven to 350 degrees F. Boil all but last two ingredients for 10 minutes. Dilute agar-agar with water and add to hot amasake mixture. Stir and simmer for 3 minutes. Remove from heat and allow to cool. Pour into bottom pie crust and cover with upper crust. (See preceding recipes for pie dough.) Bake for 40 minutes, until crust is golden.

## Saffron and Apple Pie

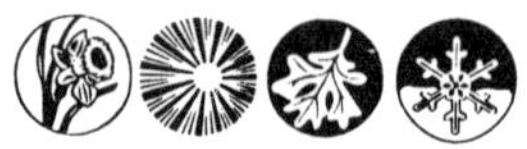

ALL TYPES

Fills two 9" pies

4 cored apples
12 strands saffron
1/4 tsp cinnamon
1/8 c apple juice concentrate

*V types: substitute peaches and peach juice concentrate.*

Preheat oven to 350 degrees F. Dice apples and combine all ingredients. Pour into bottom crust of pie. (See preceding recipes for pie dough.) Cut upper rolled crust into twelve 3/4" wide strips. Criss-cross over filling. Bake for 40 minutes, until crust is golden.

## Raspberry Gel Pie

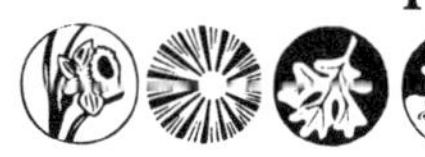

ALL TYPES

Fills one 9" pie

1/2 c cherry juice
1/4 tsp almond extract
2 tbs kudzu (or arrowroot)
1/4 c cold water
1 lb fresh raspberries
2 tbs maple syrup

Preheat oven to 350 degrees F. Boil cherry juice and add extract. Dilute kudzu in cold water; add to the boiled juice. Stir over medium heat until thickened into a gel.

Wash the raspberries and add to the mixture, along with the maple syrup. Pour into a bottom pie crust and cover with top crust. (See preceding recipes for pie dough.) Bake for 40 minutes, until crust is golden.

## Almond and Hazelnut Cream Pie

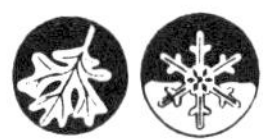

V, VP, VK
Fills one 9" pie

1/2 lb blanched almonds
1/2 lb blanched hazelnuts
1/2 tsp hazelnut extract
1/2 c certified raw cow's cream
1/2 c certified raw cow's milk
1/2 c unrefined brown sugar
2 tsp agar-agar
2 tbs warm water

Preheat oven to 350 degrees F. Using a small hand grinder, blend the almonds, hazelnuts, and extract into a coarse paste. Boil the cream and milk for 5 minutes; add brown sugar and nut paste. Dilute agar-agar in warm water and add, stirring until mixture begins to thicken. Pour into bottom pie crust and cover with top crust. (See preceding recipes for pie dough.) Bake for 40 minutes, until crust is golden.

## Popcorn Crunch Crustless Pie

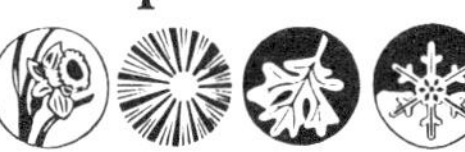

P, PV, PK, K, KV, KP
Fills one 9" pie

1 tsp sunflower oil
1/8 c popcorn kernels
1/2 c pear juice concentrate
1/4 c carob powder

Preheat oven to 400 degrees F. Heat oil in a large saucepan over medium heat for 3 minutes. Add kernels, cover, and pop over medium-low heat for about 4 minutes. Add juice concentrate and carob powder to popped corn and mix to coat. Lightly oil a pie dish and fill with popcorn mixture. Bake for 15 minutes.

# FESTIVE DESSERTS

## Clay Pot Baked Apples

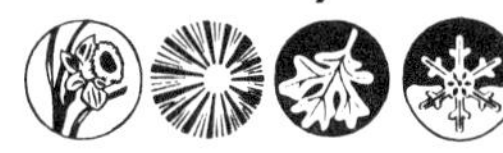

P, PV, PK
Serves 6

6 medium Granny Smith apples
8 oz ricotta cheese
3 tbs maple syrup

Presoak a clay pot in water for 10 minutes. Core the apples. Combine cheese and maple syrup and stuff into cavities. Place stuffed apples in pot, cover, and place in cold oven. Turn oven to 450 degrees F. and bake for 30 minutes.

## Cherry Strudel

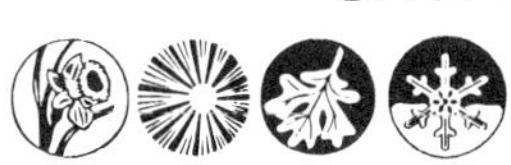

ALL TYPES
Serves 2

1/2 whole wheat pie dough (see page 311)
1 lb fresh cherries, pitted
1/8 c cherry juice
1/2 c cherry juice concentrate
1/4 tsp almond extract
1/4 tsp nutmeg powder

Preheat oven to 350 degrees F. Roll pie dough to shape of a rectangle, 1/8" thick. Combine all remaining ingredients and boil for 5 minutes; pour into center of rolled dough.

Fold sides of rectangle over each other, and press ends together with a fork. Make holes in the top with a fork to allow excess air to escape. Bake for 35 minutes, until crust is golden brown.

## Universal Trifle

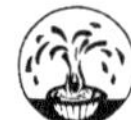

ALL TYPES
Serves 4

*Corn Base:*
1 c cornmeal
1/4 c corn oil
Pinch of sea salt
1/2 c water

Combine cornmeal, corn oil, and sea salt together. Add enough water to form a thick paste. Oil a 12" cast-iron skillet. Pour corn dough into the skillet and cook over medium heat for 15 minutes. Set aside.

*Fresh Fruit Gel:*
1/4 c each: crushed pineapple, sliced peaches, sliced strawberries
2 c cherry juice
1/4 c puréed bananas
1 tbs agar-agar
1/4 c warm water

Boil the pineapple, peaches, and strawberries in cherry juice for 3 minutes; add puréed bananas. Dilute agar-agar in warm water and stir into mixture, cooking over medium heat for 3 minutes.

Remove cornbread intact and place in the bottom of a 12" mold (preferably one that can be opened from the bottom). Pour fruit gel over cooked cornbread and chill for 2 hours.

*Almond Cream Topping:*
1 c blanched almonds
1/8 c maple syrup
1 tsp almond extract
1/2 c whipped cream (optional)

*K types: substitute 1/2 cup honey for maple syrup, and do not use whipped cream.*

Using a hand grinder, purée the almonds to a fine paste. Add maple syrup and almond extract. Pour over chilled cornbread/fruit gel and top with whipped cream. Cut like a cake and serve.

## Raspberry Tart

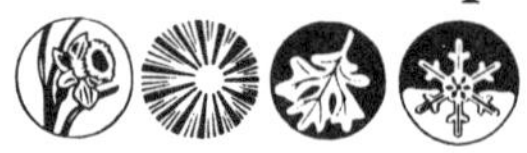

ALL TYPES
Makes twelve 3" x 3" tarts

1/2 c cherry juice
1 c fresh raspberries
12 strands saffron
1/2 tsp orange extract
2 tbs cherry juice concentrate
Pinch of sea salt
2 tsp agar-agar
2 tbs warm water
1/2 whole wheat pie dough (page 311)

Bring cherry juice to a boil and add raspberries, saffron, orange extract, fruit concentrate, and sea salt. Dilute agar-agar with warm water. Stir over medium heat until very thick. Remove from heat and allow to cool for half an hour before filling tarts.

Preheat oven to 350 degrees F. Roll pie dough into 9" x 12" rectangle, 1/8" thick. Cut into 12 equal pieces and fill center of each square with raspberry mixture.

Fold two opposite tips of a square together to form a triangle. Press folded edges with a fork to seal. Repeat process for remaining tarts. Make holes in top of each tart to allow air to escape. Bake in oiled pan for 20 minutes, until the crusts turn golden.

## Clay Pot Baked Pears

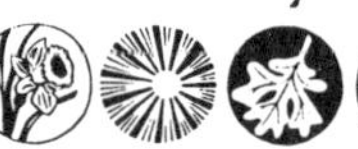

V, VP, P, PV
Serves 4

4 firm pears
4 tsp fructose
1/4 c unsweetened carob chips
1/4 tsp grated lemon rind
1/2 c pear juice
1/2 c whipping cream
1/2 tsp vanilla extract

Presoak a clay pot in water for 10 minutes. Core the

pears and put 1 teaspoon fructose in each cavity; top with carob chips and sprinkle with lemon rind. Place pears in pot and pour the pear juice over the pears. Cover and place in cold oven. Turn oven to 450 degrees F. and bake for 45 minutes or until pears are soft but not mushy. Whip the cream with vanilla until slightly stiff and serve over pears.

## Ricotta Fruit Dessert

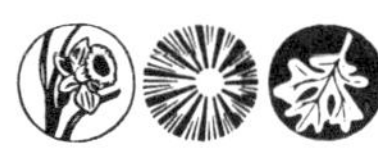

P, PV, PK
Serves 2

1 c ricotta cheese
1/2 c fresh strawberries
1/2 tbs raisins
1/4 c fresh apricots
2 tbs maple syrup
1/2 c orange juice
1/4 tsp cardamom powder

Place ricotta cheese in the center of a dessert dish. Arrange strawberries, raisins, and apricots around edges of cheese. Mix together remaining ingredients and pour over cheese and fruit.

## Mango and Melon Custard

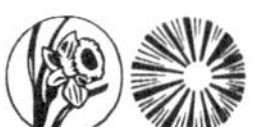

V, VP, P, PV, PK
Serves 4

2 peeled ripe mangoes
1 peeled melon (honeydew or cranshaw)
1 tsp kudzu (or arrowroot)
2 tbs cold water
2 c mango juice
1 tsp maple syrup

Pulp melon and mangoes and purée, using a food grinder. Set aside. Dilute the kudzu in cold water. Heat the mango juice in a small saucepan and simmer for 10 minutes over medium heat. Remove from heat, pour in a custard bowl, and add the puréed fruits and kudzu mixture. Stir in the maple syrup. Place in refrigerator to set for 15 minutes. Serve cool.

## Pineapple Kanten

Kanten *is sometimes used interchangeably with the term* agar-agar. Kanten *is also the Japanese name for a gelled dessert.*

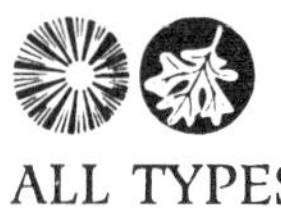

ALL TYPES
Serves 4

2 c orange juice
2 c pineapple juice
4 tsp agar-agar
1/4 c warm water
1 c pineapple chunks
1 c orange sections

Combine the juices and warm over low heat. Dilute agar-agar in warm water and add to juices. Add fruits and stir over medium heat for 2 minutes until mixture begins to thicken. Remove from heat and allow to cool for 15 minutes. Pour into a mold and refrigerate for 2 hours.

## Fruit Cobbler

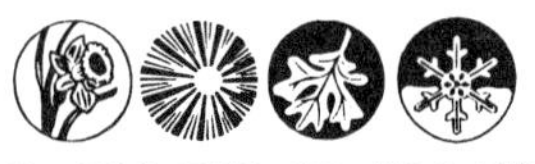

P, PV, PK, K, KV, KP
Serves 4

**1/2 c diced apples**
**1/2 c diced fresh apricots**
**1/4 c currants**
**1/4 c dried pineapple and pear pieces**
**1 c water**
**1/8 c barley flour**
**Pinch of ginger**
**Pinch of cinnamon**
**1/4 c fresh whole raspberries (if available)**
**1/8 c fruit juice concentrate**
**1/4 tsp vanilla essence**
**Garnish: 1/4 c granola**

In a medium saucepan, add all fruits, except raspberries, to water and bring to boil. Cover and simmer over medium heat for 15 minutes until fruits are cooked yet still firm.

In a cast-iron skillet, roast the barley flour until light brown. Add roasted flour, ginger, and cinnamon to cooked fruits. Gently stir in raspberries. Pour in the fruit concentrate and vanilla essence. Stir and simmer for 3 minutes. Serve warm in small bowls. Garnish with granola.

## Fresh Fruit Mold

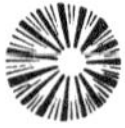

ALL TYPES
Serves 4

**3 c cranberry juice**
**2 tsp agar-agar**
**1/4 c warm water**
**1/4 c each: strawberries, orange pieces, blueberries, crushed pineapple**

Warm the cranberry juice. Dilute agar-agar in warm water and add to juice. Add fruits and stir over medium heat for 2 minutes until mixture begins to thicken. Remove from heat and allow to cool for 15 minutes. Pour into a mold and refrigerate for 2 hours.

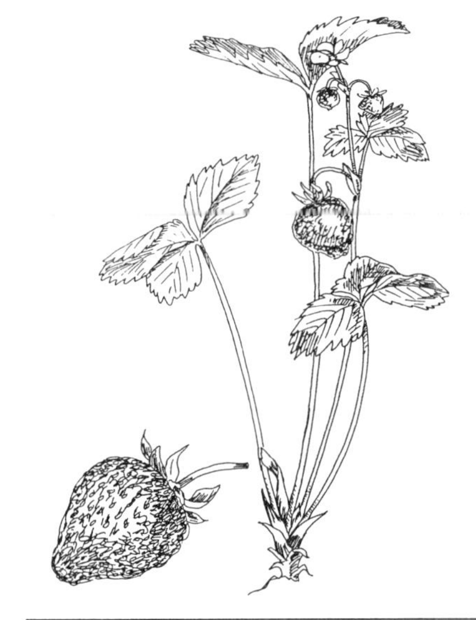

Strawberry

## Hazelnut Carob Mousse

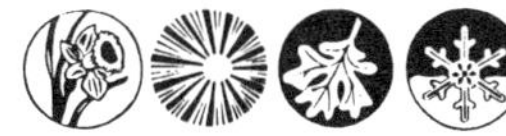

ALL TYPES, OCCASIONALLY
Serves 4

**2 tbs hazelnut butter**
**1 c amasake**
**1/4 c unsweetened carob powder**
**1/2 tsp vanilla extract**
**1 tbs kudzu (or arrowroot)**
**1/4 c cold water**
**Garnish: 6 mint leaves and 1 tbs finely grated orange rind**

Add hazelnut butter to amasake and stir until combined; stir in carob powder and vanilla extract. Simmer over low heat for 15 minutes. Dilute kudzu in cold water and add to mixture. Stir until mixture thickens. Pour into 4 small mousse dishes and chill for 2 hours. Garnish with mint leaves; sprinkle with orange rind and serve.

## Peppermint and Walnut Mousse

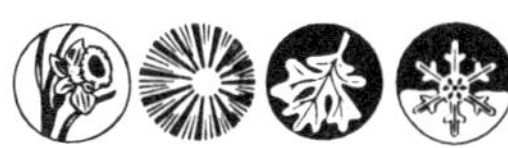

ALL TYPES, OCCASIONALLY
Serves 4

1/8 c walnuts
2 c strong peppermint tea
1 tsp walnut extract
1/4 c carob powder
2 tbs kudzu (or arrowroot)
1/4 c cold water
1/4 c honey
Garnish: 2 tbs unsweetened carob chips

*P types: substitute 1/4 c unrefined brown sugar for honey.*

Using a small food grinder, purée walnuts; combine with peppermint tea, walnut extract, and carob powder. Pour into a small saucepan and simmer over low heat for 15 minutes. Dilute kudzu in cold water and pour into peppermint mixture. Stir over medium heat until mixture thickens. Remove from heat and cool for 20 minutes. Add honey and pour into 4 mousse dishes. Chill for 2 hours. Garnish with carob chips before serving.

## Mocha Mousse

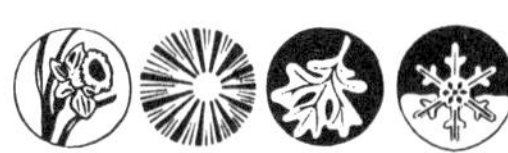

ALL TYPES, OCCASIONALLY
Serves 4

1 c almond milk (page 195)
1/4 c maple syrup
1/4 c grain beverage (such as Pero, Roma), dry measure
2 tsp agar-agar
1/4 c warm water
1/4 tsp vanilla extract
1/4 c roasted carob chips

Combine almond milk, maple syrup, and grain beverage in a small saucepan. Simmer over low heat for 12 minutes. Dilute the agar-agar in warm water and pour into mixture. Add vanilla extract and stir over medium heat until mixture thickens. Add roasted carob chips, pour into 4 mousse dishes, and chill for 2 hours.

## Rosewater Pudding

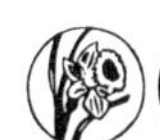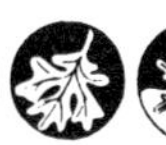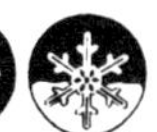

ALL TYPES
Serves 4

1/2 c cornmeal
1/2 c certified raw cow's milk
1/4 c rose water
Pinch of salt
1/4 tsp ground cardamom
1/4 tsp cinnamon
Pinch of nutmeg
1/4 c currants
1/4 c rice syrup
1/2 tsp vanilla extract
1/4 c water

*K types: substitute 1/2 cup soy milk for cow's milk.*

Preheat oven to 400 degrees F. Combine cornmeal, milk, rose water, salt, and spices, and simmer over low heat for 5 minutes. Add currants, rice syrup, vanilla extract, and water. Pour mixture onto an oiled baking dish and bake pudding for 30 minutes.

## Vanilla Flan

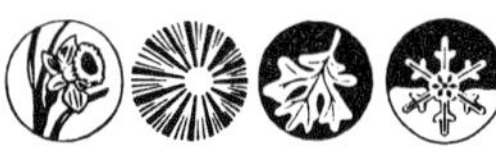

ALL TYPES, OCCASIONALLY
Serves 4

1 c almond milk
1/2 tsp vanilla extract
1 tsp ghee
1/2 c pear juice concentrate
2 tbs kudzu (or arrowroot)
1/4 c cold water

Combine milk, vanilla extract, ghee, and pear juice concentrate in a small saucepan; simmer over low heat for 15 minutes. Dilute kudzu in cold water. Pour into mixture and stir over medium heat until it thickens. Pour into 4 small dishes and chill for 2 hours. Whip with whisk and serve.

# CAKES AND PUDDINGS

## Blueberry Pudding Cake

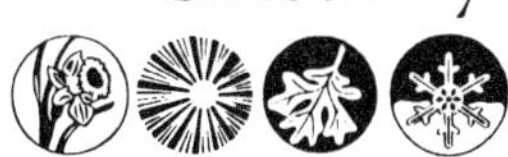

ALL TYPES
Serves 4

1 c orange juice
1 c peach juice
2 1/2 c cold water
2 c couscous
1 c blueberries
1 tsp vanilla extract
1 tbs grated orange rind
Pinch of sea salt

Combine juices and cold water; simmer in a saucepan over medium heat for 5 minutes. Add couscous and stir for a few minutes. Cover and simmer over low heat for 10 minutes. Add blueberries, vanilla extract, orange rind, and salt. Pour into a dish and chill for 1 hour.

## Fruit Cake

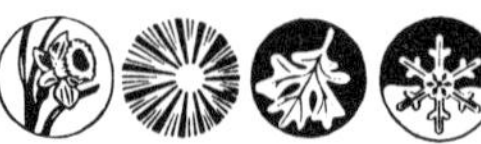

ALL TYPES, OCCASIONALLY
Serves 6

1 c dried pineapple
1/2 c dried apricots
3 c water
1 1/2 c whole wheat pastry flour
1/8 c chilled sunflower oil
Pinch of sea salt
1/4 c chopped walnuts
1 c orange juice
1 tbs grated orange rind
1/2 tsp vanilla extract
*K types: substitute 1 1/2 cup barley flour for wheat flour.*

Soak pineapple and apricots separately in 1 1/2 cups of water each overnight.

Preheat oven to 350 degrees F. In a mixing bowl, combine flour, oil, and salt. Drain the fruits and cut into small pieces. Combine the fruits, walnuts, orange juice and rind, and vanilla extract with the flour mixture and mix thoroughly but gently for 30 seconds.

Oil a loaf pan and pour in the batter. Bake for 30 minutes, or until a fork placed in the cake comes out clean.

## Date Bread Pudding

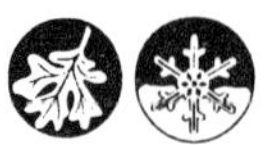

V, VP, VK, P, PV
Serves 6

1 c certified raw cow's milk
1/2 c pitted dates, finely chopped
2 c whole wheat flour
Pinch of sea salt
Pinch of baking soda
1/4 c currants

Combine milk and dates in a mixing bowl, and using a hand grinder, purée into a cream. Whip in flour, salt, baking soda, and currants. Pour into a clay pot and cover.

Place pot on rack inside a larger pot containing 6" of water. (Clay pot should be immersed in but not covered by water.) Bring water to boil; cover larger pot and simmer over low heat for 3 hours. Remove the clay pot and chill for 30 minutes before serving the pudding.

## Marzipan Date Cake

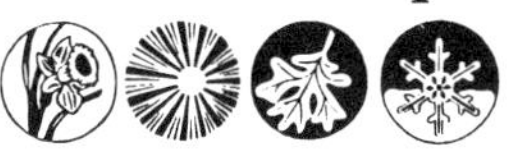

ALL TYPES, OCCASIONALLY
Serves 6

1/4 c blanched almonds
1/4 c pitted dates
1 tsp almond extract
1/2 c almond milk
2 c barley flour
Pinch of baking soda
Pinch of sea salt
1/2 c water

Preheat oven to 350 degrees F. Using a food grinder, purée the almond, dates, and almond extract with almond milk into a cream. Combine flour, baking soda, and salt, and pour in the cream. Add water and knead into a batter. Pour batter into an oiled loaf pan and bake for 35 minutes.

## Bean Pudding

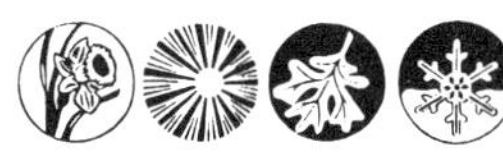

ALL TYPES
Serves 2

1/2 c overcooked aduki beans
1/2 c maple syrup
1 tsp walnut extract
1/4 c water
1 tbs kudzu (or arrowroot)
1/4 c cold water

Using a food grinder, purée the cooked beans. Stir in maple syrup and walnut extract. Add 1/4 cup water to the mixture and stir to a smooth consistency. Boil for 3 minutes over medium heat. Dilute kudzu in cold water and pour into warm bean mixture. Simmer over medium heat for 3 minutes and pour into a pudding dish. Chill for 2 hours. Whip with whisk and serve.

# PAYASAM

Payasam, which originates from South India, is a fluid nectarlike dessert that is served on special occasions. It is usually offered to the gods during religious ceremonies. While this sattvic dish may well be easily digested by the powerful *devatas*, mere mortals need to be careful not to indulge in it too frequently.

## Sago Payasam

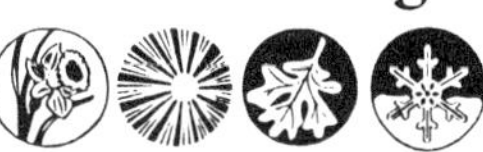

V, VP, P, PV OCCASIONALLY
Serves 6

12 strands saffron
1 tbs ghee
1 c sago (tiny tapioca)
3 c water
2 c certified raw cow's milk
1/4 c unrefined brown sugar
1/4 tsp cardamom

Soak saffron for 10 minutes in 3 teaspoons of water.

In a large skillet, melt the ghee and sauté the sago until light brown. In a separate pan, boil the water and add to sago. Simmer over medium heat for 15 minutes, stirring frequently, until sago becomes transparent.

In a small saucepan, bring the milk, sugar, saffron (and soaking water), and cardamom to a boil; add to sago. Remove from heat and allow to cool. Chill and serve.

## Amasake Payasam

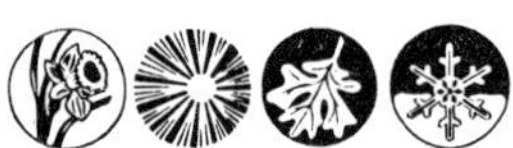

ALL TYPES, OCCASIONALLY
Serves 6

8 c water
1/2 lb bean thread noodles
1 tsp ghee
2 c amasake
1/4 tsp turmeric
1/4 c maple syrup

Boil 7 cups of the water in a large pot; break noodles into small pieces and add to water with ghee. Simmer over medium heat for 10 minutes, stirring continuously; drain noodles.

In a small saucepan, heat amasake, turmeric, and maple syrup. Add remaining cup of water and simmer for 5 minutes. Place noodles in a dessert bowl and cover with the amasake sauce. Allow to cool for 45 minutes; toss and serve.

## Pal Payasam

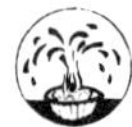

V, VP, P, PV
Serves 4

12 strands saffron
2 c certified raw cow's milk
1 c water
1/4 c unrefined brown sugar
1/4 tsp cardamom
1/2 c cooked sweet brown rice

Soak saffron in 3 teaspoons of water for 10 minutes.

Boil milk, water, sugar, saffron (with soaking water), and cardamom for 5 minutes in a medium saucepan. Add cooked rice; cover and simmer over low heat for 20 minutes. Stir occasionally to prevent sticking. Cool and serve.

## Rava Payasam

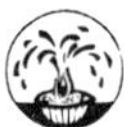

V, VP, P, PV
Serves 6

12 strands saffron
2 tbs ghee
2 tbs cashews
2 tbs golden raisins
1/2 c cream of wheat
2 c hot water
2 c fresh coconut milk (see page 194)
1/4 c unrefined brown sugar
1/2 tsp cardamom

Soak saffron in 3 teaspoons of water for 10 minutes.

Melt ghee in a skillet, and sauté cashews until light brown. Using a slotted spoon, remove cashews and sauté raisins for a few minutes. Remove raisins and add cream of wheat; toast for a few minutes. Add hot water, cover, and simmer over low heat for 10 minutes.

In a large saucepan, bring coconut milk, saffron (with soaking water), sugar, cardamom, raisins, and cashews to boil. Cook for 5 minutes over low heat and add the toasted cream of wheat. Stir until mixture becomes thick. Cool and serve.

# NURTURING BREWS AND BEVERAGES

Those people whose systems do not tolerate lactose may substitute rice, almond, or soy milk for cow's milk. Some general guidelines followed in these recipes should be applied when making other beverages as well:

Dilute all milk with an equal amount of water.
Dilute all fruit and vegetable juice with an equal amount of water.
Do not add honey to beverages until they have cooled. (Cooked honey is toxic.)
Use sandalwood powder sparingly (a pinch) and never on a daily basis.

## Cool Barley Brew

*This drink revitalizes and reinforces the nervous system.*

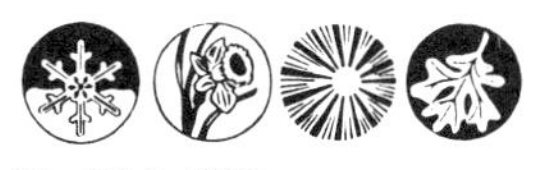

P, PV, PK
Serves 2

**2 c water**
**1/2 c hulled barley**
**Pinch of turmeric**
**1/4 tsp bala powder**
**Pinch of cinnamon**
**2 tsp maple syrup**
**1/4 c leafy green or root vegetable water (optional)**

Bring water to boil in a medium pot. Add barley, cover, and simmer over medium heat for 2 hours. Allow to cool for 10 minutes. Place a colander in an empty pan and drain barley. Combine resulting creamy barley water with turmeric, bala, cinnamon, and maple syrup. Add vegetable water, if available. Allow brew to cool for 30 minutes more. The cooked barley can be eaten as part of a regular meal. Take brew once or twice a week; make it fresh each time.

## Warm Barley Brew

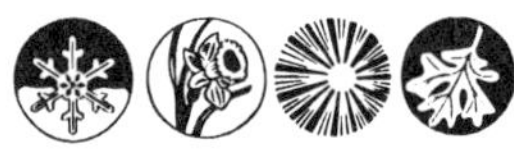

K, KV, KP
Serves 2

1/2 c hulled barley
1/4 c leafy green water
2 c water
Pinch of turmeric
Pinch of cinnamon
Pinch of cardamom
1/4 tsp bibhitaki powder
1/2 tsp honey

Bring water to boil in a medium pot. Add barley, cover, and simmer over medium heat for 2 hours. Allow to cool for 10 minutes. Place a colander in an empty pan and drain barley. Combine resulting creamy barley water with spices, herbs, and vegetable water. Simmer over medium heat for 2 minutes and allow to cool for 5 minutes; add honey. The cooked barley can be eaten as part of a regular meal. Take brew once or twice a week; make it fresh each time.

## Warm Rice Brew

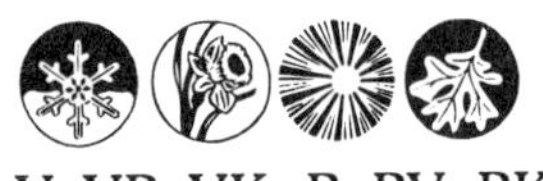

V, VP, VK, P, PV, PK
Serves 2

1/2 c sweet brown rice
2 c water
Pinch of turmeric
Pinch of black pepper
Pinch of cinnamon
Pinch of nutmeg
1/4 tsp bhringaraja powder
1/2 c sweet orange or mango juice

Bring water to boil in a medium pot. Add rice, cover, and simmer over medium heat for 2 hours. Allow to cool for 10 minutes. Place a colander over an empty pan and drain rice. Combine resulting creamy rice water with the spices and herbs. Then add fruit juice and warm over medium heat for a few minutes. The cooked sweet rice can be eaten as part of a regular meal. Take brew once or twice a week; make it fresh each time.

## Warm Spiced Tea

***Drink as a revitalizer; to relieve intestinal distension and cleanse the blood.***

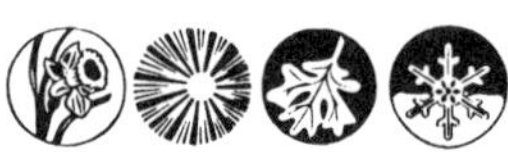

V, VP, P, PV, PK
Serves 2

1/2 tsp cardamom seeds
1/4" piece cinnamon
1/4 tsp ground cloves
1 tbs unrefined brown sugar
1 c boiling water
1 tsp black tea (optional)
2 c certified raw cow's milk
A few drops almond essence

Warm a large heavy pot by pouring hot tap water into it and letting it sit for a few minutes. Remove the water and add cardamom, cinnamon, cloves, and brown sugar. Pour the boiling water over the herbs and tea (if desired); cover and steep for 8 minutes. In a saucepan bring milk to boil and add almond essence. Strain the spices and return liquid to pot. Add the boiled milk and serve hot.

## Elder Flower Tea (variation 1)

*Elder flowers have a bitter and pungent taste with a cooling tendency. They cleanse the blood, encourage the elimination of wastes through the skin, and are a diuretic. Elder flowers may be used occasionally by all, but they are best for P and K types.*

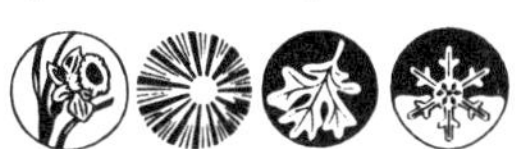

P, PV, PK
Serves 1

1 tsp elder flowers
1 c boiling water
1/2 tsp maple syrup

Steep flowers in boiling water for 5 minutes; strain and add maple syrup. (Flowers may also be steeped in 1 cup of hot certified raw cow's milk or soy milk, for occasional use only.)

## Elder Flower Tea (variation 2)

V, VP, VK
Serves 1

1 tsp elder flowers
1/8 tsp cardamom powder
1 c boiling water (or certified raw milk)
1 tsp honey

Steep flowers and cardamom in boiling water for 3 minutes. Strain and allow to cool for a few minutes before adding honey.

## Elder Flower Tea (variation 3)

K, KV, KP
Serves 1

1/2 tsp elder flowers
1/8 tsp cardamom powder
Pinch of clove powder
1 c boiling water
1/2 tsp honey

Steep the flowers, cardamom, and cloves in boiling water for 5 minutes. Strain and allow to cool before adding honey.

## Ginger, Cumin, Coriander Tea

*All three herbs used in this recipe are considered to be pungent. Cumin and coriander have a bitter taste as well; ginger has a secondary sweet taste. While ginger and cumin have a heating tendency, coriander is cooling. Ginger, a potent stimulant, relieves phlegm and mucus from the lungs, relieves gas, and encourages sweating and the elimination of wastes through the skin. Cumin synergizes well with ginger, performing most of the same functions; it cleanses the blood also. Coriander provides the cooling balance to both herbs while performing most of the same actions; it is also a diuretic.*

LATE EARLY : V, VP, VK

EARLY LATE : K, KP, KV

Serves 2

1/4 tsp roasted cumin seeds
1/4 tsp roasted coriander seeds
1/4 tsp grated dried ginger
2 c boiling water

Warm a teapot by rinsing with hot tap water. Place seeds and ginger into the warmed pot and cover with boiling water. Steep for 5 minutes, strain, and serve. When cooled, add a touch of honey for K types.

## Cardamom, Coriander, Fennel Tea

*Coriander, fennel, and cardamom combine to form the sweet, bitter, and pungent tastes. Coriander and fennel have a cooling tendency, while cardamom is heating. This combination makes a good year-round brew. In the summer, P types may substitute 1/4 teaspoon chamomile leaves for the cardamom to provide a totally cooling trinity. The actions of all three herbs are carminative (relieve intestinal gas and distension) and diuretic (promote urine flow). Fennel also relieves muscular spasms. This tea is excellent for balancing Pitta, and is a great thirst quencher to take after physical exertion.*

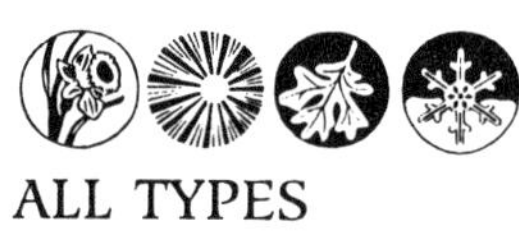

ALL TYPES
Serves 2

1/4 tsp cardamom seeds
1/4 tsp coriander seeds
1/4 tsp fennel seeds
2 c boiling water
1 tsp maple syrup or unrefined brown sugar (optional)

Warm a teapot by rinsing with hot tap water. Place all seeds into the warmed pot and cover with boiling water. Steep for 5 minutes and allow brew to cool. Strain and add maple syrup or brown sugar, if desired.

## Ginger, Cinnamon, Clove Tea

*The main ingredients in this recipe share the pungent taste. Cinnamon and ginger also share the sweet taste, with cinnamon having a secondary taste of astringency. The heating tendencies of each combine synergistically to form a potent brew. This tea is tailor-made for K types. Although best taken in the late winter and early spring, it may be used throughout the year. The combined actions relieve phlegm and mucus from the lungs, tone the intestines, relieve gas, and stimulate the digestive system, all of which set K types in motion. The cloves also add a delicate aphrodisiac energy to this heating trio.*

LATE EARLY 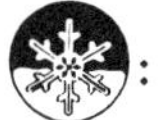: V, VP, VK

LATE 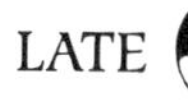 EARLY 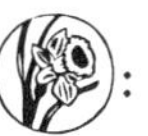: K, KV, KP

Serves 2

1/4 tsp ginger powder
4" piece cinnamon
1/4 tsp cloves
2 c boiling water
1/4 tsp honey (optional)

Warm a teapot by rinsing with hot tap water. Place ginger, cinnamon, and cloves into the warmed pot, and cover with boiling water. Steep for 5 minutes. Strain and allow to cool. Add honey and serve.

## Soy and Orange Peel Brew

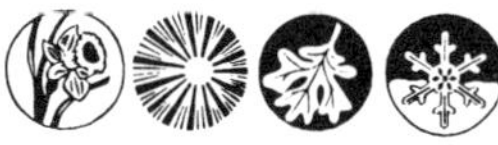

P, V, PV, VP, PK
Serves 2

1/2 c soy milk
1 c water
1 tsp grated orange peel
Pinch saffron

Bring milk and water to boil; add peel and saffron. Simmer for 10 minutes over low heat. Serve warm or cool.

## Pear Lassi

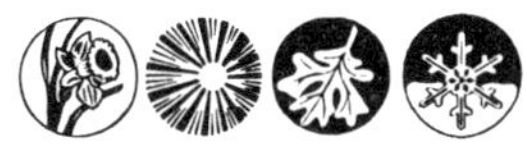

V, VP, P, PV
PK OCCASIONALLY, IN SUMMER
Serves 4

1/4 c cottage cheese
1/4 c yogurt
1 c pear juice
Pinch of saffron
1 tsp unrefined brown sugar
1/2 c milk
3 c water

*V types: use orange juice instead of pear juice.*

Place all ingredients in blender and blend for a few minutes until smooth.

## Energy Shake

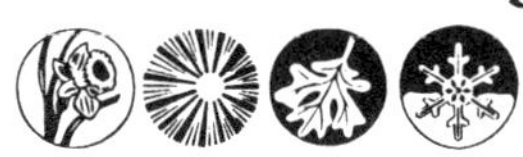

ALL TYPES
Serves 2

1/8 c raisins
2 tbs dates or figs, chopped
1/8 c prunes
1 c water
1 c milk

*K types: use 1 cup soy milk instead of cow's milk.*

Place all ingredients in blender and blend for a few minutes until semi-smooth. Use for energy.

## Morning Booster

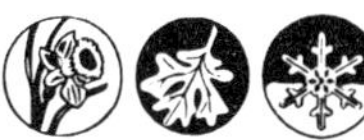

ALL TYPES
Serves 2

1 c soy milk
1 c water
1 tbs grain beverage (such as Pero, Roma)
1/2 tsp cardamom powder
Pinch turmeric
Pinch black pepper

Heat milk and water for 3 minutes. Add grain beverage and spices. Allow to come to a frothy boil. Serve hot.

## Warm Soy Chai

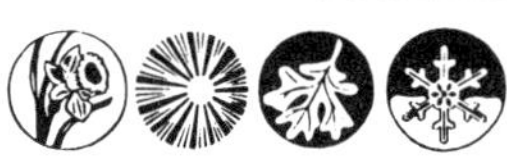

V, VK, PK, K, KV
Serves 1

1/2 c soy milk
1/2 c water
1 tsp black tea
Pinch cardamom powder
Pinch ginger powder

*PK: omit ginger in summer.*

Combine soy milk and water and bring to a boil. Add tea and steep for 20 minutes. Strain; add cardamom and ginger.

## Warm Goat's Milk with Cardamom

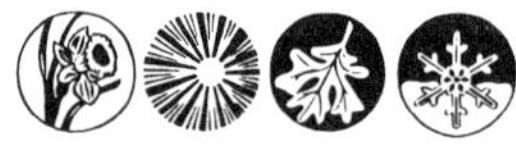

P, PK, K, KV, KP
Serves 2

1/2 c goat's milk
2 c water
1/2 tsp cardamom powder
Few strands saffron

Combine milk and water and bring to boil. Add cardamom and saffron; simmer over medium heat for a few minutes.

## Warm Almond and Nutmeg Brew

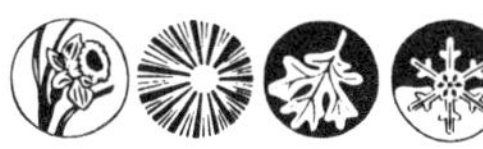

V, VP, VK
Serves 1

1/2 c almond milk (see page 195)
1/2 c water
Pinch of nutmeg
Drops of rose water

Warm milk and water over low heat for a few minutes. Sprinkle in nutmeg and add rose water. Drink warm.

## Warm Sandalwood Milk Brew

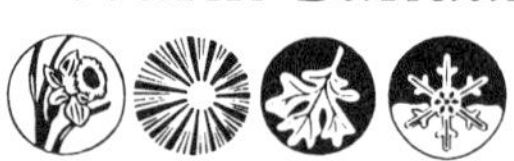

V, VP, VK,P, PV, PK
Serves 1

1/2 c almond milk (see page 195)
1/2 c water
Tiny pinch of sandalwood powder

Warm milk and water over low heat for a few minutes. Sprinkle in sandalwood powder and add sweetener, if desired. Drink warm.

## Warm Almond and Peach Nectar

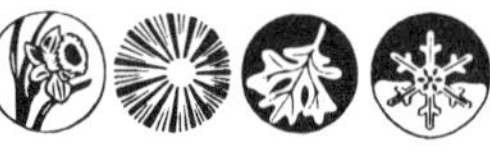

V, VP, VK, KV, KP
Serves 1

1/4 c almond milk (see page 195)
1/2 c water
1/4 c peach nectar (or concentrate)
Drops of almond essence

Warm milk, water, and nectar over low heat for a few minutes. Add essence. Drink warm.

## Warm Saffron Milk

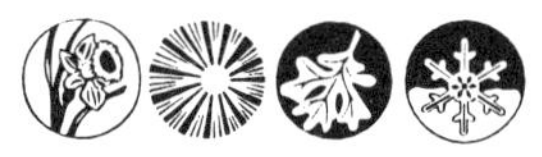

V, VP, VK, P, PV, PK
Serves 1

1/2 c certified raw milk
1/2 c water
9 strands saffron
Pinch turmeric

Warm milk and water. Add saffron and turmeric. Drink warm.

## Warm Spiced Soy Milk

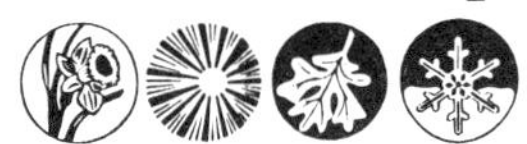

ALL TYPES
Serves 1

½ c soy milk
½ c water
¼ tsp black pepper
¼ tsp cardamom
Pinch of turmeric
Pinch of salt

Warm milk and water. Add spices and salt. Drink warm or at room temperature.

## Hot Milk Tea (Chai)

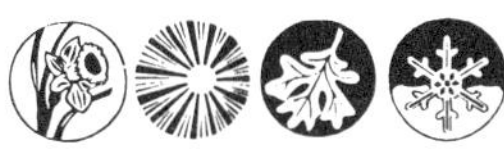

V, VK, K, KV
Serves 2

1 c certified raw milk
1 c water
1 tsp black tea
Pinch of cardamom
½ tsp unrefined brown sugar
*K types: omit sugar.*

Bring milk and water to boil. Add tea and continue to boil for another 3 minutes. Strain; add cardamom and sugar. Serve warm.

## Spiced Yogurt Drink

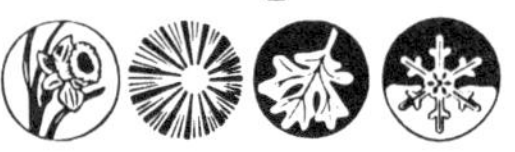

V, VP, VK
P, PV, PK OCCASIONALLY

½ c certified raw yogurt
1 c water
Pinch each black pepper, turmeric, and salt
7 curry leaves

Using a wooden spoon, combine ingredients and mix to a smooth consistency.

## Carrot, Celery, Ginger Juice

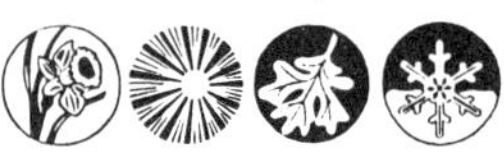

P, PK, K, KP

2 carrots
2 celery stalks
½ c water
½ tsp lime juice
Pinch of dried ginger
*P, PK: substitute a pinch of fresh mint leaves for ginger.*

Scrub carrots and celery. Slice into chunks and juice. Dilute with water; add lime juice and ginger.

## Beet, Carrot, Mint Juice

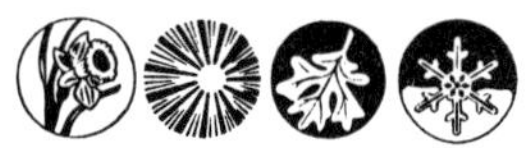

V, VK, K, KV
Serves 2

2 beets
3 carrots
6 fresh mint leaves (or 1 parsley sprig)
1/4 tsp lemon juice
1 c water

Scrub beets and carrots; slice into large chunks. Add to juicer along with mint leaves (or parsley) and lemon juice. Dilute with water.

## Carrot, Mint, Lime Juice

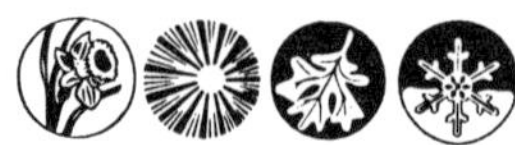

V, VP, P, PV
Serves 2

3 carrots
6 mint leaves (or cilantro leaves)
1 tsp lime juice
1 c water

Scrub carrots; slice into chunks. Add to juicer along with mint leaves and lime juice. Dilute with water.

AFTERWORD

# THE DHARMAS: UNIVERSAL VALUES

Every person is intrinsically aware of what is right and what is wrong. Dharmas are the unwritten codes of proper conduct inherent in all of life. These primal values, unchanged through the centuries, are the common-sense actions congruous to our existence with each other and with the universe. The classic story of the Bhagavad Gita began with the mention of *dharma-ksetra,* the physical place and physical body within which dharma ruled. Bharata, ancient India, was ruled by the Vedas, and thus the ruling factor of all human activity was the law of dharma. India is weaned on the tradition of dharma and was known as Bharatabhumi, the land of Bharata, whose history of dharma has survived thousands of years of exploitation and destruction.

All human pursuits should be guided by dharma; when it is violated, all accomplishments and possessions remain bereft of grace and happiness. In the Vedas, the primary dharmas are called *sattvika,* that which produces balance. Without adherence to this, we become victims of conflicts and confusion. We are all born with the basic elements of dharma, but these virtues need to be continuously invited into our lives from childhood. In time we grow to enjoy the freedom gained by right action and are able to travel within the grace of its universal protection.

The primary dharmas of love, faith, purity, compassion, truth, courage, and devotion are gained only by long years of nurturing. The mere sounds of these familiar values invoke a certain sense of goodness in all, but dharmas need to be taught and practiced before they become alive.

## SADHANA OF LOVE

*When we live gently on the earth*
*And innocence and humility are in every action*
*When the joy of universal remembrances*
*Shines through us, we are love*
*And everything we touch becomes love*
*Our beauty inspires the beauty in*
*everyone*
*In this collective love, we are one*
*We are free.*

Love is the most essential dharma on earth. After twenty billion years of universal existence, the human species was created. Every fiber of collective memory from the beginning of the cosmos is refined into the latent emergence of the human. We have walked the surface of earth for less than four billion years. In our human adolescence, we have dithered and gamboled with time and values. Now we are on the verge of maturing and discovering our essential nature to be the celebration of love.

The cosmos functions in stupendous dynamism. Continents meld and vast oceans separate, stars collide with celestial brio, and galaxies exist in a constant state of attraction. The power of infinite magnetism surrounds us. All life is born in the waters of love, which are absorbed in our being and lived through our heart.

Love is not an emotion. It is our complete state of being human. There is no wall love cannot tear down, no hate which love cannot imbue with light, no obstacle love cannot overcome. We have been miserly with love. Self-absorbed, we miss the very essence of who we are. When we express love, it brings us the solutions to all problems, the warmth and embrace and resolve of all things. When we feel anger, we must sit in the self and observe this anger. All things eventually dissolve if we remain aware.

The sadhana to encourage love is to sit in stillness in the mornings after your bath. Observe the thoughts, emotions, and pressures that arise without conversing with them. Allow them to be what they are, and just observe. Quietude in our lives is most essential to the gathering of love. Stillness is the food of love. Every moment of quiet nourishes love. The heart is the kitchen of love. When love feasts there, the memories of universal joy ebb and flow through it. When the heart is open it reflects all we need to know. It gives light to the eternal self, and we are able to transform the banalities of this finite world into idyllic bliss.

Love in itself cannot be taught. The great dramatist, Stella Adler, defines the truth within an action as something doable. To merely say the words "I love you" is meaningless if all the supporting actions are contrary, and do not communicate that love. The doable feats that inspirit the value of love are (1) sharing the things we hold dear, (2) being honest within our daily actions, (3) being alert within our activities, (4) assuming responsibility for any unpleasant results of our actions, and (5) recognizing when unpleasantries and difficulties are caused by others (and not blaming ourselves). The latter is a most arduous task when family and friends are involved. Alertness is imperative here, since our perceptions become blurred within the partialities of intimate relationships.

We cannot help others by assuming their burdens. It is necessary to exercise a discriminate tolerance of those who do not assume responsibility for their actions, and to accept the results of our own mistakes as well. Love is ojas, the quintessential essence of hard-earned practice. The nature of love is singular. It is only the expressions of love which are many. When we are thrown together in consanguinity, the bond is inevitably firmer, for the time together with family is so compact. When we spend time with those to whom we are attracted, a similar intensity sets in. Likewise when we are with a good teacher, the essence of love is there. In these and other cases of intimacy, love is the common factor, but its expressions are different. For love to exist in any situation, the elements of self-honesty, sharing, acceptance, and endurance need to be present.

Relationships are the various circumstances in which we practice our actions in order to attain certain results. It is only the actions and not the circumstances that dictate the result. More often than not, we take the intimate situations of brotherhood and friendship for granted. We presume that the nature of our karmic bond necessarily provides the desired result of love. This assumption is a fundamental, universal mistake. It is only our right actions that animate love and our wrong actions that bring infelicity. Relationships are the lesson grounds given to us to improve our practice. To be born together in a home is a blessing, to be bound together in friendship is a blessing, to be at the feet of a great teacher is a blessing. But these blessings will not live unless they are continuously nurtured. Our actions congruent to dharma are the only food for love. When the factors that foster love are diligently performed, love will reign complete. When we neglect our daily sadhanas we become unobservant and look to the circumstances of our various relationships to provide our happiness.

Every dharma provides a driver, a vehicle, and a destination. In the dharma of love, the driver is the individual's choice of actions, the vehicle is the circumstances in which the actions are performed, and the destination is the result of the actions performed. Love is arrived at only when the doer chooses the right actions of self-honesty, sharing, acceptance, and endurance within each situation. When these protocols are neglected, love is inevitably impaired and diffused into expectations. It is difficult for us to curb expectations altogether, but it is wise to note these expectations as reminders concerning the duties left undone. Disappointment always steps on the heels of expectation, and thus it becomes necessary to neutralize the advancement of expectation before the love is altogether lost. Expectations wield a double edge. We have an inevitable set of norms that teaches us to expect certain conditions, benefits, and performances from any given circumstance. We expect the promises that are made to us to be kept. It is essential to give up this pattern of living and to redefine our thoughts so as to harmonize with ourselves and others. All of our exchanges having to do with our duties in life must be clear and brisk. This is not to say that we cannot trust in promises that are made, but we must always remember that everything changes, and we must allow for even the most sacred of promises to endure change. All observations are time-bound. They are thus subject to change, and oftentimes they change radically. Truth deals with the timelessness of eternity.

Negative opinions ride loosely on the hips of sharpshooters. It is difficult not to criticize or judge others, but all opinions are temporary and need to be tempered with humor and verification. All conclusions need to remain open-ended if we are to maintain valid information in our cognitive memories. When situations become abusive, it becomes necessary to remove ourselves. It is most difficult not to be hurt by offensive behavior, but in distancing ourselves from such situations, it is easier to understand that the real victims are those who sustain anger and bitterness.

It is essential to recognize in life the factors that nurture, inform, and teach us. The attitude of regard is perhaps the greatest gift one can bring to love. Consideration is a rare and valuable asset which we must work on inviting to ourselves. We are becoming idle and neglectful, taking what we need without grace or consideration. We are eager to prove ourselves, and in the process we step on the very grounds that sustain us. When we take from a parent or teacher, we must be very aware that the graces we receive are not endless but must—if they are to continue—be properly acknowledged. According to dharma, the avatars, teachers, and rulers must never be approached with empty hands. This form, or custom, encourages the big nature of goodwill. Forms are very important to maintain for the benefit of our own growth and awareness. Gifts are a necessary acknowledgment of our own blessings. Those to whom we turn for advice, assistance, and education must be rewarded by our generosity. Spiritual leaders are not supported by the state; they are supported by *daksina*, the donations of students and devotees. Vedanta exhorts us not to charge a tuition for its teachings. But those who benefit from it must also adhere to dharma, by making it possible for their teachers to live and to continue sharing the knowledge so essential to our well-being. When the services performed for our well-being and knowledge are offered without a fee, we must respond in a conscious and giving manner. A teacher, by definition, is anyone from whom we learn something. And the great teachers are those who devote their lives to the dissemination of knowledge.

Dharmas have remained unchanged since the beginning of time. The proper conduct within the relationship of the sexes is another classic example of how far we have strayed from the basic chord of human dignity. The relationship of man and woman is the cosmic love of the deities Shiva and Shakti, the symbolic marriage of all dualities. It is the primal mating for the continued existence of karma, the vehicle that allows us to live out, in time, our eventual discoveries of the absolute nature of self and God. We have reduced much of this to the feeble antics of sensory desires. Women have forgotten their basic nature as the fundamental, nurturing, maternal force amid their external pursuit of competitive power, or their acceptance of a victimized existence. A woman's innate prowess is timeless if she is knowledgeable of her own fine nature. Men need to redefine their roles dramatically, but instead they are reacting to women by altering their own participation in the significant interplay of the sexes. The sense of chivalry has been dulled to near extinction. The generosity of a man's marvel at woman's magic has been pared down to a few gestures of accommodation. The dharmas of the sexes are greatly endangered, unless both men and women begin to evaluate the cosmic and real nature of love. The dating and mating processes are valid and need to be kindled according to dharma.

## SADHANA OF COMPASSION

The Vedic devatas were exemplars signifying the various traits of dharma. Lord Brahma is considered the embodiment of love, purity, compassion, and truth. The devatas were meditated upon in order to invoke the dharmas and as a constant reminder of our duties. If love is the mother-nectar of our survival, compassion is the base of our stability. Compassion is the long slack we extend to others in order to keep our criticisms and vituperative actions in check. The drivers of compassion are the actions of tolerance, maturity, and patience. The vehicle is the endless circumstances that are given us in which to accommodate our fellow humans, in order that we may foster the spirit of compassion.

Pity and sympathy are the uninformed step-sisters of compassion. The emotions are honorable, but the states themselves are helpless. Compassion interlaces us with each other. In order to bring this emotion alive, we need to cognize the basic values of the living love, which unites experience and study with maturity. Rasa is the essence of such maturity, and it is the single most important qualification for culling compassion. In the present age of Kali Yuga—when worlds are rife with conflict, hearts are torn asunder, and minds are bereft of peace—compassion indeed becomes the requisite word.

Love, which is the acceptance of all things, is often mistaken for compassion. Compassion contains love and is the greatest teacher of self-acceptance. It is an objective emotion, whereas love tends to be subjective. The most profound help the young may receive in their growing years is the love of their parents and family. The most profound help a cancer or drug victim may receive is that of a supportive aide who has survived a similar struggle. The first example is one of love, and the second one of compassion.

I discovered the nature of compassion during my cancer years. My first instinct was to distance myself from everyone. My family was already far away, and this made the distancing of myself from my friends much easier. I knew that in the limited and crucial time which I had, I could not deal with the fervent sympathies and helpless fears of those close to me. It was an entirely selfish act, but in the long run it gave me back my life and also helped my friends and family. I was not fortunate enough to have someone who had survived cancer available to me, but I found the privacy within my self-imposed isolation to be fundamental to my getting better. I had only the burdens of my own self-discovery to deal with. It would have been a nightmare to have my family and friends around at that time. For as a victim, I stood closer to the truth of my own being, and thus to my disease, and as such I had the intrinsic consolation of knowing that I could uncover and discover the anger within me. This distancing gave me courage, support, and the fuel to endure. In these situations, family and friends are always in a seemingly unfair position, for even their love is not an answer to the victim's problems. In such instances, it is that very love which deepens the chasms of pain and hurt, and this becomes a further burden to the patient.

Throughout my stay in hospitals, I found compassion to be the salve that helped me. I was fortunate to have in Barbara Pyle a friend with this rare quality. She delivered the necessities such as bindi *bhaji* and *samosas* (adroitly under wrap) to my room and never lingered beyond the time it took to greet me. It was years later that I realized how frightened she was for me and how courageous she was in hiding her fears. This is compassion. And it is the most selfless and divine action that we can give to those whose lives depend upon it. The suspension of norms and distancing of relationships do not infer a finality to those whom we love. These are temporary measures, and invariably we return to our relationships with inner strength and more clarity.

## SADHANA OF TRUTH

*Tavat satyam jagat bhati suktikarajtam yatha yavat na jnayate brahma sarvadhistanam advayam.*

The world of duality is real until the truth of the supreme whole is recognized by you, like even the silver on the mother of pearl.

***Atmabodha, Verse 7***

*The perception of the external world is neither direct nor immediate, but is dependent upon the sense and the mind and is always colored by them.*

***Swami Nikhilananda***

Truth is intertwined in all the dharmas, and all dharmas coalesce in the discovery that the self is the cosmic light—formless, unassailable, impenetrable, and unborn. Ultimate reality is a recognition of the One consciousness without the instruments of the senses and the mind. Our perceptions are led by our fears and desires and are conducted by the mind and senses. Our profound sense of duality creates infinite opportunities for self-deception, and so the seers established a method of cognizing the absolute truth. Vedanta does not allude to our perceptions of dualism as an illusion. It defines the observation of the senses and mind to be partial truths, since ultimate reality is that which is self-evident and nonpolemic. Through the teachers of great knowledge, it has set certain criteria for the methodical unfolding of the knowledge of the true self. We perceive a division between ourselves and the planet, the planet and the universe, and so on. These conclusions of what appear to be truth are referred to as *mithya*, that which has its basis in something else. For example, gold bangles have their primary nature in the original material of gold, and not in the many forms of the bangles. Essentially, that which we assimilate through the mind, senses, and experiential memory appears to be real to us, but these appearances are often deceiving. Ultimate truth can only be known through the cognate knowledge of the eternal self.

*To know the many without knowledge of the One is ignorance, whereas to know the One is knowledge.*

***Ramakrsna***

The method prescribed by the Vedas to determine the absolute nature of truth is threefold: through the cognition of *sruti* (scriptural authority), *yukti* (reasoning), and *anubhava* (personal experience). Any one of these three means will render a partial truth, but when all three means vivify the same conclusion we arrive at the infinite, absolute reality of truth.

*Like even the silver on the mother of pearl, what is perceived as silver by the sight may be only a sea shell.*

***Swami Dayananda Saraswati***

The seers encourage us to refrain from absolute conclusions unless we have arrived at the whole of the truth according to the three criteria of observation. In our daily lives, the closest we come to the recognition of truth is when we sit in our selves. Contemplation as a daily sadhana is essential for the truth of all situations to emerge at its own level. Since we cannot wholly depend upon our physical and emotional perceptions to guide us, it is essential to develop our instinctual self. This instinct will always direct us to contemplate all situations of incongruence. It is essential that we learn to discriminate between what is heard and what is actual; between what is a belief and what is believed.

As love exhorts us not to nurture expectations, the truth urges us not to hasten to conclusions. The open mind encourages an alert mind. And an alert mind becomes a discriminate mind, whereby we choose our daily paths of least resistance. The path of truth is always well lit when our eyes are open.

## SADHANA OF DEVOTION

If we pray for anything, it is that we remember our nature. Only then will the spirit of devotion rise in celebration.

To know ourselves to be Brahman is to gain the greatest wealth of the universe. Devotion is an attitude that is primarily influenced by the knowledge of God. It is an acceptance of the nature of all things, and not a resignation to unpleasantness. It is the firm, tangible knowing that all which comes to us is *prasada*, a gift of God.

The universe has a cosmic order, and when we are in harmony with it, the results we reap are always rewarding. When we are unobservant of its order, we are caught by surprise by its rewards. To accept the universal prasada, without anger and hurt, whether pleasant or not, is the test of trust in our attitude of devotion.

Prayers are where we begin in our spirit of devotion. We acknowledge the omniscient force of the Lord and his help to us. As we maintain a prayerful disposition, we recognize that the Lord's help is always impartial. We benefit from the grace whether or not we see the results. A *bhakta* is a devotee, one whose acceptance of the Lord as the provider and will behind everything is complete. A bhakta knows that when we tamper with God's will, we incur the just results, and that when we flow within Isvara's universal harmony, we are blessed with grace. The grace we earn may not always be what we hope for, but when we accept it as our lesson (or lessons) to bear, we are living in cosmic love.

When we make an offering to the Lord, it comes back to us, just like the fruits we place upon the alter and share with each other after prayers. When our offerings return to us, they are transformed into prasada. A devotee is not one who is exempt from wrongdoing, but one who accepts the results of his or her wrong actions with graciousness. A devotee may not recognize the wrongness of an action, but accepts the *karmaphala*, the fruits of the action, however unpleasant, without grief. The attitude of acceptance of all things that come to us is the greatest beauty of the human spirit. This does not mean that when we are being abused, we must remain in that condition. There are other factors present in these situations, and we must summon the courage to run from destructive interplay. Devotion is both the joyous acceptance of the good results and the recognition of the poor results as lessons to be learned.

No stage of spiritual growth is exempt from the spirit of devotion. The simple person who does not have the knowledge of self may be a great devotee of God. In contrast, a scholar of the scriptures cannot know the omniscient self without the spirit of devotion. With or without the knowledge of Brahman, devotion is the fundamental spirit of nature. With devotion, the poor and ignorant continue to be blessed and happy; without it the scholar could never know God.

## SADHANA OF SILENCE

*Solitude, silence, and freedom are the nourishers of life. We think we are nourishing ourselves with words, ideas, thoughts, but though these things are the content of consciousness, they are not the content of reality*

*Vimala Thakar*

As I write, I expend breath through the silent words. There are many thousands of breaths granted to each of us as we serve the mala bead of one lifetime. When this ration of breath is used, the physical body ceases to be. Even in deep silence, breath is spent. But it is spent wisely as it hums along with the universe.

The greatest sadhana of contentment and joy is to sit in the love and light of your own being. Silence is the last boon given after all the lessons of cosmic being are learned. It is difficult to begin the sadhana of silence, but we earn it as we practice the wholesome actions of the food sadhanas. When memory is waning, the mind becomes cluttered. There is no room for silence. We are shut out of existence. The penance to reenter is to sit in the self and observe the thoughts and emotions. The mind will not easily empty its sticky thoughts, but you will be able to observe them. This observation burns the invalid emotions and leaves the residue of what is real.

Observation is a celebration of our being, even when we are in trouble. By observing we become still. Stillness is the secret of the trees and mountains. They are in no hurry to accelerate the process of becoming. When you bathe in moonlight, you become moonlit; when you sit in the forest, you become the essence of the trees; when you climb a mountain like the gravity-defying goats, you become that mountain. They are all essential stillness in quiet motion. Observe nature and allow yourself to be transformed. Transformation is the fire of observation. Stillness is the gift of awareness.

Every morning take a bath. Sit within yourself for twenty minutes. Allow yourself to be vacant, to receive the love and light of the infinite. Allow the pain to pass. Allow the simple grace of your being. Allow. If there is anger, give it room to resound. Give it a field in which to play itself out. Know that it is from lack of cognition of the self that all anger appears. Direct it and dissolve it. Give in to the natural grace of your presence. Give in.

If there is fear, sit with it. Let it conjure the most devastating images. Let it show you the darkest hour. Let it turn every rope into a snake. Let it be. Sit with it until silence overcomes. Let it be.

If there is hate, allow it to rear its head. Look it in the face and confirm your hate. See your eyes reflecting in the one you hate. See your face full of hate. See your body distorted by hate. See yourself in the hated one. Hold the image as long and hard as you can. When you can no longer hold that image, there can be no more hate. Send love and light to the one you hated. Send love and light to your body. See your face in the loved one's face. See your eyes in the light of love. See your body calm and unfolding. See the love.

Sit within yourself. Sit and be still. Sit and allow the chords of remembrance to shimmer in harmonic resonance. Be still.

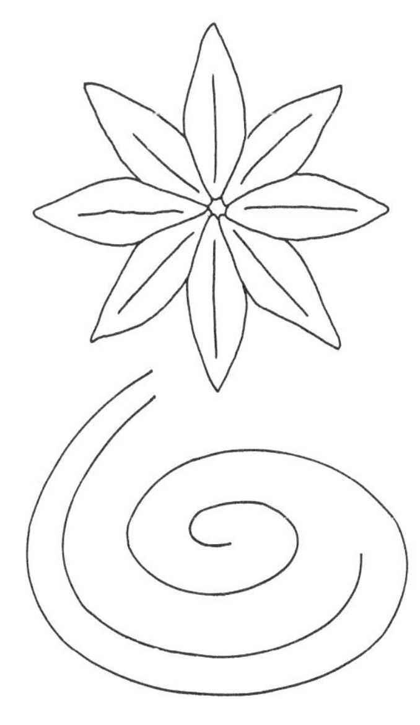

Emblem of Sound

APPENDIX

# AYURVEDIC RESOURCES AND SUPPLIERS

## AYURVEDA RESOURCES

American Institute of Vedic Studies
Attn: David Frawley
P.O. Box 8357
Santa Fe, NM 87504
(505) 983-9385

Ayurvedic Holistic Center
82A Bayville Avenue
Bayville, NY 11709
(516) 628-8200

The Ayurvedic Institute & Wellness Center
P.O. Box 23445
Albuquerque, NM 87192-1445
(505) 291-9698
Offers an Ayurveda correspondence course, "Lessons and Lectures in Ayurveda" by Dr. Robert E. Svoboda

Himalayan Institute
RR1, Box 400
Honesdale, PA 18431
(800) 822-4547

Lotus Ayurvedic Center
4145 Clares Street, Suite D
Capitola, CA 95010
(408) 479-1667

Wise Earth Institute
(Vedic studies)
Attn: Bri Maya Tiwari
25 Howland Road #R8
Asheville, NC 28804
(704) 258-9999

## AYURVEDIC HERBAL SUPPLIERS

The Ayurvedic Institute & Wellness Center
11311 Menaul N.E., Suite A
Albuquerque, NM 87112
(505) 291-9698

Auromere Inc.
1291 Weber Street
Pomona, CA 91768
(800) 925-1371

Ayush Herbs Inc.
10025 N.E. 4th Street
Bellevue, WA 98004
(800) 925-1371

Raven's Nest
Attn: Brian and Terry Craft
4539 Iroquois Trail
Duluth, GA 30136
(404) 242-3901

Bazaar of India Imports, Inc.
1810 University Avenue
Berkeley, CA 94703
(510) 548-4110

Frontier Herbs
P.O. Box 299
Norway, IA 52318
(800) 669-3275

Herbalvedic Products
Ayur Herbal Corporation
P.O. Box 6054
Santa Fe, NM 87502
(414) 889-8569

Kanak
P.O. Box 13653
Albuquerque, NM 87192-3653
(505) 275-2469

Lotus Brands
P.O. Box 325
Twin Lakes, WI 53181
(414) 889-8561

Lotus Herbs
1505 42nd Avenue, Suite 19
Capitola, CA 95010
(408) 479-1667

Maharishi Ayurveda Products Int'l, Inc.
417 Bolton Road
P.O. Box 541
Lancaster, MA 01523
(800) 843-8332 X903

## AYURVEDIC PANCHAKARMA CENTERS

Ayurveda at Spirit Rest
P.O. Box 3538
Pagosa Springs, CO 81147-3538
(303) 264-2573

The Ayurvedic Institute & Wellness Center
P.O. Box 23445
Albuquerque, NM 87192-1445
(505) 291-9698

Diamond Way Health Associates
214 Girard Boulevard, N.E.
Albuquerque, NM 87106
(505) 265-4826

Dr. Lobsang Rapgay
2931 Tilden Avenue
Los Angeles, CA 90064
(310) 477-3877

Lotus Ayurvedic Center
4145 Clares Street, Suite D
Capitola, CA 95010
(408) 479-1667

Swami Sada Shiva Tirtha
Ayurvedic Holistic Center
82A Bayville Avenue
Bayville, NY 11709
(516) 628-8200

Tej Beauty Enterprises, Inc.
162 West 56th Street, Room 201
New York, NY 10019
(212) 581-8136

## KITCHEN EQUIPMENT

Earth Fare
Attn: Roger Derrough
66 Westgate Parkway
Asheville, NC 28806
(704) 253-7656
Carries hand grinders and clay pots

Garber Hardware
49 Eighth Avenue
New York, NY 10014
Carries hand grinders, but no mail order. (Also check old-fashioned hardware stores.)

## ORGANIC/CERTIFIED RAW MILK

Organic milk comes from cows that are given organic grain feed free of antibiotics, pesticides, and growth hormones. It is pasteurized at the minimum allowable temperature but is not homogenized. Certified raw milk is equally healthful. It is neither pasteurized nor homogenized. Most health food stores will order these products for you if they don't already carry them. The following suppliers can be contacted by your local health food store. In some cases, they can deliver to you directly.

Alta Dena Certified Raw Milk
P.O. Box 388
City of Industry, CA 91747
(818) 964-6401
Non-pasteurized, non-homogenized milk

Natural Horizons, Inc.
7490 Clubhouse Road
Boulder, CO 80301
(303) 530-2711
Organic/pasteurized, non-homogenized milk—whole, low-fat, skim, buttermilk, and cream

# GLOSSARY OF UNCOMMON INGREDIENTS

For definitions of spices and herbs, see Vedic Herbs, Spices, and Accents, page 295; for a discussion of grains and dhals, see pages 160–173. Many unfamiliar terms are defined as they appear in the text.

### Agar-agar (*see also* Kanten)

A buff-colored, translucent seaweed available in 12-inch bars or in flakes. Indigenous to India, agar-agar has been used since Vedic times as a food thickener and to make gels (use warm water or other liquid to dissolve). Available in most health food stores and in Indian and Oriental grocery stores.

### Ajwan (Ajwain)

Also known as bishopweed, this spice seed is related to caraway and cumin. Its delicate flavor resembles the combined tastes of lemon, pepper, and thyme. Available in Indian and Oriental grocery stores and occasionally in health food stores.

### Amasake

Traditional to Japan, amasake is a sweet milk made from fermented sweet rice. Available in health food stores.

### Arame seaweed

The size of tobacco leaves when freshly harvested, this seaweed is generally shredded before it is sold. Like most seaweeds, it is a staple in Oriental cuisines. It is deep brown in color and has a mildly sweet, salty, and pungent taste. Available in health food stores and Oriental grocery stores.

### Arrowroot
The root of the arrowroot plant is best known for its starch which is used as a food thickener (use cold water or other liquid to dissolve).

### Arugula
The bitter green leaves of this plant resemble dandelion leaves and are used in salads. Available in health food stores and farmer's markets.

### Aspic
A light, gelatinous dish that is served cold and usually in the summer.

### Bamboo shoots
These young, tender shoots that sprout from the base of the bamboo tree are a delicacy in Oriental cuisines. They are peeled and used in stir-fries, soups, and other dishes. Occasionally available fresh in health food stores and bottled in Oriental grocery stores.

### Besan
Chickpea flour

### Bijun noodles
A transparent rice noodle, traditional to Oriental cuisines. Available in Oriental grocery stores and health food stores.

### Broccoli rabe
A leafy variety of the broccoli family. Available in farmer's markets and health food stores, especially on the East Coast.

### Brown bean sauce
A tangy paste generally made from aduki beans and available in Oriental grocery stores and occasionally in health food stores.

### Burdock root
This dark brown root of the burdock plant is long, thin, and wiry and has medicinal properties. Available in health food stores.

### Cassava
Also known as *yuca* and *manioc,* this tuber is a native of Africa and South America. It has a thin, waxy, light brown skin that is peeled off before the starchy tuber is used. Cassava is sweet and drying in nature and delicious in soups and root vegetable dishes. It is also processed to yield the tapioca pearls known as sago. Available in Indian, Oriental, and Latin American grocery stores.

### Daikon radish
Native to India, where it is called *mula,* this long, white, tapered root is very pungent. Available in health food stores, Oriental grocery stores, and farmer's markets.

### Dulse
A soft, dark green seaweed native to coastal countries such as Japan, Ireland, and the United States, dulse is mildly pungent and very salty. Available in health food stores and Oriental grocery stores.

### Ghee
Best made fresh (see pages 182–183), this Indian clarified butter is also available in health food stores and Indian grocery stores.

### Gourd squash
One good variety, called bottle gourd or *loukie,* is known in Oriental stores as *hula.* Traditional to India, this squash is cooked when young and tender, with a light green skin. It is watery, cooling, and sweet. Available in Indian and Oriental grocery stores.

### Grain brew
Several different grain teas or brews are made from roasted, sometimes crushed, grains such as barley or rice. Available in health food stores.

### Halvah
A pudding of soft fudge consistency made from grain flours mixed with milk, ghee, nuts, seeds, fruits, and sometimes shredded sweet vegetables.

### Hijiki

A dark brown (almost black), nubby seaweed with two-inch strands that are string-like and very pungent. Available in health food stores and Oriental grocery stores.

### Hot chili pepper

Native to tropical and semi-tropical climates, chili peppers come in an infinite variety of hotness. Those recommended in this book are the medium-hot variety, such as the one-inch-long red or green chilies found in Indian, Oriental, and Latin American grocery stores. You can reduce the heat of a pepper by deseeding it: cut off the stem and slice the pepper in half lengthwise. Use a dinner knife to scrape the seeds off. Alternatively, remove the stem by cutting around it and twisting/pulling it out of the pepper; most of the seeds should come out with the stem intact.

### Jicama

Native to Mexico, this root vegetable is hard and round and slightly flatter than a rutabaga. After peeling the thin, tan skin, the vegetable is cooked to a soft, watery consistency. Available in Latin American grocery stores and occasionally in health food stores.

### Karhi

Traditional to India, this yogurt soup may be prepared with a variety of spices chaunked in oil or ghee.

### Kanten

Sometimes used interchangeably with the term *agar-agar,* kanten is also the Japanese name for a gelled dessert.

### Karela

Also known as bitter melon, this unusual vegetable is a native of India and South America. It is six to eight inches long with medium-green skin that is ridged and bumpy. Extremely bitter when eaten raw, it becomes sweet-bitter when cooked. In South India, it is served in a popular dish cooked with yogurt. Available in Indian and Oriental grocery stores.

### Kohlrabi

A light green, bulbous vegetable that grows above ground. It resembles broccoli in taste and bears shoots of large leaves that may also be eaten. Kohlrabi is generally peeled before using. Available in farmer's markets and health food stores.

### Kombu

A two-inch wide seaweed that generally hardens after it is dried. Used widely in Japan, it is recommended in this book for cooking with beans to soften them and reduce their gas-producing effect. Like most seaweeds, kombu is pungent and salty. Available in health food stores and Oriental grocery stores.

### Kudzu

The root of the kudzu plant is best known for its starch, which is used medicinally in Oriental medicine. Similar to *guducci,* a root starch used in Ayruvedic medicine, kudzu is sweet and cooling in nature. It is used as a food thickener for culinary purposes. (Dissolve in cold water or other cold liquid.)

### Kuttu

From the Tamil word meaning "combinations," this dish is a combination of dal, vegetables, and spices cooked into a fairly thick stew. Kuttu is often served at weddings.

### Ladoo

A fudge-like confectionery ball popular in northern India, usually made from chickpea flour, milk, ghee, and jaggery.

### Landcress

Native to the southern terrain of the United States, this tender leafy green is a member of the watercress family. It grows on land, however, instead of in water.

### Lassi

A thick, spiced yogurt drink traditional to India and taken after a meal as a titillating digestive aid.

### Mirin

Traditional to Japanese cuisine, mirin is a sweet, slightly fermented vinegar made from rice. One of the mildest of vinegars, it is available in health food stores and Oriental grocery stores.

### Miso

A fermented, salty paste made from grains such as rice and barley and legumes such as soybeans and chickpeas. A staple of Japanese cuisine, it is available in health food stores and Oriental grocery stores.

### Mochi

A pounded sweet rice that is a traditional dessert and special occasion food of Japan. Available in health food stores.

### Osha

A bitter and pungent herb, osha is used by Kapha types as a stimulant and to relieve congestion and colds, and by Vata types to prevent bacterial infection and as a digestive stimulant. It is grown in the United States and is available in health food stores (see also Ayurvedic Resources and Supplies, page 336).

### Peera

A fudge made from milk and jaggery popular in northern India.

### Pippali

A hot and pungent red pepper, two to three inches long, that is one of the three ingredients in the Ayurvedic formula known as *trikatu.* It is excellent for Kapha types (and occasionally for Vata types) to provide heat to the body and to stimulate digestion.

### Plantain

Known as green banana in the United States and *kacha kela* in India, plantain is actually considered a vegetable. Used in the cuisines of South India and South and Central America, it is available in most Indian and Latin American grocery stores.

### Pokeroot

A smaller-leaf green than spinach, pokeroot is grown mostly in the southern and southeastern regions of the United States. While still young and tender, it is excellent in salads. When it matures and the stems become purple, it is no longer palatable. Available in farmer's markets and health food stores in regions mentioned above.

### Pudina

The Sanskrit term for mint, pudina is mentioned as a vital tridoshic herb in ancient Ayurvedic texts. Especially pleasing to Pitta types, it is available fresh or dried in health food stores and farmer's markets.

### Radicchio

Widely used as a salad vegetable in Europe, this bitter leaf is available in most health food stores and farmer's markets.

### Riverweeds

These weeds are harvested from rivers just as seaweeds are from the sea. They contain less saline than seaweeds and have a more delicate taste.

### Rock salt

Primarily mined in crystalline form from the seabeds of the Sindh Mountain region in Pakistan, this salt has been used since ancient times in Ayurvedic foods and medicines (where it is known as *sendha namak*). It may be used by all the types and substituted for sea salt in any of the recipes in this book. Its sister salt, known as *kala namak,* is a deep purple, highly pungent rock crystal that has a volatile taste and a smell resembling hardboiled eggs. It may be used occasionally (in small quantity) by Vata and Kapha types. Rock salt may be ordered through Ayurvedic Resources and Supplies (see page 336). A clear rock salt comparable to the sendha namak is readily available in Jewish kosher markets.

### Salsify

A brown root resembling burdock, it is white and milky inside when cooked. Available in health food stores.

### Sansho leaves

An herb with purple leaves resembling basil and used in Japan in the preparation of pickled umeboshi plums. Available in Oriental grocery stores and some health food stores.

### Seaware

A curly seaweed about six inches long and 1/2 inch in width, seaware has a mild taste and chewy texture. Like kombu and wakame, it is now harvested off the West Coast of the United States. Available in health food stores.

### Shiitake

The Japanese name for a mushroom that is grown in the bark of trees. These mushrooms are known for their delicious flavor as well as their medicinal properties. Available in health food stores and Oriental grocery stores.

### Soba

The Japanese name for noodles made from a combination of buckwheat and whole wheat flours. (also available in 100% buckwheat). Delicious and mildly sweet tasting, soba noodles are available in health food stores and Oriental grocery stores.

### Soursop

A sour, pulpy fruit native to India and South and Central America. Occasionally available in Latin American and Caribbean grocery stores.

### Tamarind

The pulp of the tamarind pod, used since ancient times in India. The tamarind tree is considered auspicious in Indian mythology, and its fruit is known as *imli.* Fresh tamarind is available in the tropics. Dried tamarind is packed in the shape of bricks or slabs that can be prepared as a pulp. Dried tamarind, tamarind pulp (or paste), and a gel-like tamarind concentrate are all available in Indian grocery stores.

### Taro

A small, brown, potato-like root with fuzzy skin, this vegetable grows in hot climates. Cooked in soups and other dishes in African, Indian, Japanese, and Caribbean cuisines, it is also used to make poultices in Oriental medicine.

### Udon noodles

Japanese whole wheat noodles resembling linguine. They are off-white in color and have a soft, silken texture when cooked. Available in health food stores and Oriental grocery stores.

### Umeboshi plums

Traditional to Japan, these once-sweet plums are pickled in sea salt and seasoned with sansho leaves. They have a strong flavor and are popular in macrobiotic cuisine. Available in health food stores and Oriental grocery stores.

### Wakame

A seaweed used predominantly in Japanese cooking as an accent to miso soup. It resembles kombu in shape and taste but has a softer texture. Available in dried form in health food stores and Oriental grocery stores.

### Wasabi

A Japanese horseradish mixed with green mustard. It is generally used as a condiment with nori rolls and sushi. Its highly pungent taste clears the head and brings water to the eyes if more than a pinch is taken at once. Available in health food stores and Oriental grocery stores.

# BIBLIOGRAPHY


*Animals of the Soul: Sacred Animals of the Ogala Sioux.* Joseph Epis Brown. Longmead, Shaftsbury, Dorset, U.K.: Element Books, 1989.

*The Art of Indian Vegetarian Cooking.* Yamuna Devi. New York: E.P. Dutton, 1987.

*Atma Bodha of Sri Sankaracharya.* 2d ed. Vidyaratna T.N. Menon. Palghat, India: The Educational Supplies Depot, 1964.

*Ayurvedic Medicine, Past and Present.* Pandit Shiv Sharma. Calcutta, India: Dabur Publications, 1975.

*Ayurveda, the Science of Self-Healing: A Practical Guide.* Dr. Vasant Lad. Sante Fe: Lotus Press, 1984.

*Basic Principles of Ayurveda.* Bhagwan Dash. New Delhi, India: Concept Publishing Co., 1980.

*Brother Eagle, Sister Sky.* Susan Jeffers. New York: Dial Books, 1991.

*Caraka Samhita.* P. V. Sharma. Delhi, India: Chaukhambha Orientalia, 1981.

*Chakras, Energy Centers of Transformation.* Harish Johari. Rochester, Vt.: Destiny Books, 1987.

*Companion Planting.* Gertrud Franck. Wellingborough, Northamptonshire, U.K.: Thorsons Publishers, Ltd., 1983.

*Diet for Natural Beauty.* Maya Tiwari, Wendy Esko, and Aveline Kushi. Japan: Japan Publication, 1990.

*Doctrines of Pathology in Ayurveda.* Vidyavilas Ayurveda Series, #3. Prof. K. R. Srikantha Murthy. Varanasi, India: Chaukhambha Orientalia, 1987.

*The Edited Works of Ramana Maharshi.* Edited by Arthur Osborne. London: Rider, 1986.

*The Eloquence of Living.* Vimala Thakar. San Rafael: New World Library, 1989.

*A Handbook of Ayurveda.* Vaidya Bhagwan Dash and Acarya Manfred M. Junius. New Delhi, India: Concept Publishing Co, 1983.

*Holy Bible.* The New King James Version. Nashville: Thomas Nelson, 1982.

*Madhava Nidanam (Roga Viniscaya) of Madhavakara: A Treatise on Ayurveda.* Jaikrishnadas Ayurveda Series, #69. Prof. K. R. Srikanta Murthy. New Delhi, India: Chaukhambha Orientalia, 1987.

*May All Be Fed: Diet for a New World.* John Robbins. New York: William, Morrow, & Co., 1992

*Prakruti: Your Ayurvedic Constitution.* Robert E. Svoboda. Albuquerque: Geocom Press, 1988.

*The Ramayana of Tulsidasa.* Translated by F.S. Growse. New Delhi, India: Motilal Banarsidass Publishers, Private Ltd.

*The Ramayana of Valmiki.* New Delhi, India: Chaukhambha Orientalia, 1984.

*Returning to Eden.* Michael A. Fox. New York: Viking Press, 1980.

*The Sadhana and the Sadhya.* Swami Dayananda. Purani Jhadi, Rishikesh, India: Sri Gangadhareswar Trust, 1984.

*Srimad Bhagavad Gita: Bhasya of Sri Sankaracharya.* Sri Ramakrishna Math. (Sanskrit edition). Madras, India: Mylapore, 1983.

*State of the World, 1990.* Edited by Lester R. Brown. New York: W.W. Norton & Co., 1989.

*A Study in Consciousness.* Annie Besant. Adyar, Madras, India: The Theosophical Society, 1947.

*Sushruta Samhita.* Translated by K.L. Bhishagratna (Sanskrit series). Varanasi, India: Chaukhambha, 1981.

*The Universe is a Green Dragon.* Brian Swimme. Sante Fe: Bear & Co. Publishing, 1984.

*Upadesha Sahasri of Sri Sankaracharya.* Sri Ramakrishna Math. (Sanskrit/English edition). Madras, India: Mylapore, 1984.

*Upanisad Bhasyam,* vol.1. (Sri Shankara Bhagavatpada's version), (Sanskrit edition). Varanasi, India: Mahesh Research Institute, 1949.

*The Value of Values.* Swami Dayananda Saraswati. Purani Jhadi, Rishikesh, India: Sri Gangadhareswar Trust, 1984.

*Viveka Chudamani of Sri Sankaracharya.* Swami Madhavananda. Calcutta, India: Aovaita Ashram, 1982.

*The Yoga of Herbs: An Ayurvedic Guide to Herbal Medicine.* Dr. David Frawley and Dr. Vasant Lad. Sante Fe: Lotus Press, 1988.

# INDEX

***Bold italic page numbers indicate charts***